Recent Results in Cancer Research 127

H.-J. Senn R.D. Gelber A. Goldhirsch
B. Thürlimann (Eds.)

Adjuvant Therapy of Breast Cancer IV

With 37 Figures and 71 Tables

Springer-Verlag
Berlin Heidelberg New York
London Paris Tokyo
Hong Kong Barcelona
Budapest

Prof. Dr. med. Hans-Jörg Senn
Department of Medicine C, Kantonsspital
CH-9007 St. Gallen, Switzerland

Richard D. Gelber, Ph.D.
Division of Biostatistics
Dana Farber Cancer Institute,
44, Binney Street,
Boston, MA 02115, USA

Prof. Dr. med. Aron Goldhirsch
Ospedale Civico
CH-6900 Lugano, Switzerland

Dr. med. Beat Thürlimann
Department of Medicine C, Kantonsspital
Ch-9007 St. Gallen, Switzerland

ISBN 3-540-55304-5 Springer-Verlag Berlin Heidelberg New York
ISBN 0-387-55304-5 Springer-Verlag New York Berlin Heidelberg

Typesetting: Best-set Typesetter Ltd., Hong Kong
19/3130/SPS-5 4 3 2 1 – Printed on acid-free paper

Preface

Advances in breast cancer research, achieved through the progress of knowledge and development of new therapies, have been translated into improved quality of care for breast cancer patients. Clinical investigations and clinical trials have made the largest contribution to the body of knowledge that finds its way to the patient. Never before during the past decades of management of breast cancer has there been such a fruitful intellectual cross-fertilization of ideas among individuals involved in the generation of hypotheses, basic research, development of drugs and treatments, conduct of clinical trials, and statistical evaluation – the results of all of which are now translated into progress in clinical care. Even issues such as the quality of life of breast cancer patients, once the domain for few, are now being openly addressed by trials and discussed in a much broader forum.

The IVth International Conference on the Adjuvant Therapy of Primary Breast Cancer, also known as the St. Gallen Conference, was again attended by more than 800 scientists and clinicians interested in this broad spectrum of breast cancer research and the interactions between such diverse fields of interest and specialties as cancer pathology, molecular biology, and psychosocial oncology.

This volume collects findings and conclusions presented at the conference. No attempt has been made to provide the reader with an encylopedic list of facts and definitions about the current management of primary breast cancer; the book should instead be considered as an excursion into the innovative, still partly controversial and fast-evolving research in this field. The reader will find that many chapters contain not only hypothetical approaches to biological and clinical issues, but also try to present a state-of-the-art summary of our knowledge about primary, multimodal therapy of breast cancer. Details of surgical and radiotherapeutic approaches and of adjuvant systemic treatments are summarized by internationally recognized experts, intended to gradually change attitudes toward clinical routine in managing primary breast cancer worldwide. For this reason, the closing session of the conference was structured as an "international concensus on risk-adapted adjuvant therapy of breast cancer," greatly appreciated by the audience from more than 27 countries around the world.

A clear message emerges from most of the presentations at the conference: The primary treatment of breast cancer, despite the considerable progress achieved, still remains largely unsatisfactory. Hence, much more has to be done to improve current therapies. Conducting rational and critically evaluated clinical trials seems by far the best way to identify superior treatments in order to provide them to the patients of today and tomorrow.

Boston, MA, USA — Richard. D. Gelber
Lugano, Switzerland — Aron Goldhirsch
St. Gallen, Switzerland — Hans-Jörg Senn
St. Gallen, Switzerland — Beat Thürlimann
September, 1992

Contents

*List of Contributors**

* The addresses of the authors are given on the first page of each contribution.

[1] Page on which contribution begins.

I. Biological Mechanisms and Models

Kinetic Concepts in the Treatment of Breast Cancer

L. Norton

Breast and Gynecologic Cancer Medicine Service Memorial Sloan-Kettering Cancer Center, NY, USA

A great puzzle of modern medical oncology is why the survival times of patients with advanced breast cancer have not improved significantly over several decades [1]. Although most patients' tumors respond to modern high-dose chemotherapies, median survival times have advanced by mere months [2]. Indeed, prolongation of life to the length of a "natural" lifespan *sans* cancer is rarely achieved. Even ultrahigh-dose chemotherapy with autologous bone marrow reinfusion is of major benefit only to the unusual patient whose cancer is being exquisitely responsive to conventional chemotherapy [3].

Our best kinetic models of tumor growth and regression do not adequately explain these results. In Skipper's model [4] murine leukemia grows exponentially: If it takes x days for 10^2 mouse leukemia cells to grow into 10^3 cells, it takes x days for 10^6 cells to grow into 10^7. Furthermore, each administration of chemotherapy kills a percentage of the leukemia cells present, regardless of their absolute number: If one cycle of treatment Z would reduce the number of cells from 10^6 to 10^5 over y days (a log-kill of 1), then two cycles of Z would result in 10^4 cells over $2y$ days (a log-kill of 2). Each reduction in tumor volume results in a consistent increase in survival: If it takes 10^6 unperturbed cells $3x$ days to kill the mouse at 10^9 cells, each log-kill of 1 increases the duration of life by $x + y$ days.

Deviations from the rule of "more chemotherapy, longer survival" can be due to drug resistance [5]. That is, if some cells in the population will not die in response to therapy Z, once all Z-sensitive cells are killed the tumor will grow in spite of continuation of Z. For his reason, the only hope of using Z to cure the cancer is to treat at a time when there are no Z-resistant cells. According to the theory of Delbruck and Luria [6], extended to murine cancer by Law [7] and more generally to neoplasia by Goldie and Coldman [8], this is only possible in tiny cancers. Mutants resistant to Z will certainly arise by the time 10^5 cells, uniformly sensitive to Z, grow into 10^7 cells.

Recent Results in Cancer Research, Vol. 127

This concept has been used to make two specific predictions: (1) chemotherapy must start at as small a tumor size as possible [9]; (2) as many drugs as possible must be used as early as possible lest cells that could be killed by a drug are left to grow to mutate to resistance to the drug [10]. True combination chemotherapy, using many drugs simultaneously, would be best [11]. If this is precluded by overlapping toxicity, then the alternation of different regimens would be better than using the drugs or drug combinations sequentially. The worst plan would be to use a single drug initially, since that would delay the use of combination chemotherapy.

Remarkably, clinical experience has not confirmed either prediction. The International (Ludwig) Group randomized node-positive patients to either six months of a cyclophosphamide, methotrexate, and 5-fluorouracil (CMF) variant starting about 1 month after surgery or 7 months of a similar regimen starting within 1.5 days of surgery [12]. Both treatments gave identical results regarding disease-free and overall survival! The Cancer and Leukemia Group B (CALGB) randomized node-positive postsurgical patients to one of two treatment arms: The first arm gave a CMF variant for about 1 year; The second gave about half a year of the same CMF variant followed by about half a year of the vinblastine, doxorubicin, thiotepa, and fluoxymesterone (VATH) combination [13]. The results were that the VATH conveyed a significant advantage in disease-free survival, in spite of its being started more than half a year after surgery! Hence, it is not necessary to start chemotherapy immediately after surgery to obtain maximum benefit.

Neither is alternating chemotherapy unequivocally superior to other schedules. The Italian National Cancer Institute [14, 15] randomized stage II patiens with more than three involved axillary lymph nodes to eight cycles CMF and four of doxorubicin (Adriamycin, A) given either as arm I,

CMF–CMF–A–CMF–CMF–A–CMF–CMF–A–CMF–CMF–A,

or arm II,

A–A–A–A–CMF–CMF–CMF–CMF–CMF–CMF–CMF–CMF.

Arm I applied combination chemotherapy early, and used both CMF and doxorubicin as soon as possible after surgery. Arm II delayed the use of combination chemotherapy. Yet, against expectations, arm II was superior to arm I in both disease-free and overall survival!

What is the source of this divergence between theory and experience? One problem may be that failure to cure is not becasue drug-resistant cells are the only ones that escape the treatment. Both the Cancer and Leukemia Group B [16] and the Italian National Cancer Institute [17] have found that patients relapsing more than a year after they received adjuvant chemotherapy have tumors that are as responsive to subsequent chemotherapy as do chemotherapy-naïve patients. Hence, their recurrent tumors cannot be comprised entirely of drug-resistant mutants! Another problem may be in our assumption of exponential growth, which is not applicable to human breast cancer. Data from the nineteenth century concerning survival with untreated breast cancer [18] and from the recent worldwide overview concerning disease-free and overall survival [19] are fit best by a family of curves which are Gompertzian [20]. In the overview, for node-positive patients not treated with adjuvant polychemotherapy, the median time to relapse after primary surgery is about 4 years, and the median survival time is 7–8 years. Hence, letting N represent the cell number at t months, if relapse occurs at 10^{11} cells and death 10^{12} cells, then

$$N = 10^7 \exp[12.65(1 - e^{-0.02732t})].$$

Since 73% of node-positive patients not receiving adjuvant polychemotherapy had relapsed by 10 years, the median metastatic case is at the 36.5th percentile of all cases. For this individual the proper Gompertzian equation is

$$N = 10^7 \exp[12.65(1 - e^{-0.04504t})].$$

Using these equations, the supposition that the volume of tumor is reduced by polychemotherapy from 10^7 cells immediately after surgery to 6.7×10^3 cells at 7 months after surgery (6 months of chemotherapy starting 1 month after surgery) gives a median time to relapse of about 6 years and a median survival of about 9 years, which closely match the real data.

The special characteristic of Gompertzian growth is that the relative growth rate – the growth rate divided by the tumor size – decreases steadily as the tumor grows larger [21]. Since the rate of tumor regression after effective chemotherapy is positively related to the rate of growth, a therapy that causes a log-kill of 4 at 10^7 cells would cause a log-kill of just over 1 at 10^{11} cells. Nevertheless, the rate of regression of a cancer should increase as we increase the intensity of chemotherapy. A log-kill of 1, from 10^{11} to 10^{10} cells, will increase survival by 45 weeks. An additional 1 log-kill, to bring the 10^{11} cells down to 10^9 cells, will increase survival by only another 30 weeks. That is, the smaller tumors that could result from more intensive therapy would regrow more quickly with each increment in cytoreduction. Hence, higher response rates to more intensive chemotherapy might not be reflected in greatly improved survival times.

For similar reasons, patients might be relapsing after adjuvant chemotherapy because sensitive cells are left even after treatments of high intensity [22]. The above cancer would take 29 months to grow from 10^7 cells to 10^{11} cells. If 6 months of chemotherapy (started 1 month after surgery) could reduce the tumor to 6.7×10^3 cells, the time of relapse would be postponed by 17 months (to 46 months after surgery). If we improve the efficacy of the chemotherapy so that only 67 cells remained at 7 months, this would bring the total relapse-free duration to only 51 months! When these cells grow to relapse, they may respond again to chemotherapy since they were never drug-resistant!

Our analysis leads us away from the question of how to prevent drug resistance from developing during treatment, and toward the question of how to eradicate sensitive cells in a collection of cells heterogeneous in drug sensitivity at the time when treatment is initiated [23]? We might already be numerically closer to disease eradication than our survival statistics would lead us to believe. Since resistance does not emerge rapidly over the first few postoperative months, we should probably use our various different therapies as intensively as possible during their time of exposure, rather than dilute them by alternating them with other therapies. That is, imagine that a postoperative micrometastatic breast cancer is comprised of some cells sensitive to either CMF or doxorubicin, some cells sensitive only to CMF, and the remainder sensitive only to doxorubicin. The cells sensitive to either therapy will be killed equally by any temporal combination that gives eight CMF and four doxorubicin cycles in 33 weeks. The CMF-sensitive cells will be killed just a bit more efficiently by arm I in the Milan trial, which gives eight CMF cycles over 30 weeks, than by arm II which gives the same amount of CMF over 33 weeks. However, the doxorubicin-sensitive cells will experience a much greater log-kill from arm II, which gives four cycles over 9 weeks, than from arm I, giving the same amount of doxorubicin over 33 weeks. Hence, arm II should be and is superior!

At Memorial Sloan-Kettering Cancer Center we are piloting, in stage II patients with four or more involved axillary lymph nodes, a regimen which uses the concept of sequential chemotherapy to significantly increase dose intensity [24]. We are using doxorubicin as in Milan, but followed by three cycles of cyclophosphamide at $3\,g/m^2$ each for 2 weeks, as permitted by granulocyte-colony stimulating factor. Other applications of the sequential concept are using induction chemotherapy followed by ultrahigh-dose combination chemotherapy with autologous bone marrow rescue [25].

In an effort to increase cell-kill further, we are exploring in the laboratory the combination of chemotherapy with monoclonal antibodies directed against growth factor receptors. The division of breast cancer cells is driven by growth factors interacting with transmembrane receptors [26]. Tamoxifen is thought to kill cancer cells by interfering with estrogen-mediated growth factor loops [27]. We have hypothesized that chemotherapy disrupts growth factor loops as well [28]. Hematopoietic cells deprived of their growth factors die by apoptosis [29, 30]. Cancer cells undergo apoptosis in response to chemotherapy as if they were deprived of growth factor activity [31]. This would explain high degrees of log-kill in tumors with low S phases. In a human tumor cell line with high expression of the epidermal growth factor receptor (EGFR) low doses of doxorubicin cause up-regulation of the receptor and, transiently, its autocrine ligand transforming growth factor alpha [32, 33]. When xenographs in nude mice are treated with doxorubicin or with an anti-EGFR antibody, their growth is inhibited, but the combination is profoundly synergistic, causing tumor disappearance in most cases. If such an augmentation of cell-kill can be accomplished clinically, it is our hope that optimally designed chemotherapy sequences will improve survival times as well as response rates in advanced breast cancer, and cure more patients in the postoperative setting.

References

1. Norton L (1991) Metastatic breast cancer – length and quality of life (editorial). N Engl J Med 325:1370–1371
2. Hryniuk WM (1988) The importance of dose intensity in the outcome of chemotherapy. In: DeVita VT Jr, Hellman S, Rosenberg SA (eds) Important Advances in Oncology 1988. Lippincott, Philadelphia, pp 121–141
3. Peters WP (1991) High dose chemotherapy and autologous bone marrow support for breast cancer. In: DeVita VT Jr, Hellman S, Rosenberg SA (eds) Important Advances in Oncology 1991. Lippincott, Philadelphia, pp 135–150
4. Skipper HE (1986) Laboratory models: the historical perspective. Cancer Treat Rep 70:3–7
5. Skipper HE (1986) Analyses of multiarmed trials in which animals bearing different burdens of L1210 leukemia cells were treated with two, three, and four drug combinations delivered in different ways with varying dose intensities of each drug and varying average dose intensities. South Res Inst Booklet 7(42): 87–92
6. Luria SE, Delbruck M (1943) Mutations of bacteria from virus sensitivity to virus resistance. Genetics 28:491
7. Law LW (1952) Origin of resistance of leukaemic cells to folic acid antagonists. Nature 169:628–629
8. Goldie JH, Coldman AJ (1979) A mathematic model for relating the drug sensitivity of tumors to their spontaneous mutation rate. Cancer Treat Rep 63:1727–1733
9. Goldie JH (1987) Scientific basis for adjuvant and primary (neoadjuvant) chemotherapy. Sem in Oncol 14:1–7
10. Goldie JH, Coldman AH (1986) Application of theoretical models to chemotherapy protocol design. Cancer Treat Rep 70:127–131
11. DeVita VT Jr, Young RC, Canellos GP (1975) Combination vs. single agent chemotherapy: a review of the basis for selection of drug treatment of cancer. Cancer 35:98–110
12. Ludwig Breast Cancer Study Group (1988) Combination adjuvant chemotherapy for node-positive breast cancer. N Engl J Med 319:677–683
13. Perloff M, Norton L, Korzun A, Wood W, Carey R, Weinberg V, Holland JF (1986) Advantage of an adriamycin combination plus halotestin after initial CMFVP for adjuvant therapy of node-positive stage II breast cancer. Proc Am Soc Clin Oncol 70:273
14. Buzzoni R, Bonadonna G, Valagussa P, Zambetti M (1991) Adjuvant chemotherapy with doxorubicin plus cyclophosphamide, methotrexate and fluorouracil in the treatment of resectable breast cancer with more than three positive axillary nodes. J Clin Oncol 9:2134–2140
15. Bonadonna G, Valagussa P, Zambetti M, Buzzoni R (1992) Sequential adriamycin-CMF in the adjuvant treatment of breast cancer with more than three positive axillary nodes. Proc Am Soc Clin Oncol 70
16. Kardinal CG, Perry MC, Korzun AH, Rice MA, Ginsberg S, Wood WC (1988) Responses to chemotherapy or chemohormonal therapy in advanced breast cancer patients treated previously with adjuvant chemotherapy: a subset analysis of CALGB study 8081. Cancer 61:415–419

17. Valagussa P, Tancini G, Bonadonna G (1986) Salvage treatment of patients suffering relapse after adjuvant CMF chemotherapy. Cancer 58:1411–1417
18. Bloom H, Richardson M, Harris B (1962) Natural history of untreated breast cancer (1804–1933): comparison of treated and untreated cases according to histological grade of malignancy. BMJ 2:213–221
19. Early Breast Cancer Trialists Collaborative Group (1992) Systemic treatment of early breast cancer by hormonal, cytotoxic, or immune therapy. Lancet 339:1–15, 71–85
20. Norton L (1988) A Gompertzian model of human breast cancer growth. Cancer Res 48:7067–7071
21. Norton L, Simon R (1977) Tumor size, sensitivity to therapy, and the design of treatment schedules. Cancer Treat Rep 61:1307–1317
22. Norton L, Simon R (1986) The Norton-Simon hypothesis revisited. Cancer Treat Rep 70:163–169
23. Norton L (1985) Implications of kinetic heterogeneity in clinical oncology. Semin Oncol 12:231–249
24. Hudis C, Lebwohl D, Crown J, Gilewski T, Surbone A, Hakes T, Reichman B, Seidman A, Harrison M, Bellettieri R, Hamilton N, Yao TJ, Weiselberg L, Moore A, Greenberg S, Norton L (1992) Feasibility of adjuvant dose-intensive cyclophosphamide with G-CSF after doxorubicin in women with high-risk stage II/III resectable breast cancer. Proc Am Soc Clin Oncol 48
25. Peters WP, Ross M, Vredenburgh J, Meisenberg B, Rosner G, Marks L, Mathias B, Henderson C, Hurd D, Budman D, Norton L, Weiss RB (1992) High-dose alkylating agents and autologous bone marrow support for stage II/III breast cancer including 10 or more axillary lymph nodes. Proc Am Soc Clin Oncol 59
26. Lippman ME, Dickson RB, Bates S, Knabbe C, Huff K, Swain S, McManaway M, Bronzert D, Kasid A, Gelman EP (1986) Autocrine and paracrine growth regulation of human breast cancer. Breast Cancer Res Treat 7:59–70
27. Lippman ME (1987) Hormonal stimulation and chemotherapy for breast cancer (editorial). J Clin Oncol 5:331–332
28. Norton L (1990) Biology of residual breast cancer after therapy: A kinetic interpretation. In: Ragaz J, Simpson-Herren L, Lippman ME, Fisher B (eds) *Effects of therapy on biology and kinetics of the residual tumor, part A: pre-clinical aspects*. Wiley-Liss, New York, pp 109–132
29. Koury MJ, Bondurant MC (1990) Erythropoietin retards DNA breakdown and prevents programmed death in erythoid progenitor cells. Science 248:378–381
30. Williams GT, Smith CA, Spooncer E, Dexter TM, Taylor DR (1990) Haemopoietic colony stimulating factors promote cell survival by suppressing apoptosis. Nature 343:76–79
31. Barry MA, Behnke CA, Eastman A (1990) Activation of programmed cell death (apoptosis) by cisplain, other anticancer drugs, toxins and gyperthermia. Biochem Pharmacol 40:2353–2362
32. Norton L, Baselga J, Masui H, Hyman J, Kumar R, Mendelsohn J (1991) Growth factor perturbation: a therapeutically exploitable mechanism for chemotherapy action. Proc Am Soc Clin Oncol 208
33. Baselga J, Norton L, Miller W, Masui H, Mendelsohn J (1992) Synergistic antitumor effects of adriamycin and anti-epidermal growth factor receptor meonclonal antibodies. Proc Am Soc Clin Oncol 238

Tumor Stem Cells and the Curability of Early Human Breast Cancer

C. Jasmin

Department of Hematooncology, Hôpital Paul Brousse, 14 Av. P.V. Couturier, 94800 Villejuif, France

The Dual Tumor Stem Cell Concept

Stem cell models of malignant tumors have been based on the existence of three categories of cells within the total tumor cell population: (a) proliferating, self-renewing stem cells, (b) proliferating, non-self-renewing (transitional) cells and (c) non-proliferating, differentiated (end) cells. In 1984 we introduced the concept of two subpopulations of tumor stem cells (TSC; Fig. 1) [1]. One of these we refer to as the primitive or ancestral TSC (ATSC), which can remain out of cycling in G_o for prolonged periods of time. ATSC have a very long life span (almost unlimited). We hypothesized that late metastases, arising clinically more than 5 years after removal of the primary tumor, derive from these. The second we have called the committed TSC (CTSC), which has a restricted and transient development potential (limited to 4–5 years). In 1984 it was believed that a committed precursor could not retain its stem cell capacity. Indeed, normal stem cells were defined only by their very high reproductive capacity and multilineage differentiation potential.

The existence of at least two subpopulations of hematopoietic stem cells has been demonstrated in mice by using bone marrow transplantation after lethal irradiation. These experiments have allowed recognition of an early phase of a few months during which multiple stem cell clones with a transient and restricted development potential are active, and a later stage with a stable contribution from one or two pluripotent stem cells with long life span [2, 3]. We believe that the postulated 4- to 5-year survival of CTSC matches well the 2- to 3-month life span of hematopoietic committed stem cells. Therefore, our original model of tumor stem cells is compatible with the well-defined model of normal hematopoiesis. Human hematopoietic stem cells with high repopulating ability display the following characteristics: (a) presence of CD34 antigen, (b) absence of differentiation markers and HLA-DR antigens, and (c) resistance to 4-hydroxy-peroxycyclophosphamide.

Recent Results in Cancer Research, Vol. 127

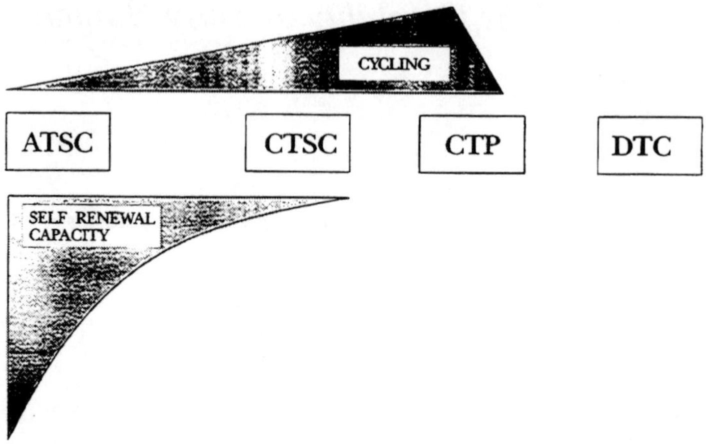

Fig. 1. Malignant stem cells of breast cancer. *ATSC*, ancestral tumor stem cell; *CTSC*, committed tumor stem cell; CTP, committed tumor progenitors (transitional); DTC, differentiated (end) tumor cells

Similarly, ATSC may be also protected from the direct cytotoxic effect of cycle-dependent therapeutic agents unless they are triggered into cycle.

Effect of Treatment on Tumor Stem Cells

The cycling effect of surgical removal of the primary tumor has been demonstrated in experimental tumor models [4–6]. The existence of growth-inhibiting factors, for example, transforming growth factor-β (TGF-β), may explain why the removal of the main source of production of the factors which keep the ATSC in G_o may stimulate the cycling of ATSC contained in micrometastatic deposits. Unopposed estrogens may constitute a second signal to promote the proliferation and committment of ATSC. Other growth factors produced either by the tumor cells and/or the micrometastatic stroma may also participate in the promotion of CTSC clones [7]. This mechanism of commitment of micrometastatic ATSC may also explain the stimulation of early metastases observed in premenopausal women after removal of the primary tumor during the unopposed estrogenic phase of the menstrual cycle [8–10].

According to our scheme, ovarian ablation in premenopausal patients could reduce the development of both early and late metastases by removing a growth-promoting signal acting on the cycling of ATSC induced by removal of the primary tumor. It is also understandable why ovarian ablation has no indication in postmenopausal patients.

Tamoxifen displays complex mechanisms of action. Tamoxifen has been shown to be mediated entiredly by the antiestrogen receptors present within thses cells. The induced TGF-β in the hormone-responsive breast cancer cell line MCF-7. This induction appears to be mediated entirely by the antiestrogen receptors present within these cells. The induced TGF-β was predominantly in the active form and could thus act directly on the cells, eliminating the need to propose a mechanism of activation. Based on this model one can see how tamoxifen would be of use even in a heterologous tumor composed of both estrogen-responsive and -unresponsive cells: the unresponsive cells would be growth inhibited in a paracrine manner by the TGF-β secreted by adjacent estrogen-positive cells [11]. To explain the finding that the benefit from tamoxifen is very dependent on the presence or absence of tumor estrogen receptors, it has been proposed that tamoxifen induces the secretion of TGF-β by the stroma of micrometastatic tumor cells. Indeed, Coletta has shown that tamoxifen causes a 5- to 25-fold increase in de novo active TGF-β secretion from two human fetal fibroblast cell lines both devoid of estrogen receptors [12]. Thus, even tumor cells that are unable to generate their own autocrine TGF-β loop could still benefit from the paracrine synthesis of TGF-β by tumor stromal fibroblasts. However, tamoxifen may also stimulate the secretion of epidermal growth factor and/or TGF-α within the tumor and increase its growth rate.

Chemotherapy can destroy cycling CTSC and committed tumor progenitors both in pre- and in postmenopausal patients. In premenopausal patients part of the antitumor effect of chemotherapy may be attributed to a chemical castration.

Current Results of Adjuvant Treatments of Human Breast Cancer and Predictions of the Dual Stem Cell Model

In Premenopausal Patients

The results of the Early Breast Trial Collaborative Group [13] (reprinted in part in this volume) clearly show that ovarian ablation produces a reduction in the annual death rate of about 25%. Interestingly, ovarian ablation continues to yield a reduction in annual recurrence rate even after 10 years of follow-up. These findings support the hypothesis that ovary secretion regulates the cycling and promotion of ATSC, the only stem cells with a very long survival capacity. Meta-analysis also suggests a further benefit of the combination of ovarian ablation with chemotherapy [13], a result which fits with the hypothesis of two types of TSC: ATCS which are the targets of ovarian ablation and CTSC which are chemosensitive. The results of the International Breast Study Collaborative Group [14], showing a specific effect of ovarian ablation on bone metastases, indicates that micrometastatic ATSC located in the bones and hormone-sensitive clones are the major targets of oophorectomy.

Tamoxifen (for 2 years at least) produces a significant reduction in recurrence during years 0–4 but does not (yet) reduce mortality. If confirmed, the antagonistic effects of ovarian secretions and tamoxifen could explain these results.

It is not surprising that polychemotherapy produces a significant reduction in recurrence during years 0–4. Polychemotherapy can destroy CTSC which give rise to early metastases. Its effects can be mediated partially by its ablative effect on ovarian function. This chemical ovarian ablation could explain its prolonged effect on survival; indeed, the ovary can no longer be stimulated and promote the multiplication of already activated ATSC. It is of importance to test directly whether there is an additive effect from the combination of chemotherapy with ovarian ablation or tamoxifen [13].

In Postmenopausal Patients

Tamoxifen reduces both the annual rate of recurrence by 20% and the 10-year mortality rate by 8%. The length of tamoxifen administration seems to be of importance. A 2-year treatment is superior to a 1-year treatment. Longer administration might be needed. As expected, Tamoxifen is more active in the absence of ovarian hormonal production.

Polychemotherapy reduces both the annual rate of recurrence and the mortality rate, although the latter is reduced only slightly. According to our model, classical adjuvant chemotherapy beginning 2–4 weeks after removal of the primary tumor has little chance of increasing the cure rate very significantly because ATSC which are not triggered by surgery and promoted by ovarian secretion are not sensitive to cycle-dependent cytotoxic agents.

The striking additive or synergistic effect of tamoxifen and chemotherapy, if confirmed by direct comparative trials, would suggest that tamoxifen could promote the transition of triggered ATSC into the CTSC compartment, a possibility which has been demonstrated in experimental tumors [15].

Perioperative Chemotherapy

Our model predicts that perioperative chemotherapy should reach greatest efficacy if administered when the primary tumor has been removed during the unopposed estrogenic phase.

Conclusions

We have attempted to match a model of breast cancer stem cells with the results of adjuvant therapy of breast cancer. Our model fits well with the observed results of surgical, hormonal, and cytotoxic therapy. Our model differs from all previous models by the presence of a compartment of committed stem cells endowed with a self-renewal capacity limited to a few years. The lifespan of this compartment, which is intermediate between the ATSC, well-protected from cycle-dependent therapeutic agents, and the committed tumor progenitors, constitutes the main target of treatments which act by direct destruction, inactivation or differentiation of tumor cells. This model takes into account the role of stromal cells which constitute the niche of TSCs. The identification of factors able to modulate the entry into cycle of ATSC would provide a potentially powerful therapeutic tool.

References

1. Jasmin C, Judde JG, Georgoulias V, Smadja-Joffe F, Poupon MF (1984) Models for adjuvant therapy. In: Jones SE, Salmon SE (eds) Adjuvant therapy of cancer. Grune and Stratton, Philadelphia, pp 35–45
2. Keller G, Snodgrass R (1990) Life span of multipotential hematopoietic stem cell in vivo. J Exp Med 171:10–47
3. Moore MAS (1991) Clinical implications of positive and negative hematopoietic stem cell regulators. Blood 78:1–19
4. Simpson-Herren L, Standford AH, Holmquist JP (1976) Effect of surgery on the cell kinetics of residual tumor. Cancer Treat Rep 60:1749–1760
5. Gunduz N, Fisher B, Saffer EA (1979) Effect of surgical removal on the growth and kinetics of residual tumor. Cancer Res 39:3861–3865
6. Fisher B, Gunduz N, Saffer EA et al. (1983) Influence of their interval between primary tumor removal and chemotherapy on kinetics and growth of metastasis. Cancer Res 43:1482–1488
7. Diskson RB, Huff KK, Spencer EM, Lippman ME (1986) Induction of epidermal growth factor-related polypeptides by 17-oestradiol in MCF-7 human breast cancer cells. Endocrinology 118:138–141
8. Hrushesky WJM, Bluming AZ, Gruber SA, Sothern RB (1989) Menstrual influence on surgical cure of breast cancer. Lancet 2:949–952
9. Senie RT, Rosen PP, Rhodes P, Lesser ML (1990) Prognosis of primary breast cancer in relation to time of diagnostic surgery during the menstrual cycle. Breast Cancer Res Treat 16:14–16
10. Badwe RA, Fentiman IS, Saad Z, Bentley A, Richards MA, Gregory W, Chaudary MA, Rubens RD (1991) Surgical procedures, menstrual cycles phase, and prognosis in operable breast cancer. Lancet 338:815–816
11. Knabbe C, Lippman ME, Wakefield LM et al. (1987) Evidence that transforming growth factor beta is a hormonally regulated negative growth factor in human breast cancer cells. Cell 48:417–428
12. Fisher B, Redmond C, Brown A et al. (1986) Adjuvant chemotherapy with or without tamoxifen in the treatment of primary breast cancer: five-year results from the NSABP trial. J Clin Oncol 4:459–471
13. Early Breast Cancer Trialist's Collaborative Group (1992) Systemic treatment of early breast cancer by hormonal, cytotoxic, or immune therapy: 133 randomised trials involving 31 000 recurrences and 24 000 deaths among 75 000 women. Lancet 1–15, 71–84

14. The International Breast Cancer Study Group (1990) Late effect of adjuvant oophorectomy and chemotherapy upon premenopausal breast cancer patients. Ann Oncol 1:30–35
15. Fendl KC, Zimniski J (1992) Role of tamoxifen in the induction of hormone-independent rat mammary tumors. Cancer Res 52:235–237

A New Paradigm for Breast Cancer

M.W. Retsky, D.E. Swartzendruber, P.D. Bame, and R.H. Wardwell

University of Colorado, Colorado Springs, CO 80933, USA

Introduction

Adjuvant chemotherapy extends disease-free survival in breast cancer, but it is usually not curative. Naturally, one must ask why. The main reasons often cited for treatment failure are drug resistance and host toxicity. Much research is directed to understanding and combating these effects, which have been known for some years. Although complex strategies for overcoming these obstacles are being developed, the problems have thus far not been resolved. When there is lack of progress, all assumptions need to be questioned, including generally accepted characteristics of tumors. One must examine the current paradigm for breast cancer and consider the experimental and theoretical basis of the paradigm. Most current therapies are based upon the original animal model studies of Skipper and Schabel [31], the kinetic studies of Laird [13], and the theoretical studies of Goldie and Coldman [3]. Our research of the past 10 years has given us reason to seriously doubt the validity of this paradigm [17, 18, 22, 26, 29, 32].

Discussion

In 1982 we determined that with the long time scale in the disease process, empirical methods to optimize therapy are not practical. If it takes 15 years to determine the results of treating a patient, traditional trial and error techniques cannot be carried out in one researcher's lifetime. We decided that computer modeling could reduce the time to a manageable scale. Our modeling started by trying to fit well-accepted [3a, 4, 9, 15, 16] Gompertzian kinetics to two natural history studies. One is that of data collected by Bloom et al. [1] on survival of untreated women with diagnosed breast cancer. The other is the Heuser et al. [10] data of serial mammography on 10000 women. These data provided information on tumor size at two

Recent Results in Cancer Research, Vol. 127

different times. Thus growth could be determined. We assumed that these two studies would be sufficient to quantify the Gompertzian parameters, and that we could then proceed to model the more interesting aspects of breast cancer such as chemotherapy.

We could not reconcile these data with the Gompertzian model. This could have been done if we had selectively discarded discordant data that were impossible to fit [22], but this was not considered an acceptable option to us since those data were as valid as any other data. Of the growth rates measured by Heuser et al. [10], 28% (9/23) were discordant to Gompertzian kinetics. Instead, a program was developed that would allow some variations in the Gompertzian model and agree with natural history data. That is, it would start off as Gompertzian and evolve into a different configuration that would provide a better fit to all the data. The program was complex and would run for several days on a mainframe computer. The program predicted that tumor growth was not Gompertzian but rather showed a biologically distinct irregular growth pattern, with alternating periods of growth and periods of little or no growth. The growth plateaus would last from a fraction of a year to perhaps 8 years. Figure 1 shows three typical growth curves on a semi-log plot. One milliliter is normally associated with 10^9 cells and 1 l with 10^{12} cells. The initial growth plateau occurs at 620 000 cells, which would be a sphere approximately 1 mm in diameter. Our model predicts that every tumor passes through this phase before kinetic heterogeneity is established.

There is an interesting biological relationship between the first growth plateau in our model and the tumor angiogenesis studies of Folkman [7]. The first growth plateau is the same size that a tumor can achieve before it induces the host to vascularize the tumor, as shown in the schematic figure

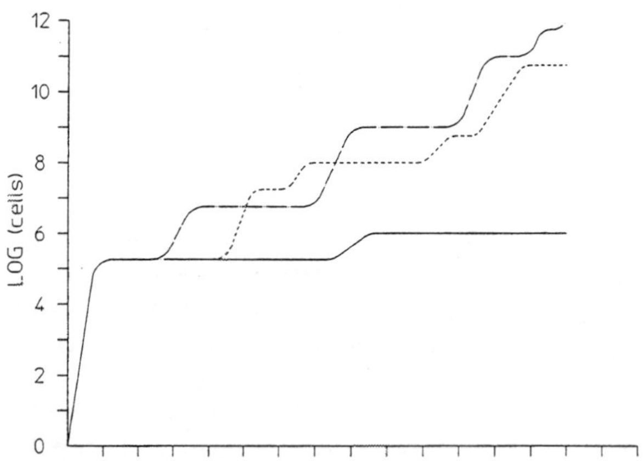

Fig. 1. Three typical breast cancer growth curves based on the computer model

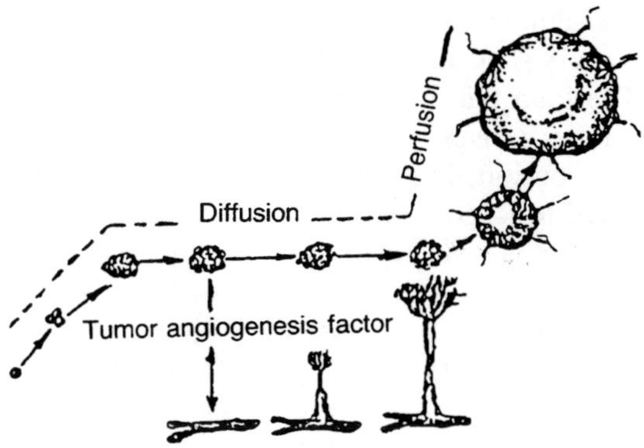

Fig. 2. Folkman's [7] stylized illustration of the concept that most solid tumors may exist as tiny cell populations living by simple diffusion in the extracellular space. Further growth requires vascularization, and the tumor then maintains itself by perfusion. Tumor angiogenesis factor may be the mediator of neovascularization. (Reprinted with permission)

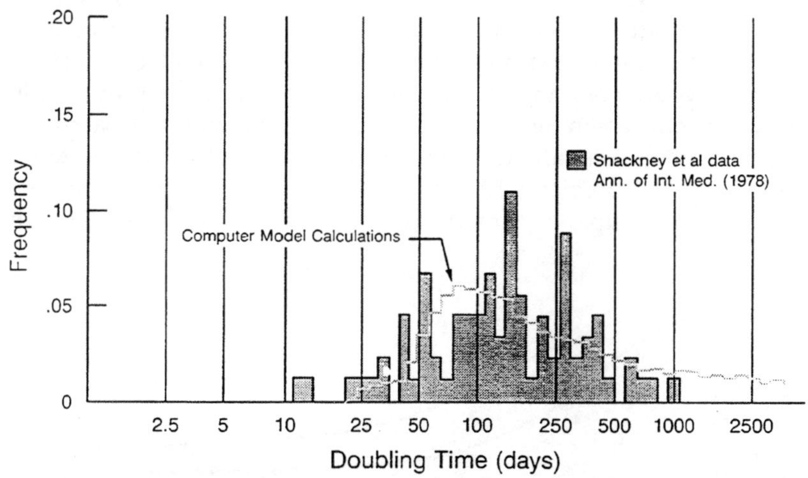

Fig. 3. Data reviewed by Shackney et al. [30] on the distribution of breast cancer doubling times for 91 tumors. Also shown is the result of simulated measurement of doubling times using our model for 30000 tumors [19]

from Folkman (Fig. 2). Prior to host vascularization, tumors achieve a diffusion-limited size of 1–4 mm. After angiogenesis, tumors have a growth spurt similar to our model. Our model also agrees with measured tumor doubling times. The shaded area in Fig. 3 refers to data reviewed by Shackney et al. [30] on the distribution of breast cancer doubling times for 91 tumors. The data ranged from 10 to 1000 days with a mean of 129 days.

We simulated measurement of doubling times using our model for 30 000 tumors [19]. Our resulting mode was 90 days, and the median was 175 days. The long tail in the distribution corresponding to some very slowly growing tumors causes the mean to be inappropriate. However, as can be seen, the distributions are quite similar. Thus tumors in our model usually grow from small to large size with doubling times consistent with data.

Next we incorporated chemotherapy into the model [18]. Once again, clinical data were used to develop the chemotherapy model. Later, in collaboration with Salmon [20], we determined that our calculated chemosensitivities are consistent with clonogenic assay data from the University of Arizona. We calculate that log cell kill per dose in clinical trials is limited by toxicity and drug resistance to 0.2–0.3 typically. This we estimate is about a factor of 2 from curative levels of 0.5 log. In contrast, animal models have 0.3–6 logs, [31] and Goldie and Coldman used 2 logs [8] in their calculations. We have used the model to predict disease-free survival for individual patients. The model is well calibrated and has been tested with an independent large data base. The average error in disease-free survival prediction has been measured as 4% [21].

We predict that only a small minority of premenopausal patients will be cured with adjuvant chemotherapy [27, 28]. We are referring to true cures, not just temporary extension of survival. This would be most apparent in patients with small aneuploid primaries and a few positive nodes. Figure 4 shows our computer simulation of treated and untreated disease-free survival for such a patient. There is a difference of approximately 10% at 15 years; thus we predict a 10% cure rate for a patient with one positive node and 0.8 cm aneuploid primary. In other cases, such as negative nodes and

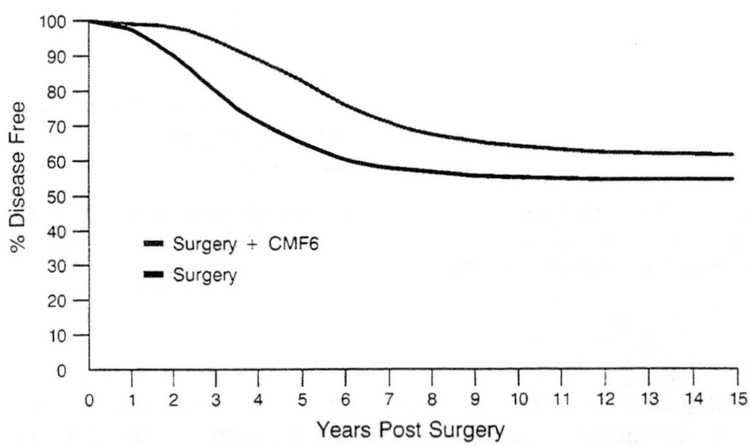

Fig. 4. Computer simulation of treated and untreated disease-free survival for a patient with one positive node and 0.8-cm aneuploid primary. *CMF6*, six-course treatment with cyclophosphamide, methotrexate, and 5-fluorouracil

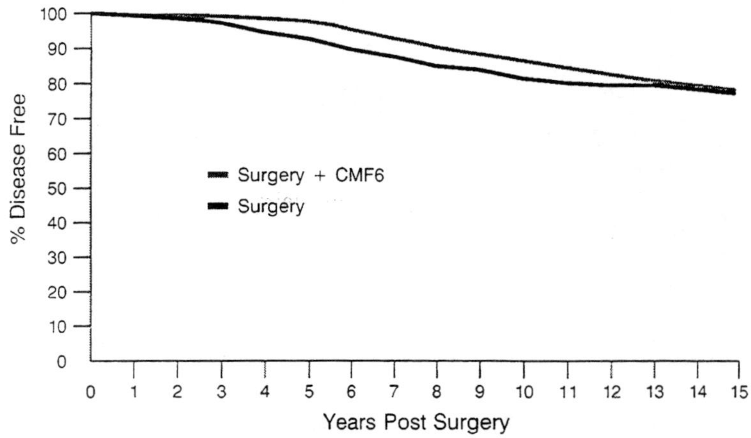

Fig. 5. Computer simulation of treated and untreated disease-free survival for a patient with negative nodes and a 0.8-cm, low %S, diploid primary. *CMF6*, six-course treatment with cyclophosphamide, methotrexate, and 5-fluorouracil

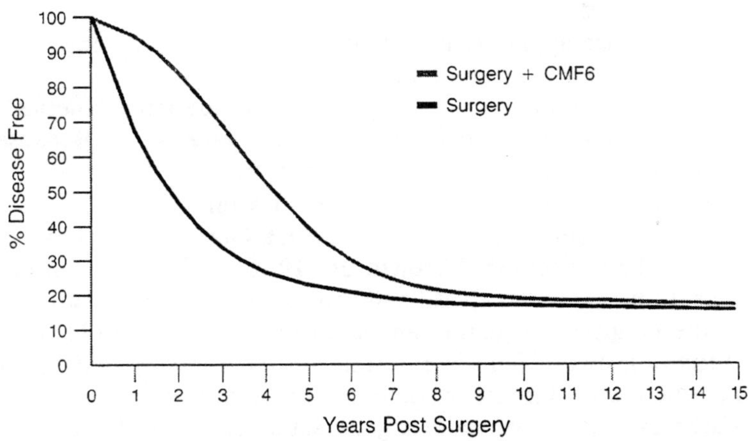

Fig. 6. Computer simulation of treated and untreated disease-free survival for a patient with ten positive nodes and a 3.0-cm aneuploid primary. *CMF6*, six-course treatment with cyclophosphamide, methotrexate, and 5-fluorouracil

small size, low %S, diploid primaries, as seen in Fig. 5, some cures occur but would be difficult to observe because there are so few relapse events. In the opposite case of many nodes and large aneuploid primaries, cures very rarely occur because the tumor burden is too large as seen in Fig. 6. These predictions are in some agreement with trial B-05, a clinical study from the NSABP [6] which indicates that long-term survival advantage from treat-

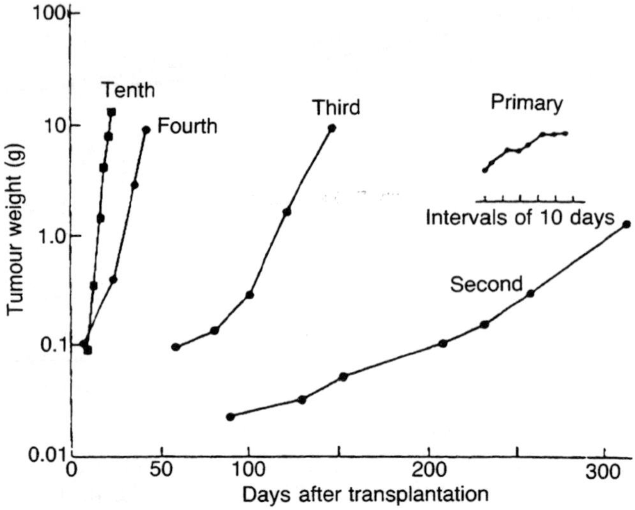

Fig. 7. Data from Steel [33] that show the growth of an original spontaneous animal tumor and how it changes as it is successively passaged through animals. From [33]

ment is most apparent in patient populations with one to three positive nodes and poorly differentiated primary tumors.

Since our studies seriously question Gompertzian kinetics, we must ask what the hard evidence for Gompertzian kinetics is. Because of limits of human experimentation, there are unfortunately few data.

Studies that use Gompertzian kinetics directly [9, 15, 16] or indirectly [3a, 4] cite Laird [13] as evidence that Gompertzian kinetics is valid for tumors. Laird measured growth of "19 examples of 12 different tumors of the rat, mouse, and rabbit" and concluded: "The pattern of growth defined by the Gompertz equation appears to be a general biological characteristic of tumor growth." This is a far-reaching statement based on only 18 rodents and one rabbit. Implicit in Laird's conclusion is the tenuous assumption that multipassaged animal models grow similarly to human tumors. Indeed, this is a poor assumption. Consider data from Steel [33], shown in Fig. 7. These data show the growth of an original spontaneous animal tumor and how it changes as it is successively passaged through animals. It originally grows in an erratic manner with a 50-day doubling time, and it gradually becomes Gompertzian and rampant, with 1 day doubling time. There is obviously a selection process. It is quite remarkable that Laird is so frequently cited as evidence that human tumors grow in a Gompertzian manner. There is no foundation for the common claim that breast cancer grows in a Gompertzian manner [26]. We suggest that the tumors on the left in Fig. 7 grow similarly to those that Laird measured and upon which Skipper and Schabel [31] experimented, while Steel's [33] primary tumor grows as our model has predicted, and as breast tumors actually grow.

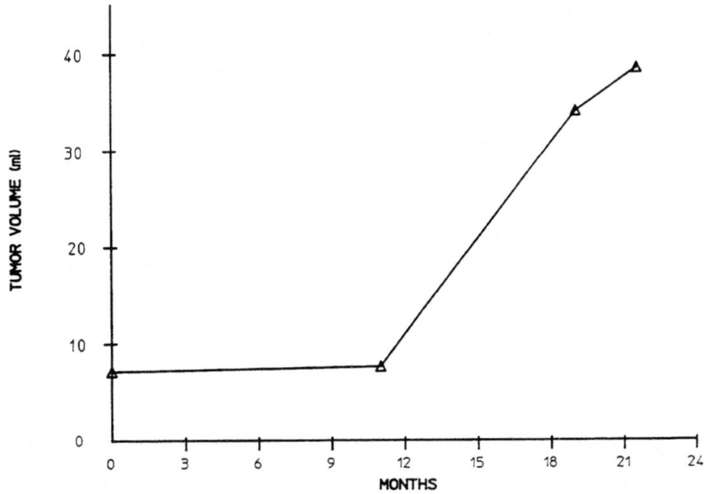

Fig. 8. Data of Ingleby and Moore [11] on growth of an untreated primary human breast cancer. Data were reported as tumor cross-sectional areas measured from X-ray films but are plotted as volumes here

If tumors grow as our model predicts, there should be some supporting evidence perhaps in older papers, when watchful waiting was an accepted practice. There are such data on multi-year observations of untreated malignancies which we have reviewed [26], and the literature is rich in examples of dormancy. For reviews, see Meltzer [14] and Stewart et al. [34]. One especially well-documented example of primary breast dormancy and subsequent regrowth is from Ingleby and Moore [11] and is shown in Fig. 8. This 78-year-old patient refused any treatment except for occasional breast X-rays over a 2-year period. The tumor was detected essentially in a growth plateau with 20-year doubling time for almost a year, and then it began to grow with a 180-day doubling time before it was removed and examined after another year. If this tumor grew with a constant doubling time of 20 years, it would lead to the unacceptable result that it started growing 650 years earlier. This clearly is not reconcilable with Gompertzian growth. However, it is consistent with our model.

What are the biological and clinical implications of non-Gompertzian kinetics? One can speculate on the biological processes in a temporarily nongrowing tumor [36]. Is there an equilibrium between death and division of cells, or can cells just go into temporary dormancy? Jasmin et al. [12] have discussed temporarily dormant stem cells in a "microenvironmental niche or ecosystem." Thomlinson [35] discussed sequestered cells with blood supply just sufficient to maintain them in G_1 and thus spared from cytotoxic agents. He thinks that it may be a very long time before a blood supply occurs that is good enough to cause reproliferation. He believes that the sequestered cell is the dominant cause of recurrence. J.S. Meyer (personal communication), who has published on tumor growth and thymidine labeling index, is convinced that growth is intermittent. He does not accept cell dormancy but thinks that there can be equivalency between cell proliferation and death in a tumor cell deposit. Considering the results of this research, J. Goldie (personal communication) has recently agreed that the most probable explanation is the ability of cancer cells to enter some sort of dormant state from which they randomly reemerge over a long time. He believes that it is difficult to imagine an alternative hypothesis to explain continuous and late recurrence in breast cancer. We suspect that all these processes, which are non-Gompertzian, are possible and do occur.

Conclusions

Most importantly, our work suggests that the mechanisms of treatment failure are different for Gompertzian models and adjuvant breast cancer. Treatments optimized on animal models are successful on animals but have not translated into breast cancer success. A Gompertzian tumor overruns the host without hesitation if it is not treated as soon as possible with all the drugs that the animal can tolerate. Our work suggests that may not be the case for breast cancer. There may be other mechanisms of treatment failure and therefore better treatment schemes particularly in the therapy of early stage breast cancer. The non-Gompertzian processes mean that the log cell kill approximation is not valid for breast cancer. This may partially explain why 12 months of therapy is not much more effective than 6 months of therapy [5].

Our studies suggest that short-course intensive chemotherapy serves mainly to reduce metastasis size, thus delaying early relapse. This improves disease-free survival but has less impact on survival. This is consistent with a recent meta-analysis showing that recurrence-free survival advantage from chemotherapy occurs mainly in the first 5 years after treatment and is not significantly increased or decreased after that point [5]. Our studies further suggest that therapy is too ineffective by a factor of 2 to be considered curative. However, if used judiciously, these same drugs may be effective enough to retain tumors at small size [23, 24]. We believe that this is true even considering acquired drug resistance. It is like a boxer going for the decision rather than the knockout. We suggest that our paradigm can be used to design pilot studies especially for poor prognosis stage II patients [2] and stage IV patients in complete remission [25].

References

1. Bloom H, Richardson M, Harries B (1962) Natural history of untreated breast cancer (1804–1933): comparison of untreated and treated cases according to histological grade of malignancy. BMJ 2:213–221

2. Buzdar AU, Kan SW, Hortobagyi GN et al. (1992) Clinical course of patients with breast cancer with ten or more nodes who were treated with doxorubicin-containing adjuvant therapy. Cancer 69:448–452
3. Coldman AJ, Goldie JH (1985) Role of mathematical modeling in protocol formulation in cancer chemotherapy. Cancer Treat Rep 69:1041
3a. Cooper MR, Cooper MR (1991) Principles of medical oncology. In: Holleb AI, Fink DJ, Murphy GP (eds) The American Cancer Society textbook of clinical oncology American Murph. Cancer Society, Atlanta, p 50
4. DeVita V (1983) The relationship between tumor mass and resistance to chemotherapy. Cancer 51:1209–1220
5. Early Breast Cancer Trialists Collaborative Group (1992) Systemic treatment of early breast cancer by hormonal, cytotoxic, or immune therapy: 133 randomised trials involving 31000 recurrences and 24000 deaths among 75000 women. Lancet 339:71–85
6. Fisher B, Redmond C, Fisher ER, Wolmark N (1986) Systemic adjuvant therapy in treatment of primary operable breast cancer: National Surgical Adjuvant Breast and Bowel Project experience. Natl Cancer Inst Monogr 1:35–43
7. Folkman J (1971) Tumor angiogenesis: therapeutic implications. N Engl J Med 285/21:1182–1186
8. Goldie JH, Coldman AJ, Gudauskas GA (1982) Rationale for the use of alternating non-cross-resistant chemotherapy. Cancer Treat Rep 66:439–449
9. Hellman S, DeVita VT Jr (1982) Principles of cancer biology: kinetics of cellular proliferation. In: DeVita VT Jr, Hellman S, Rosenberg S (eds) Cancer: principles and practices of oncology. Lippincott, Philadelphia, p 13
10. Heuser L, Spratt J, Polk H (1979) Growth rates of primary breast cancer. Cancer 43:1888–1894
11. Ingleby H, Moore L (1956) Periodic roentgenographic studies of a growing mammary cancer. Cancer 9:749
12. Jasmin C, Poupon MF, Smadja J et al. (1986) Tumor stem cells and their ecosystem: therapeutic implications of a new concept. In: Local immunity in cancer. Regensberg and Biermann, Münster
13. Laird A (1969) Dynamics of growth in tumors and in normal organisms. Natl Cancer Inst Monogr 30:15–28
14. Meltzer A (1990) Dormancy and breast cancer. J Surg Oncol 43:181–188
15. Norton L (1988) A Gompertzian model of human breast cancer growth. Cancer Res 48:7067–7071
16. Prehn RT (1991) The inhibition of tumor growth by tumor mass. Perspectives in cancer research. Cancer Res 51:2–4
17. Retsky M, Wardwell R, Speer J (1984) A computer simulation of breast cancer growth and treatment. American Association for Medical Systems and Informatics Proceedings 453–457
18. Retsky M, Wardwell R, Swartzendruber D, Headley D (1987) Prospective computerized simulation of breast cancer: a comparison of computer predictions with nine sets of biological and clinical data. Cancer Res 47:4982–4987
19. Retsky MW, Bame PD, Wardwell RH, Swartzendruber DE (1988) Clinical implications and supporting evidence for a computer model of breast cancer. 3rd international conference on adjuvant therapy of breast cancer, March 1988, St. Gallen
20. Retsky M, Swartzendruber D, Wardwell R, Bame P, Salmon S (1988) Chemosensitivity correlation between a breast cancer computer model and clonogenic assay. Proc Meet Am Assoc Cancer Res 29:477
21. Retsky MW, Bame PD, Wardwell RH, Swartzendruber DE (1988) Predicting the results of new therapies with an accurate breast cancer computer model. Proc Meet Am Assoc Cancer Res 29:335

22. Retsky M, Swartzendruber D, Wardwell R, Bame P, Petrosky V (1989) Correspondence re: Larry Norton. A Gompertzian model of human breast cancer growth. Cancer Res 48:7067–7071, 49:6443–6444
23. Retsky MW, Swartzendruber DE, Wardwell RH, Bame PD (1989) Predictions of effective treatment plans for very poor prognosis breast cancer patients using a computer model. Proc Annu Meet Am Assoc Cancer Res 30:627
24. Retsky MW, Swartzendruber DE, Wardwell RH, Bame PD (1989) Computer predicted therapy plans for very poor prognosis breast cancer patients. In: 12th annual San Antonio breast cancer symposium, Dec 1989
25. Retsky MW, Swartzendruber DE, Wardwell RH, Bame PD (1989) Thiotepa in maintenance therapy of metastatic brain cancer; comparison to computer model predictions. International symposium on effects of therapy on biology and kinetics of surviving tumor, Feb 1989, Vancouver
26. Retsky M, Swartzendruber D, Wardwell R, Bame P (1990) Is Gompertzian kinetics a valid description of individual tumor growth? Med Hypotheses 33:95–106
27. Retsky MW, Swartzendruber D, Bame PD, Wardwell RH (1990) Modified conclusions from a computer model of breast cancer regarding chemotherapeutic cure. Sixth international conference on the adjuvant chemotherapy of cancer, Tucson, March 1990
28. Retsky M, Swartzendruber D, Bame P, Wardwell R (1990) Computer model predictions of chemotherapeutic cure in breast cancer. 81st Proc Am Assoc Cancer Res, Washington, May 1990
29. Retsky M, Swartzendruber D, Bame P, Wardwell R (1991) Tenuous link between Gompertzian kinetics and breast cancer. 14th annual San Antonio breast cancer symposium, Dec 1991
30. Shackney SE, McCormack GW, Cuchural GJ Jr (1978) Growth rate patterns of solid tumors and their relation to responsiveness to therapy – an analytic review. Ann Intern Med 89:107–121
31. Skipper H, Schabel F Jr (1982) Quantitative and cytokinetic studies in experimental tumor systems. In: Holland JF, Frei E III (eds) Cancer medicine. Lea and Febiger, Philadelphia, pp 663–685
32. Speer J, Petrosky V, Retsky M, Wardwell R (1984) A stochastic numerical model of breast cancer growth that simulates clinical data. Cancer Res 44:4124–4130
33. Steel GG (1977) Growth kinetics of tumours; cell population kinetics in relation to the growth and treatment of cancer. Clarendon, Oxford
34. Stewart THM, Hollinshead AC, Raman S (1991) Tumour dormancy: initiation, maintenance and termination in animals and humans. Can Soc Cardiovasc Thorac Surg 34:321–325
35. Thomlinson RH (1982) Measurement and management of carcinoma of the breast. Clin Radiol 33:481–493
36. Uhr JW, Tucker T, May RD et al. (1991) Cancer dormancy: studies of the murine BCL1 lymphoma. Cancer Res [Suppl] 51:5045s–5053s

A Laboratory Model To Explain the Survival Advantage Observed in Patients Taking Adjuvant Tamoxifen Therapy

D.M. Wolf and V.C. Jordan

Department of Human Oncology, University of Wisconsin Comprehensive Cancer Center, Madison, WI 53792, USA

Introduction

The nonsteroidal antiestrogen tamoxifen was first described in 1967 [1]. It was initially intended, based on its activity in rodents, for use as an antifertility agent. It was found, however, that tamoxifen actually induces ovulation in subfertile women. The antitumor effects of tamoxifen were more promising. The drug first entered clinical trials in the United Kingdom in 1971 [2] and was approved for use in the United States in 1978. It was initially used as a palliative treatment for advanced breast cancer in postmenopausal, primarily elderly, women. In a randomly selected sample of patients with advanced breast cancer, about 30%–40% have a favorable response to tamoxifen therapy. However, among patients whose primary tumors are estrogen and progesterone receptor positive response rates to tamoxifen are in the range of 70%–80% [3].

Since its initial introduction as a palliative treatment for advanced disease, the use of tamoxifen has been broadened to include treatment for all stages of breast cancer in both pre- and postmenopausal women. Indeed, a trial is under way in the United Kingdom evaluating the use of tamoxifen as a breast cancer preventive [4, 5], and another is being planned in the United States. An overview analysis of the treatment for early breast cancer, combining the results from 40 adjuvant tamoxifen trials with a total of nearly 30000 women, was published recently [6] (reprinted in part in this volume). This report demonstrated that patients treated with adjuvant tamoxifen had highly significant increases in both disease-free and overall survival. This benefit was observed in women with either stage I or stage II disease. Interestingly, the beneficial effect of tamoxifen on prolonging absolute survival appears to be maintained long after tamoxifen administration is stopped. In addition, it appears that tamoxifen is beneficial for premenopausal women as well, although the reductions in odds ratios for either recurrence or mortality are not as great as those for postmenopausal

Recent Results in Cancer Research, Vol. 127

women, and do not reach statistical significance. The overview analysis [6] demonstrated that better results were achieved by longer term administration of tamoxifen. More than 2 years (up to 5) of tamoxifen was better than 2 years, and 2 years was better than 1, in terms of improvements in both disease-free and overall survival.

Is it plausible to postulate that, since benefits derived from more than 2 years of tamoxifen treatment are greater than those observed when the drug is administered for shorter periods, the best course would be to administer tamoxifen for an indefinite duration? Recent data from our laboratory indicate that this may not be the case. Both Gottardis and Jordan [7] and Osborne et al. [8, 9] have reported that when hormone-dependent MCF-7 human breast cancer cells inoculated into athymic mice are exposed to tamoxifen for prolonged periods, tumors eventually develop which are growth stimulated by either tamoxifen or estradiol. We now report that after several years of continuous tamoxifen-stimulated growth, these tumor variants (MCF-7 TAM) have further altered their phenotype such that the administration of estradiol now produces a massive cytotoxic response. We discuss the implications of this data with respect to the overview analysis and, in particular, to the observation that tamoxifen-treated patients experience a continued survival benefit long after treatment has stopped.

The Primary Action of Tamoxifen Is Tumoristatic

Most of the laboratory data generated in the past three decades indicate that the antitumor action of tamoxifen is cytostatic rather than cytotoxic. Tamoxifen is thought to act primarily by occupying the estrogen receptor and blocking the growth-stimulatory action of estradiol. For example, estradiol stimulates the proliferation of the human mammary tumor derived cell line MCF-7 either in culture [10, 11] or when the cells are inoculated into athymic mice [12–16]. This estrogen-induced proliferation can be blocked by simultaneous treatment with tamoxifen [11, 12, 15, 16]. However, if tamoxifen is removed, and the estrogenic stimulus is maintained, growth recurs – indicating that cells treated with tamoxifen are held in nonproliferative stasis but not killed [15, 16]. Similarly, continuous treatment with tamoxifen can block the development of mammary tumors in rats treated with dimethylbenzanthracene [17–20] and in mice infected with mouse mammary tumor virus [21, 22]. Removal of tamoxifen in these systems is also accompanied by the development of mammary tumors. This indicates that tamoxifen is preventing initiated cells from proliferating, but not actually eliminating any tumor cells.

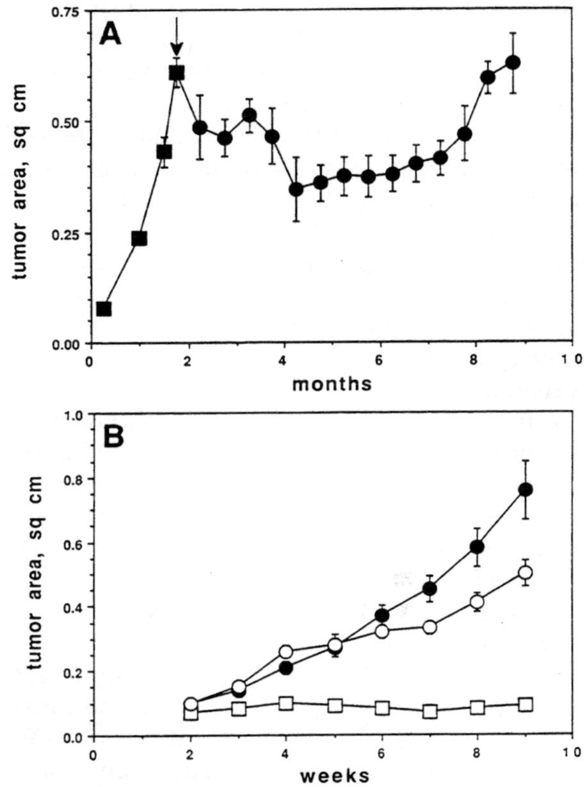

Fig. 1. A Development of tamoxifen-stimulated growth. MCF-7 tumors were implanted into athymic nude mice treated with estradiol (■). After 2 months, estradiol was removed (*arrow*) and replaced with tamoxifen (●). **B** Growth characteristics of MCF-7 TAM tumors. A tamoxifen-stimulated tumor from **A** was harvested and minced, and pieces were implanted into 4- to 5-week-old athymic nude mice, treated with either estradiol (○), TAM (●), or no treatment (□)

After Prolonged Exposure, Tumors Become Growth Stimulated by Tamoxifen

If MCF-7 breast cancer cells (or pieces of a previously established MCF-7 solid tumor) are inoculated into the flanks of athymic mice, estrogen-dependent, tamoxifen-inhibited tumors develop [11, 12, 15, 16]. If these tumors are treated with tamoxifen instead of estradiol, initially no growth occurs. However, two laboratories [7–9] have shown that after a period of several months, tamoxifen-stimulated tumors begin to grow (Fig. 1a). These tumors (MCF-7 TAM), when transplanted into new athymic mice, can be stimulated to grow by either estradiol or tamoxifen, but do not grow in untreated control animals (Fig. 1b). Further, the tamoxifen-or estradiol-stimulated growth of these tumors can be inhibited by treatment with the pure antiestrogen ICI 164384 [23].

There is currently some controversy as to the mechanism by which tamoxifen-stimulated growth in this model is achieved. One current hypothesis is that the tumor somehow acquires the ability to metabolize tamoxifen to an estrogenic compound, to a compound with minimal antiestrogenic activity, or to both [9]. One of the principal metabolites of tamoxifen is 4-hydroxytamoxifen (4-OHT), a potent antiestrogen with high affinity for the estrogen receptor [24]. It is the Z isomer of 4-OHT which is produced by the metabolism of tamoxifen. It may be that a tamoxifen-stimulated tumor could convert this compound to the E form, which is a weak, low-affinity antiestrogen [24]. Removal of the aminoethoxy side chain of tamoxifen generates the Z isomer of metabolite E [(Z) met E], a weak estrogen [24]. In order to produce an estrogen with enough potency to overcome growth inhibition by tamoxifen, the tumor would also have to be able to isomerize (Z) met E to the E isomer [(E) met E] which is a potent estrogen [24]. The tumor would have to produce this compound in an amount sufficient to overcome the growth-suppressive effects of tamoxifen and its antiestrogenic metabolites which would still be present.

Data from our laboratory indicate that altered metabolism of tamoxifen is not a likely explanation for the occurrence of tamoxifen-stimulated growth in our MCF-7 TAM model. We have shown that a fixed-ring nonisomerizable analog of tamoxifen (FRT [25]) is as efficacious as tamoxifen in stimulating the growth of MCF-7 TAM tumors (Wolf, Langan-Fahey, Parker, McCague, and Jordan, in preparation). Since this compound can form neither the weak antiestrogen (E) 4-OHT nor the potent estrogen (E) met E, it seems unlikely that isomerization of the ligand in tamoxifen-stimulated cells is a relevant contributor to tamoxifen-stimulated growth, at least in our model. An alternative hypothesis is that the tumor cells have developed the ability to retain the weak estrogenic metabolites or actively excrete the antiestrogenic metabolites of tamoxifen [9]. We have used a sensitive HPLC assay [26, 27] to detect tamoxifen and its metabolites in the serum and tumors of treated animals. We have shown that there are no significant differences between the levels of tamoxifen and its metabolites (or FRT and its metabolites) found in either wild-type MCF-7 tumors or tamoxifen-stimulated MCF-7 TAM tumors (Wolf, Langan-Fahey, Parker, and Jordan, in preparation).

Estradiol Induces the Rapid Regression of Tumors Grown for Long Periods in the Presence of Tamoxifen

The MCF-7 TAM tumors described above were transplanted serially into athymic mice treated with tamoxifen alone for roughly 4 years (16 passages). When the tumor was transplanted for passage 17 (late-passage MCF-7 TAM), all mice were implanted with a subcutaneous tamoxifen capsule as

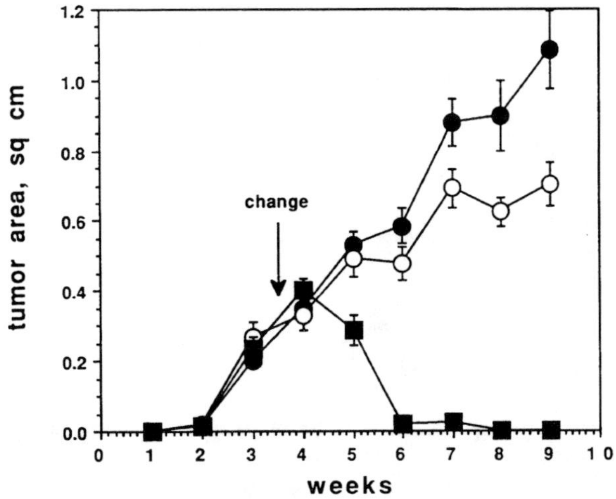

Fig. 2. Estradiol-induced regression of late-passage MCF-7 TAM tumors. Late-passage MCF-7 TAM tumors were transplanted into 4- to 5-week-old athymic nude mice and treated with tamoxifen until the point marked change (*arrow*) in the figure. At this point tamoxifen was continued (●), removed (○), or removed and replaced with estradiol (■)

usual. When the tumors had reached a cross-sectional area of approximately $0.3\,cm^2$, tamoxifen capsules were removed from six of the mice and replaced with estradiol. In 2 weeks all but two (of 12) tumors had disappeared, and the remaining two were markedly decreased in size. Within 4 weeks there was no evidence of tumor on any of the animals (Fig. 2). One of the mice was sacrificed, and the area that had previously borne tumors was examined. No evidence of gross tumor was detectable, but a few small calcified nodules were present. These nodules were presumed to be the remains of the necrotic core that forms at the center of most tumors grown in this model system.

This experiment was repeated, with similar results. Three weeks after treatment was switched from tamoxifen to estradiol we observed complete remission of all but one tumor. In addition, when MCF-7 TAM tumor pieces were implanted into animals treated with estradiol instead of tamoxifen, no growth occurred, indicating that with this tumor estradiol is more detrimental to tumor growth than the complete absence of ligand.

Tumors that Recur After Estrogen-Induced Remission Are Growth Stimulated by Estradiol but not by Tamoxifen

Five weeks after complete estradiol-induced remission had taken place (see Fig. 2), two tumors began to grow back from a possible ten sites (Fig. 3). In order to further analyze these recurrent tumors, one of them was harvested

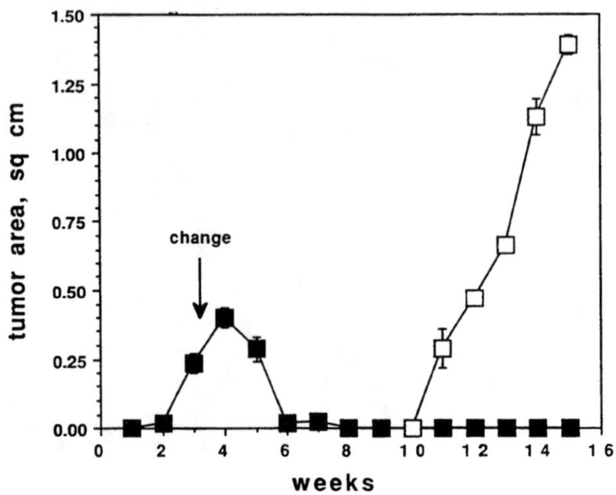

Fig. 3. Estradiol-stimulated recurrence of MCF-7 TAM after estradiol-induced regression of the original tumors. Estradiol-treated animals from Fig. 2 (○) were maintained on estrogen, and eventually two tumors from ten sites regrew (□)

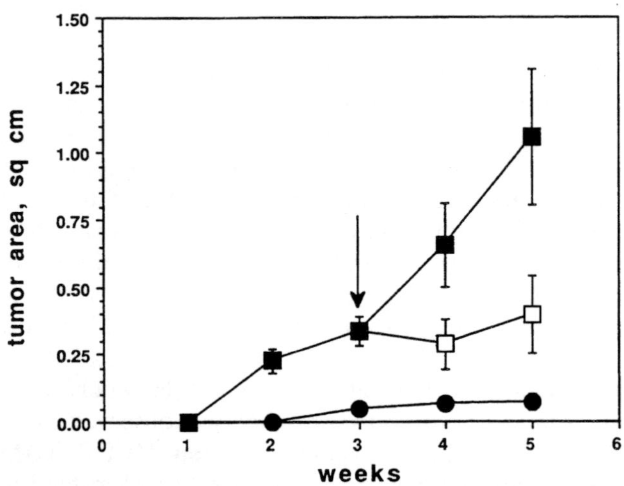

Fig. 4. Growth characteristics of estradiol-stimulated MCF-7 TAM recurrence. One of the recurrent tumors from Fig. 3 was transplanted into a new group of athymic nude mice and treated with estradiol (■) or TAM (●) or switched (*arrow*) from estradiol to tamoxifen (□) after 2 weeks of growth

and minced, and pieces were implanted into 14 recipient mice, 7 of which were treated with estradiol and 7 with tamoxifen. As can be seen in Fig. 4, estradiol stimulated the growth of these tumors, whereas tamoxifen did not. Further, when we removed the estradiol from three of the animals and

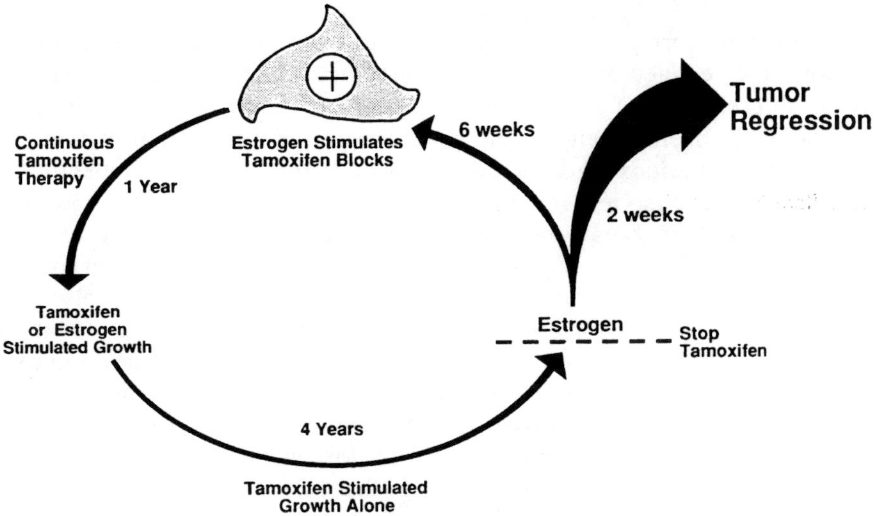

Fig. 5. A model to describe the apparently cyclical behavior of the MCF-7/MCF-7 TAM tumor model

replaced it with tamoxifen, tumor growth stopped, indicating that the tumor phenotype had changed, and that tamoxifen was no longer sufficient to stimulate growth.

Summary and Hypotheses

We have developed a model that explains the results observed with the late-passage MCF-7 TAM (Fig. 5), and we feel that this model has clinical relevance, based on the results of the Early Breast Cancer Trialists' Collaborative Group analysis [6]. As shown in Fig. 5, endocrine responsive tumor cells start out as estrogen receptor positive and are dependent upon the presence of estrogens for growth stimulation. Their growth can be inhibited by antiestrogens such as tamoxifen. If the tumor cells are exposed to tamoxifen continuously (for about 1 year in our system) tamoxifen-stimulated growth results, although the tumor cells are still responsive to estrogen as a growth stimulus. After an extended period of time during which tamoxifen is the only growth stimulus provided, a population of tumor cells hypersensitized to the weak estrogenic stimulus provided by tamoxifen is selected. When these tumor cells are exposed to estradiol, a massive and ultimately cytotoxic overstimulation results. The recurrence of a small number of tumors that have endocrine responses similar to the original cell line occurs due to the heterogeneous nature of the tumor. It is probable that a fraction of the total cells in the MCF-7 TAM tumor are of the original MCF-7 phenotype and have been maintained in a very slowly dividing state during the propagation of this tumor. When the majority of tumor cells are killed by estradiol administration, the few estrogen-responsive cells still present have a selective advantage and can grow into a new tumor.

There has been a trend in the clinic toward administration of tamoxifen for extended periods. Additional support for this trend has recently been provided in an overview meta-analysis of adjuvant therapy for early breast cancer [6]. This analysis demonstrates that tamoxifen administered for longer than 2 (up to 5) years results in both improved disease-free survival and overall survival than a shorter period of tamoxifen treatment. It also shows that the tamoxifen-associated benefits in overall survival are maintained for at least 10 years after the start of treatment – long after tamoxifen administration has been stopped. This effect is somewhat paradoxical since it has generally been supposed that the action of tamoxifen is primarily cytostatic, and that the benefit would be lost when treatment is stopped. Our model may, at least in part, explain this observation.

Figure 6 shows what may be occurring in patients receiving adjuvant tamoxifen therapy. Following removal of the primary tumor, a patient may be left with small, estrogen receptor positive, endocrine-responsive micrometasteses (cross-hatched cells shown on the far left in Fig. 6). Adjuvant tamoxifen suppresses the growth of these cells, but eventually clones of cells are selected that can respond to tamoxifen as a growth stimulus (represented by the light gray cells in Fig. 6). The tumor containing this mixed cell population can be stimulated to grow by either tamoxifen or estradiol. If tamoxifen is stopped at this point, estrogen-stimulated recurrent disease might be expected to occur. Continued exposure to tamoxifen would result

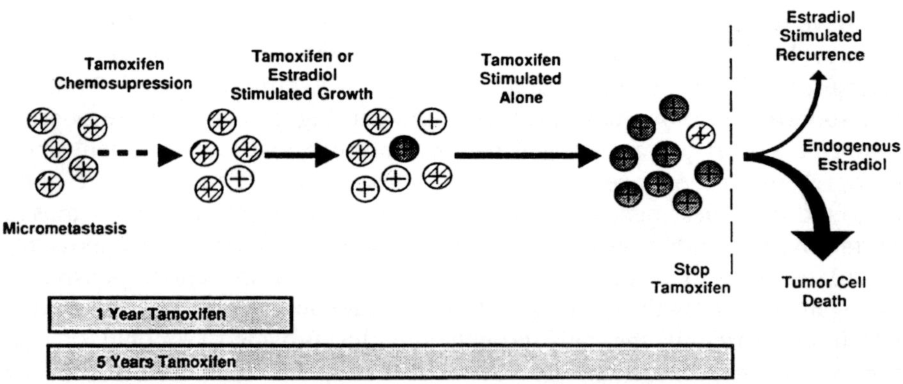

Fig. 6. A model to explain the sustained survival benefit observed in patients treated with adjuvant tamoxifen, which persists even after tamoxifen administration is stopped. *Cross-hatched cells*, estrogen-stimulated, tamoxifen-inhibited; *light gray cells*, cells stimulated by estrogen or tamoxifen; *dark gray cells*, cells stimulated by tamoxifen but killed by estradiol

in the selection of cells that are hypersensitized to take full advantage of the weak estrogenic stimulus provided by tamoxifen (dark gray cells in Fig. 6), and these cells would eventually become the dominant cells type in the (still subclinical) metastasis. If tamoxifen is stopped at this point, the patient's circulating estrogens cause a massive and ultimately lethal overstimulation of these hypersensitized cells. Even the low levels of estrone and estradiol produced by peripheral aromatization of adrenal steroids in postmenopausal women may be sufficient to cause this effect.

We are left with the question of the most beneficial course of adjuvant treatment for the patient with early breast cancer. It must be remembered that in addition to its antitumor activity, tamoxifen has other beneficial systemic effects. Tamoxifen has been show to prevent losses in bone density [5, 28] and to decrease serum cholesterol and low-density lipoprotein levels [4, 29]. In addition, one trial has actually demonstrated that tamoxifen is associated with a decrease in the incidence of fatal myocardial infarction [30]. Since node-negative patients are primarily at risk for non-breast cancer related mortality and are not eligible for postmenopausal hormone replacement therapy, it seems that the non-breast cancer related benefits associated with tamoxifen treatment outweigh the small risk of developing a tamoxifen-stimulated recurrence in this population. We therefore suggest that node-negative patients electing to receive tamoxifen be treated indefinitely; if disease recurrence is detected, the tamoxifen can be stopped at this point in an attempt to achieve an estrogen-induced cytotoxic response. On the other hand, the primary threat to the well-being of the node-positive patient is the possibility of a recurrence of her disease. In this case, the greatest benefit to the patient may be derived from the administration of a limited, yet long-term course of tamoxifen (2–5 years in duration), after which tamoxifen could be withdrawn in hope of incurring an additional beneficial estrogen-induced cytotoxic withdrawal response.

Acknowledgements. D.M.W. is a graduate student in the Department of Human Oncology and is the recipient of a Susan B. Komen scholarship. These studies were supported by the Komen foundation.

References

1. Harper MJK, Walpole AL (1967) A new derivative of triphenylethylene: effect on implantation and mode of action in rats. J Reprod Fertil 13:101–119
2. Cole MP, Jones CJA, Todd IDH (1971) A new antioestrogenic agent in late breast cancer. Br J Cancer 25:270–275
3. Jordan VC, Wolf MF, Mirecki DM, Whitford DA, Welshons WV (1988) Hormone receptor assays: clinical usefulness in the management of carcinoma of the breast. CRC Crit Rev Clin Lab Sci 26:97–152
4. Powles TJ, Hardy JR, Ashley SE, Farrington GM, Cosgrove D, Davey JB, Dowsett M, McKinna A, Nash AG, Sinnett HD, Tillyer CR, Treleven JG (1989)

A pilot trial to evaluate the acute toxicity and feasibility of tamoxifen for prevention of breast cancer. Br J Cancer 60:126–131

5. Powles TJ, Tillyer CR, Jones AJ, Ashley SE, Treleven J, Davey JB, McKenna JA (1990) Prevention of breast cancer with tamoxifen – an update on the Royal Marsden Hospital pilot programme. Eur J Cancer 26:680–684
6. Early Breast Cancer Trialists' Collaborative Group (1992) Systemic treatment of early breast cancer by hormonal, cytotoxic, or immune therapy: 133 randomized trials involving 31 000 recurrences and 24 000 deaths among 75 000 women. Lancet 339:1–15, 71–85
7. Gottardis MM, Jordan VC (1988) Development of tamoxifen-stimulated growth of MCF-7 tumors in athymic mice after long-term antiestrogen administration. Cancer Res 48:5183–5187
8. Osborne CK, Coronado E, Allred DC, Wiebe V, DeGregorio M (1991) Acquired tamoxifen resistance: correlation with reduced breast tumor levels of tamoxifen and isomerization of trans-4-hydroxytamoxifen. J Natl Cancer Inst 83:1477
9. Osborne CK, Coronado EB, Robinson JP (1987) Human breast cancer in the athymic nude mouse: cytostatic effects of long term antiestrogen therapy. Eur J Cancer Clin Oncol 23:1189
10. Lippman ME, Bolan G (1975) Oestrogen-responsive human breast cancer in long-term tissue culture. Nature 256:592
11. Lippman ME, Bolan G, Huff K (1976) The effects of estrogens and antiestrogens on hormone-responsive breast cancer in long term culture. Cancer Res 36:4595–4601
12. Shafie SM, Grantham FH (1981) Role of hormones in the growth and regression of human breast cancer cells (MCF-7) transplanted into athymic nude mice. J Natl Cancer Inst 67:51–56
13. Soule HD, McGrath CM (1980) Estrogen responsive proliferation of clonal human breast cancer cells in athymic mice. Cancer Lett 10:177–189
14. Huseby RA, Maloney TM, McGrath CM (1984) Evidence for a direct growth-stimulatory effect of estradiol on human MCF-7 cells in vivo. Cancer Res 44:2654–2659
15. Osborne CK, Hobbs K, Clark GM (1985) Effect of estrogens and antiestrogens on growth of human breast cancer cells in athymic nude mice. Cancer Res 45:584–590
16. Gottardis MM, Robinson SP, Jordan VC (1988) Estradiol-stimulated growth of MCF-7 tumors implanted in athymic mice: a model to study the tumoristatic action of tamoxifen. J Steroid Biochem 30:311–314
17. Jordan VC (1975) The anti-tumour effect of tamoxifen in the dimethylbenzanthracene-induced rat mammary carcinoma model. In: Proceedings of the symposium on the hormonal control of breast cancer, Alderley Park. ICI Pharmaceuticals Division PLC, Macclesfield, pp 11–17
18. Jordan VC (1976) Antiestrogenic and antitumor properties of tamoxifen in laboratory animals. Cancer Treat Rep 60:1409–1419
19. Jordan VC (1976) Effect of tamoxifen (ICI 46474) on initiation and growth of DMBA-induced rat mammary carcinoma. Eur J Cancer Clin Oncol 12:419–424
20. Jordan VC (1978) Use of the DMBA-induced rat mammary carcinoma system for the evaluation of tamoxifen treatment as a potential adjuvant therapy. Rev Endocrine-related Cancer. Oct Suppl: 49–55
21. Jordan VC, Lababidi MK, Mirecki DM (1990) Anti-oestrogenic and anti-tumour properties of prolonged tamoxifen therapy in C3H/OUJ mice. Eur J Cancer 26:718–721
22. Jordan VC, Lababidi MK, Langan-Fahey S (1991) Suppression of mouse mammary tumorigenesis by long-term tamoxifen therapy. J Natl Cancer Inst 83:492–496

23. Gottardis MM, Jiang S-Y, Jeng M-H, Jordan VC (1989) Inhibition of tamoxifen-stimulated growth of an MCF-7 tumor variant in athymic mice by novel steroidal antiestrogens. Cancer Res 49:4090–4093
24. Murphy CS, Langan-Fahey S, McCague R, Jordan VC (1990) Structure-function relationships of hydroxylated metabolites of tamoxifen that control the proliferation of estrogen-responsive T47D breast cancer cells in vitro. Mol Pharmacol 38:737–783
25. McCague R, Kuroda R, LeClerq G, Stoessel S (1986) Synthesis and estrogen receptor binding of 6,7-dihydro-8-phenyl-9-[4-[2-(dimethylamino)ethoxy] phenyl] 5H-benzocyclo-heptene, a nonisomerizable analogue of tamoxifen. X-ray crystallographic studies. J Med Chem 29:2053
26. Langan-Fahey SM, Tormey DC, Jordan VC (1990) Tamoxifen metabolites in patients on long-term adjuvant tamoxifen therapy for breast cancer. Eur J Cancer 26:883–888
27. Robinson SP, Langan-Fahey SM, Johnson DA, Jordan VC (1991) Metabolites, pharmacodynamics and pharmacokinetics of tamoxifen in rats and mice compared to the breast cancer patient. Drug Metab Dispos 19:36
28. Turken S, Siris E, Seldin D, Foster E, Hyman G, Lindsay R (1989) Effects of tamoxifen on spinal density of women with breast cancer. J Natl Cancer Inst 81:1086–1088
29. Love RR, Newcomb PA, Wiebe DA, Surawicz TS, Jordan VC, Carbone PP, DeMets DL (1990) Lipid and lipoprotein effects of tamoxifen therapy in postmenopausal patients with node negative breast cancer. J Natl Cancer Inst 82:1327–1332
30. Breast Cancer Trials Committee, Scottish Cancer Trials Office (MRC) (1987) Adjuvant tamoxifen in the management of operable breast cancer: the Scottish Trial. Lancet 2:171–174

Growth Factors and Angiogenesis in Breast Cancer

A.L. Harris and E. Horak

Molecular Oncology Laboratory, Imperial Cancer Research Fund Laboratories, Institute of Molecular Medicine, John Radcliffe Hosptial, Oxford OX3 9DU, UK

Introduction

An overview of adjuvant therapy in breast cancer has shown the long-term survival benefits in node-positive and-negative cases [1] (reprinted in part in this volume). However, these treatments have still made only a relatively small impact on mortality, i.e. an increase in 10-year survival from 45% to 51.3% overall and from 39.8% to 46.6% in node-positive cases. Thus, the majority still die from their cancer. Greater understanding of the mechanisms of tumour growth and metastasis may enable the rational development of new agents to complement the achievements of hormone and chemotherapy.

This chapter reviews some areas currently under study to develop prognostic markers to select patients for more intensive therapy and exploit tumour angiogenesis.

Tumour Angiogenesis: Quantification with Anti-CD31 Antibodies

Folkman [2] has shown that angiogenesis is an important step in tumour progression and has recently demonstrated [3] that quantitating angiogenesis is possible in breast cancers. Staining endothelium with anti-factor VIII antigen (VIIIag) antibodies allowed the counting of blood vessels in primary tumours and showed a correlation with node metastasis. However, in a survey of antigens expressed by different vascular endothelial beds, it was found that factor VIIIag was not always expressed by endothelium [4]. Thus, to quantitate angiogenesis it may be desirable to use a monoclonal antibody that shows all endothelial cells. The survey (of ten monoclonals) showed that anti-CD31 antibodies are optimum for staining all vascular beds. CD31 is a cell adhesion molecule, expressed to a high level on endothelial cells.

Recent Results in Cancer Research, Vol. 127

Table 1. Vascularization by tumour type, grade and lymph node (LN) status

	n	Vascular count (per mm^2)	*p*
Ductal type	80	138.9	
Grade I	11	97.8	
LN−	9	64.7	0.001
LN+	2	247.0	
Grade II	39	123.3	
LN−	27	89.9	0.001
LN+	12	198.6	
Grade III	30	174.3	
LN−	17	132.5	0.007
LN+	13	206.3	
Lobular type	11	90.5	
LN−	9	76.7	0.08
LN+	2	152.0	

The Antibody JC70 [5] was used to quantitate angiogenesis in 103 primary breast cancers. Three high-power fields were selected that showed the greatest angiogenesis and were counted. JC70 staining was compared to anti-factor VIIIag staining and found to give approximately 20% greater counts. Vascular counts per square millimetre (VC) were then compared to lymph node status, tumour size and Bloom and Richardson grade.

Angiogenesis: Correlation with Lymph Node Metastases Independent of Tumour Size and Grade

VC values were significantly higher in node-positive (mean 201, $n = 29$) versus node-negative cases (mean 94, $n = 62$; $p<0.0001$). There was no significant correlation of number of nodes versus vascular counts. For each grade of tumour, vascular counts increased (Table 1). However, when grade was stratified by node status, in each category those with positive nodes had a higher VC. Thus, an increase in VC was more closely associated with the presence of node metastases than with grade. Similarly with tumour size there was a significant increase in VC from tumours with a diameter of less than 2 cm, 2–4 cm, and greater than 4 cm. Again, stratifying by lymph node status showed that it was lymph node positive cases that had the highest VC values in each category. There was no difference between lobular or ductal carcinomas in terms of VC. Only 4% of cases with VC under 99 had node metastasis, in contrast to 79% of cases with VC above 140.

These results suggest that angiogenesis is a critical rate-limiting step in breast cancer metastasis, and that a switch-on of angiogenesis occurs with larger tumour size and poorer differentiation. However, the association of the latter features with node metastasis is due to the induction of angiogenesis rather than to poor differentiation or size per se.

Angiogenesis and EGFr Status as Markers of Early Relapse and Death

We have previously shown that epidermal growth factor receptor (EGFr) status is associated with early relapse and death and with hormone resistance [6]. In a new series of patients studied since founding our unit in Oxford, a similar poor survival has been found (137 EGFr-negative cases, relapse-free survival at 2.5 years 85%; 106 EGFr-positive patients 55%; $p = 0.05$). In the earliest sequential group of these patients angiogenesis was assessed. In 42 patients with low VC (<100) there was a significantly better survival than in 43 with high VC (100 or greater; $p = 0.036$). Combining EGFr and angiogenesis status provided a particularly poor prognosis group, with a relapse-free survival of 67% at 18 months, versus 100% for low-EGFr, low-VC patients, and 85% for high-EGFr, low-VC or low-EGFr, high-VC patients ($p = 0.02$).

These data provide the basis for assessing growth factors that are important in angiogenesis and selecting patients for antiangiogenic therapy [7]. Current work involves assessment of antiangiogeneic suramin derivatives and phosphoinositol kinase inhibitors.

Hypoxia and Mitomycin C Resistance

Tumour angiogenesis is often insufficient to provide adequate oxygen delivery to tumours, and areas of necrosis are commonly seen in poor-prognosis breast cancers. This abnormal vasculature provides a therapeutic opportunity to exploit tumour hypoxia.

Mitomycin C (MMC) has a broad spectrum of activity in solid tumours, but resistance frequently develops. It is a standard component of therapy in pancreatic (fluorouracil, doxorubicin and methotrexate), non-small cell lung cancers (MMC, ifosfamide, *cis*-platinum) and many breast cancer protocols (MMC, methotrexate and mitoxantrone). It is activated via several different pathways to generate free radicals and also to cross-link DNA. It is activated differently under hypoxic conditions compared to oxygenated conditions and shows increased toxicity under hypoxia in some cell lines [8]. Hypoxic activation of anticancer drugs is an area under intensive study by many groups [9], but MMC remains the only clinically available drug. To investigate the mechanisms of MMC resistance, a CHO cell line was made resistant in vitro to MMC [10]. It showed cross-resistance to a monofunctional analogue of MMC, but a new analogue more easily activated overcame resistance. Further study showed a defect in an activation mechanism [11], cytochrome P-450 reductase. The above experiments were carried out in normal oxygen conditions, but when repeated under hypoxic conditions, the resistant cell line was as sensitive as the initial wild-type cells. This showed that there are at least two main mechanisms of MMC activation, cytochrome P-450 reductase under oxygenated conditions and another under hypoxia. These experiments provide the rationale for an approach to modifying MMC resistance by inducing selective hypoxia in tumours.

"Left Shifting" To Modify MMC Resistance

"Left-shifting"agents modify the oxygen saturation curve for haemoglobin and reduce oxygen release under low oxygen tension [12]. They are in use for treatment of sickle cell disease. Potential selectivity against tumour oxygenation could occur because effects on haemoglobin oxygen delivery in normal tissues would be compensated by increased cardiac output, tachycardia and vasodilation. Tumour blood supply is less able to respond to these influences, and a "steal" may also occur. Tumours have areas which are intermittently hypoxic, and the left-shifting effect is more severe at the lower oxygen pressures.

A phase 1 study of the agent BW12C, which covalently binds haemoglobin-α chains, has been conducted in combination with MMC [13]. A 1-h loading intravenous infusion of BW12C was followed by a maintenance infusion for 5 h. MMC was given by intravenous bolus ($6\,mg/m^2$) 1 h after the loading dose. This was repeated every 3 weeks for four courses. The maximum tolerated dose of BW12C was 50 mg/kg. Mild headache was the only side effect, although at higher doses vomiting occurred. Approximately 50% of the haemoglobin was covalently modified. Magnetic resonance spectroscopy was used to monitor in vivo effects on normal and tumour tissue. In exercising calf muscle pH was lower after BW12C infusion than before, and phosphocreatine took longer to recover. There were marked drops in ATP over liver metastases. This shows the feasibility of modulating oxygen delivery to synergize with hypoxic-activated drugs. Once more selective drugs of the latter class are available, integration of therapies with radiation and use of antiangiogenic agents may further enhance selectivity and cytotoxicity.

Signal Transduction and Drug Resistance

Many growth factor receptors are transmembrane tyrosine kinases [e.g., EGFr, *erbB2*, follicle-growth factor (FGF) receptors, platelet-derived growth factor (PDGR) receptors]. Secondary signalling systems include activation of protein kinase C (PKC) activated via phospholipase Cγ [14]; *ras* activation also partly involves signalling via PKC. Thus drugs modifying PKC may antagonize these pathways. There is increasing evidence that changes in signalling transduction may also interact with drug resistance pathways. Thus, PKC activation can increase drug resistance in multidrug-resistance (MDR) cells [15], and epidermal growth factor receptors increase in some drug-resistant breast cancer cells [16]. Increases in transcription factors have also been described, as has modulation of *cis*-platinum resistance by PKC activators and cyclic AMP analogues [17]. Since these pathways are also used by activating oncogenes, approaches designed to block growth via these pathways may also interact with cytotoxic agents in a favourable way. Several tyrosine kinase inhibitors or other kinase inhibitors also modify MDR [18], although this may be because the complex structures have multiple sites of action.

The first PKC partial agonist, bryostatin 1, has recently entered phase 1 study [19]. It can inhibit the effects of phorbol esters that stimulate PKC (antagonist action) [20] but can activate PKC when there is a low level of endogenous activation (agonist activity). Many oncogenes increase activity of the protein kinase C pathway [21], for example, Ha-*ras*, *erbB2*, receptor tyrosine kinases including EGF, FGF, PDGF, colony-stimulating factor receptors, bombesin. Activation of lymphocytes can occur partially via PKC. Thus, potential antagonist effects on transformed cells and positive effects on lymphocytes and neutrophils could occur. Since bryostatin is so potent, the phase 1 study started at $50\,\mu g/m^2$ and is currently at $50\,\mu g/m^2$ every 2 weeks. Initial toxicity was phlebitis, but this has been overcome by saline infusion to dilute the drug. Effects on platelet counts and interleukin-2 receptor expression by peripheral T-lymphocytes have occurred in some patients [22]. Pharmacodynamic monitoring is an essential part of development of these new classes of drug since tissue levels and effects are the important endpoint. These types of drug are often lipophilic, and it is the amount bound to receptor and its duration of binding rather than plasma levels which is important. Further studies are planned to assess schedule and dose.

Conclusions

The increase in basic knowledge on cancer now provides a firm basis for rational drug development. Approaches from many different areas are likely to be necessary for long-term control, and this review highlights some areas, particularly angiogenesis and signal transduction pathways, that are under clinical investigation. It needs to be recognized that such approaches should be integrated into the ongoing care of cancer patients, to optimize existing treatments and offer them the chance of therapeutic benefit with new agents. In this respect quality-of-life measurements will play an increasing role in drug evaluation.

References

1. Early Breast Cancer Trialists' Collaborative Group (1992) Systemic treatment of early breast cancer by hormonal, cytotoxic, or immune therapy. Lancet 339: 71–85
2. Folkman J (1990) What is the evidence that tumours are angiogenesis dependent? J Natl Cancer Inst 82:4–6
3. Weidner MD, Semple JP, Welch WR, Folkman J (1991) Tumour angiogenesis and metastasis – correlation in invasive breast carcinoma. N Engl J Med 324:1–8
4. Kuzu I, Bicknell R, Harris AL, Jones M, Gatter KC, Mason DY (1992) The heterogeneity of vascular endothelial cells with particular relevance to the diagnosis of vascular tumours. J Clin Pathol 45:143–148
5. Parums DV, Cordell JL, Micklem K, Heryet AR, Gatter KC, Mason DY (1990) JC70: a new monoclonal antibody that detects vascular endothelium associated antigen on routinely processed tissue sections. J Clin Pathol 43:752–757
6. Nicholson S, Sainsbury RC, Halcrow P, Kelly P, Angus B, Wright C, Henry J, Farndon JR, Harris AL (1991) Epidermal growth factor receptor (EGFr); results of a 6 year follow-up study in operable breast cancer with emphasis on the node negative subgroup. Br J Cancer 63:146–150
7. Bicknell R, Harris AL (1991) Novel growth regulatory factors and tumour angiogenesis. Eur J Cancer 27:781–784
8. Hughes CS, Irvin CG, Rockwell S (1991) Effect of deficiencies in DNA repair on the toxicity of mitomycin C and porfiromycin to CHO cells under aerobic and hypoxic conditions. Cancer Commun 3:29–35
9. Coleman CN (1988) Hypoxia in tumors: a paradigm for the approach to biochemical and physiologic heterogeneity. J Natl Cancer Inst 80:310–317
10. Hoban PR, Walton MI, Robson CN, Godden J, Stratford IJ, Workman P, Harris AL, Hickson ID (1988) Mitomycin C resistance under aerobic but not hypoxic conditions in a mammalian cell line: association with impaired drug activation and decreased NADPH: cytochrome P-450 reductase activity. Cancer Res 50:775–778
11. Bligh HFJ, Bartoszek A, Robson CN, Hickson ID, Kasper CB, Beggs JD, Wolf CR (1990) Activation of mitomycin C by NADPH: cytochrome P-450 reductase. Cancer Res 50:7789–7792
12. Wireko FC, Abraham DJ (1991) X-ray diffraction study of the binding of the antisickling agent 12C79 to human hemoglobin. Proc Natl Acad Sci USA 88:2209–2211
13. Philip P, Harris AL, Rea D, Carmichael J, Rajagopalan B, Bedford P, Thompson C, Radda GK (1992) Phase I/II trial of left shifting agent BW12C and mitomycin C. Monitoring by magnetic resonance spectroscopy (MRS). Proc ASCO II:137
14. Review Issue (1991) Cell 64:235–364
15. Yu G, Ahmad S, Aquino A, Fairchild CR, Trepel JB, Ohno S, Suzuki K, Tsuruo T, Cowan KH, Glazer RI (1991) Transfection with protein kinase Cα confers increased multidrug resistance to MCF-7 cells expressing P-glycoprotein. Cancer Commun 3:181–189
16. Nuti M, Zupi G, D'Agnano I, Turchi V, Candiloro A, Frati L (1991) Antigenic expression changes occurring in Adriamycin resistant MCF-7 mammary carcinoma cells. Anticancer Res 11:1225–1230
17. Andrews PA, Howell SB (1990) Cellular pharmacology of cisplatin: perspectives on mechanisms of acquired resistance. Cancer Cells 2:35–43
18. Kawada M, Imoto M, Umezawa K (1991) Suppression of multidrug resistance by inostamycin in cultured human carcinoma KB cells. J Cell Pharmacol 2:138–142

19. Gschwendt M, Furstenberger G, Rose-John S, Rogers M, Kittstein W, Pettit GR, Herald CI, Marks F (1988) Bryostatin 1, an activator of protein kinase C, mimics as well as inhibits biological effects of the phorbol ester TPA in vivo and in vitro. Carcinogenesis 9:555–562
20. Nutt JE, Harris AL, Lunec J (1991) Phorbol ester and bryostatin effects on growth and the expression of oestrogen responsive and TGF-β1 genes in breast tumour cells. Br J Cancer 64:671–676
21. Cantley LC, Auger KR, Carpenter C, Duckworth B, Graziani A, Kapeller R, Soltoff S (1991) Oncogenes and signal transduction. Cell 64:281–302
22. Rea D, Prendiville J, Harris AL, Wolf P, Philip P, Carmichael J, Lewis C, Dallman M, Walker T, Sri-Pathmanathan R, Thatcher N, Crowther D (1992) A phase I study of bryostatin 1 – a protein kinase C partial agonist. EORTC-NIH, New Drugs Conference, Amsterdam

Mechanisms of Treatment Failure

M.H.N. Tattersall

Department of Cancer Medicine, University of Sydney, NSW 2006, Australia

Introduction

The recently published overview of systemic treatment of patients with early breast cancer provides the best information available concerning the impact of these treatments on disease-free and overall survival [4] (reprinted in part in this volume). The modest reduction in risk of relapse achieved by these treatments may translate into major community health benefits when viewed in the context of a common disease affecting hundreds of thousands of women in the world each year. However, these results also indicate that many women who have received adjuvant systemic treatments die of metastatic breast cancer, presumably because some cells in the micrometastatic disease present before treatment survive after adjuvant treatment is ceased, and these cells later grow to cause advanced disease and premature death. Strategies to improve these results must include, on the one hand, the development of techniques to identify women with early breast cancer who have a normal life expectancy without adjuvant systemic therapy, i.e., either no metastases or metastases which will not cause symptoms during life, and, on the other, to establish the therapy which eliminates micrometastases or prevents their growth.

The development of new therapies which may improve the outcome for women with early breast cancer has drawn on experience treating patients with advanced breast cancer and on the application of approaches designed to reduce the emergence of drug resistant cells. Surprisingly few studies have taken as their starting point for new treatment an analyses of the biological or genetic characteristics of breast cancer cells in the primary tumour and that of metastases which develop without, during and after adjuvant systemic therapy. An understanding of the ways in which adjuvant systemic therapies fail to control micrometastases would be a major advantage in the development of new approaches to improve the outcome of systemic therapies in early breast cancer.

Recent Results in Cancer Research, Vol. 127

Comparison of Primary Breast Cancers and Their Metastases that Develop Later With or Without Adjuvant Systemic Treatment

Few direct comparisons of the characteristics of primary breast cancers and their metastases have been reported. Hormone receptor measurements on primary tumours have been found to be a useful guide to the probability of tumour regression with endocrine treatment within the primary tumour and in metastases which develop subsequently. Muss et al. [13] observed a tamoxifen response rate of 26% in breast cancer patients who presented with metastatic disease after ceasing adjuvant tamoxifen treatment. These findings suggest that selection by adjuvant tamoxifen treatment of a resistant cell population is not necessarily the usual means by which adjuvant tamoxifen treatment fails. More detailed comparisons, including information about the hormone receptor levels in primary tumours and in metastases with and without adjuvant therapies, are required.

Rutquist et al. [16] have considered that second breast cancers developing in women who have received adjuvant tamoxifen treatment for their first cancer are more likely to be oestrogen receptor negative than tumours developing without tamoxifen. However, the number of contralateral cancers (seven in the control group versus three in the tamoxifen-treated group) is too small for firm conclusions. Information about the receptor content of tumours which develop in women taking tamoxifen as a preventive therapy will be of considerable biological importance [5].

Cell kinetic parameters of primary breast cancers have prognostic significance, but comparison of the properties of the primary tumour and of subsequent metastases have rarely been reported [18, 19]. The use of paraffin blocks to examine cell kinetic parameters retrospectively provides one means of examining this question more thoroughly, so long as biopsy material is available from relapsed tumours.

P-glycoprotein is a membrane protein which acts as an efflux pump for several anticancer drugs. The gene for this protein has been cloned, and transfection of cloned *mdr* sequences transmits multidrug resistance to sensitive cells. Expression of P-glycoprotein is faint in the normal cells lining the breast ducts, but data on the expression of P-glycoprotein in breast cancers at the time of diagnosis and relapse are mixed [6, 12, 17].

Drug Treatment of Recurrent Disease in Patients Who Have Had or not Had Adjuvant Systemic Therapy

The survival after relapse of patients who have received adjuvant systemic therapy is somewhat reduced compared to that of patients who received no adjuvant therapy [7]. This observation supports the notion that adjuvant treatment may select for resistant tumours which may have a shorter doubling time, and hence shorter median survival after relapse. In addition, bone marrow reserve may be permanently reduced by some adjuvant systemic therapies, making further myelotoxic therapy after relapse less easy to deliver.

Studies of chemosensitivity of metastatic tumours developing after adjuvant therapies have revealed that early relapse is usually not sensitive to retreatment with the failed adjuvant therapy. However, if relapse occurs later, retreatment with endocrine or cytotoxics given as adjuvant achieves tumour response at a similar rate to that in untreated patients [2, 13, 20].

The latter observations raise the possibility that failure of adjuvant systemic therapy is not always due to the emergence of drug resistance. Rather, relapse may be due to insufficient therapy directed at what is fundamentaly a sensitive tumour or to the persistence of non-dividing or dormant cells that survive chemotherapy [8]. The possible mechanisms underlying failure of adjuvant systemic therapies include the following:

- Micrometastases containing drug-resistant cells
- Regrowth of drug-sensitive cells between treatment cycles
- Persistence of dormant drug-sensitive cells during therapy
- Existence of drug-sensitive cells in micrometastases located in drug-sanctuary sites
- Antagonistic drugs in the adjuvant regimen

A variety of strategies can be proposed which may improve the effectiveness of existing adjuvant treatments:

Increase in dose intensity
- Reduce tumour regrowth between cycles
- Increase fractional cell kill of sensitive tumour cells

Late reintroduction of adjuvant treatment
- Reduce proportion of relapses due to sensitive cells

Recruitment of dormant cells into cycle with growth factor
- Reduce proportion of relapses due to sensitive cells

Elimination of antagonistic drugs in regimen
- Tamoxifen/cytotoxic sequence (?)
- Methotrexate/fluorouracil (?)

Adding non-cross-resistant drugs to regimen
- Overcome resistance and maintain cell kill of sensitive cells

The possible importance of dose intensity in the optimal use of adjuvant cytotoxic drugs has been highlighted by retrospective analyses of treatment outcomes in patiens receiving standard treatment and by comparison of results of regimens with differing dose intensity [1, 10]. No prospective randomized trials have compared adjuvant regiments with different dose intensity in patients with primary breast cancer. In metastatic breast cancer the results of randomized trials addressing this question have been mixed [9].

Several current trials are evaluating the effects of the late reintroduction of adjuvant therapy in the hope that drug-sensitive cells dormant during the initial treatment period will enter the cell cycle subsequently and be eliminated by late-reintroduction treatments. The timing of these later cycles is guess-work. The alternative approach of recruiting dormant cells into the cell cycle using oestrogen-priming or other growth factors is being considered in adjuvant therapy, but concerns that the outcome might be worsened (because of recruiting into cycle tumour cells which are resistant to the current adjuvant therapies) has delayed testing of this strategy [3].

The possibility that existing adjuvant drug regimens contain antagonistic components which promote the survival of some sensitive cells has been raised in regard to the cell cycle effects of endocrine treatments protecting cells from cytotoxicity by chemotherapy. The complex biochemical perturbations/interactions of methotrexate and 5-fluorouracil also have the potential to be antagonistic in certain tumour cells, depending on their environment and the sequence/timing of drug treatment [15].

The existence of drug-resistant cells in micrometastases at the time of clinical presentation is one argument for promoting, for example, mammographic screening programs as a means of reducing breast cancer mortality in women aged over 50 years. The recent reports of mechanisms of tamoxifen resistance in human breast cancer xenografts also indicate the potential benefits of combination endocrine adjuvant therapy. Moreover, these results highlight the potential advantages of tamoxifen analogues, which are resistant to metabolism to oestrogen agonist derivatives [11, 14].

Conclusion

The 15%–30% reduction in 10-year mortality produced by adjuvant systemic therapies in women with early breast cancer implies that failure of adjuvant treatment to control micrometastatic disease remains a substantial cause of treatment failure. Strategies to improve the results of adjuvant treatment should build on an understanding of the causes of failure of current treatments. More information about the characteristics of primary tumours and of relapsed tumours after adjuvant treatments will point the way to rational approaches to improve the efficacy of treatment. The fact that many patients relapse with tumours which on rechallenge are found to be responsive to the adjuvant treatment indicates that some manipulation of existing treatments may lead to improved outcomes.

References

1. Bonadonna G, Valagussa P (1981) Dose-response effect of adjuvant chemotherapy in breast cancer. N Engl J Med 304:10–15

2. Castiglione M, Hacking A, Tattersall MHN et al. (1989) Proc ASCO 8:41
3. Davidson NE, Lippman ME (1987) Stimulation of breast cancer with estrogens: how much clinical value. Eur J Cancer Clin Oncol 23:897–900
4. Early Breast Cancer Trialists' Collaborative Group (1992) Systemic treatment of early breast cancer by hormonal, cytotoxic, or immune therapy: 133 randomized trials involving 31 000 recurrences and 24 000 deaths among 75 000 women. Lancet 339:1–15, 71–85
5. Fisher B, Redmond C (1991) New perspective in cancer of the contralateral breast: a marker for assessing tamoxifen as a preventive agent. J Natl Cancer Inst 83:1278–1289
6. Gerlach JH, Bell DR, Karakousis C (1987) P-glycoprotein in human sarcoma: evidence for multidrug resistance. J Clin Oncol 5:1452–1456
7. Goldhirsch A, Gelber RD, Simes RJ et al. (1989) Costs and benefits of adjuvant therapy in breast cancer: a quality adjusted survival analysis. J Clin Oncol 7:36–44
8. Goldie JH (1989) New information on drug resistance. Implications for the adjuvant treatment of breast cancer. Recent Results Cancer Res 115:8–16
9. Gurney H, Dodwell D, Thatcher N, Tattersall MHN (1992) Escalating drug delivery: a review of concept and practise. Ann Oncol (in press)
10. Hr yniuk W, Levine M (1976) Analyses of does intensity for adjuvant chemotherapy trials in stage II breast cancer. J Clin Oncol 4:1162–1170
11. Katzenellenbogen B (1991) Antiestrogen resistance: mechanisms by which breast cancer cells undermine the effectiveness of endocrine therapy. J Natl Cancer Inst 83:1454–1454
12. Merkel DE, Fugua SAW, Tandon A et al. (1989) Electrophoretic analysis of 248 clinical breast cancer specimens for P-glycoprotein overexpression or gene amplification. J Clin Oncol 7:1129–1133
13. Muss HB, Smith LR, Cooper MR (1987) Tamoxifen rechallenge: response to tamoxifen following relapse after adjuvant chemohormonal therapy for breast cancer. J Clin Oncol 5:1556–1558
14. Osborne CK, Coronado E, Allred DC et al. (1991) Acquired tamoxifen resistance: correlation with reduced breast tumour levels of tamoxifen and isomerisation of trans-4-hydroxytamoxifen. J Natl Cancer Inst 83:1477–1482
15. Piper A, Nott SE, MacKinnon WB, Tattersall MHNN (1983) Critical modulation by thyomidine and hypoxanthine of sequential methotrexate-fluorouracil synergism in murine L1210 cells. Cancer Res 43:5701–5705
16. Rutquist LE, Cedermark B, Glas U et al. (1992) Contralateral primary tumours in breast cancer patients in a randomised trial of adjuvant tamoxifen therapy. J Natl Cancer Inst 83:1299–1306
17. Schneider J, Bak M, Efferth T et al. (1989) P-glycoprotein expression in treated and untreated breast cancer. Br J Cancer 60:815–820
18. Silvestrini R, Diadone MG, Gasparia G (1985) Cell kinetics as a persistent prognostic marker in node negative breast cancer. Cancer 56:1982–1987
19. Tubiana M (1982) Cell kinetics and radiation oncology. Int J Radiat Oncol Biol Phys 8:1471–1489
20. Valagussa P, Tancini G, Bonadonna G (1986) Salvage treatment of patients suffering relapse after adjuvant CMF chemotherapy. Cancer 58:1411–1417

Expression of the MDR*1 Gene (P-Glycoprotein) in Breast Cancer*

R.S. Weinstein, K.K. Hansen, R.B. McBeath, and W.S. Dalton

Departments of Pathology, Surgery, and Internal Medicine, and the Arizona Cancer Center, Tucson, AR 85724, USA

Introduction

Of the many types of drug resistance reported in the literature, one of the best characterized is classic multidrug resistance, a genetically determined type of resistance to chemotherapy [1, 2]. Cancers exhibiting intrinsic multidrug resistance mediated by P-glycoprotein, the product of the *MDR*1 gene, do not respond to chemotherapy upon primary exposure to "natural product" lipophilic drugs such as colchicine, vinblastine, and doxorubicin. Characteristics of multidrug resistance in cancer cells include: (a) increased levels of P-glycoprotein, a 170-kDa membrane transporter, (b) decreased drug accumulation and enhanced drug efflux, (c) chemoresistance to multiple natural product agents, and (d) chemosensitization by transporter inhibitors (e.g., verapamil). Other cancers that respond initially to drugs may subsequently become resistant to these and other drugs to which the patient has had no previous exposure. This is multidrug resistance in the acquired form. Tumors with either intrinsic or acquired multidrug resistance mediated by P-glycoprotein usually are not cross-resistant to alkylating agents, most antimetabolites, or heavy metals. Often, intrinsic multidrug resistance occurs in tumors derived from organs that normally express P-glycoprotein, such as intestine, liver, kidney, and adrenal [3]. The multidrug resistance phenotype also occurs in the absence of P-glycoprotein, reflecting the multiplicity of mechanisms that produce this phenomenon [4].

The Mdr1 isoform of P-glycoprotein, a 170-kDa integral membrane protein, confers multidrug resistance by preventing the intracellular accumulation of drugs. Reduction of the intramembrane concentration of drugs may also play a role [5]. Many of the drugs that have been implicated in multidrug resistance do not share a common intracellular target. This observation focused the attention of early investigators on the role of the plasma membrane in multidrug resistance and led to the discovery of P-glycoprotein, by Juliano and Ling [6]. It is now well established that P-glycoprotein provides

Recent Results in Cancer Research, Vol. 127

protection against lipophilic drugs by functioning as an efflux transporter with exceptionally broad specificity [2]. Drugs in the extracellular space cross the cell membrane by Fickian diffusion or carrier-mediated passive transport. P-glycoprotein ejects the drugs from the cell in a process that is energized by hydrolysis of ATP at nucleotide binding sites on the P-glycoprotein polypeptide [2].

Two closely related genes *MDR*1 and *MDR*2 encode for highly homologous integral membrane proteins. Both of these genes have been labeled as multidrug resistance genes because of their structural similarities, but only the *MDR*1 gene has been linked to multidrug resistance. No transport function has been ascribed to the product of the *MDR*2 gene. This is of clinical importance since the expression of the irrevelant *MDR*2 gene in human tissues can complicate laboratory testing for the Mdr1 isoform of P-glycoprotein.

Chemosensitization as a Therapeutic Strategy

The discovery of the Mdr1 transporter opened the door for the development of new strategies to overcome P-glycoprotein mediated multidrug resistance. A crucial observation was that chemosensitivity to various drugs can be reestablished by blocking efflux transporter activity with competitive inhibitors. Inhibitors such as the calcium channel blocker verapamil can function as effector-inhibitors of P-glycoprotein [7]. Clinical applications based on this finding are under investigation. Early clinical trials using combinations of chemotherapeutic drugs and P-glycoprotein inhibitors in patients with lymphoma and myeloma have been associated with some remissions in patients with advanced disease [8, 9]. These studies seem to warrant more trials in patients with solid tumors.

P-Glycoprotein Laboratory Measurements

Approaches used to detect and quantify P-glycoprotein include: (a) measuring protein, (b) measuring *MDR*1 mRNA, and (c) assessing *MDR*1 gene amplification [10]. Quantification of the protein by immunoblotting or immunocytochemistry is more direct but often less sensitive and specific than measuring *MDR* message. Measurement of *MDR*1 gene amplification is of interest to researchers but of limited value as a clinical test, since increased expression of the human *MDR*1 gene does not require gene amplification. Choice of methodology for detecting and quantifying P-glycoprotein must take into account the expression of P-glycoprotein in stromal cells, lymphocyte subsets, and endothelial cells. The presence of P-glycoprotein expressing stromal cells in surgical pathology specimens could complicate the interpretation of results obtained on bulk tissue specimens.

Table 1. Measurements of *MDR*1 mRNA in breast

Method	Expression[a]	Reference
Normal		
Quantitative PCR	1/1	Noonan et al. [18]
Carcinoma		
Slot blot	9/57	Goldstein et al. [3]
In situ hybridization	9/16	Kacinski et al. [11]
Quantitative PCR	0/1	Noonan et al. [18]
	18/74 (Av. 24%)	

PCR, Polymerase chain reaction.
[a] Number positive/total.

*MDR*1 mRNA and P-Glycoprotein in Normal Breast and Carcinomas

Before P-glycoprotein chemosensitivity testing is introduced into routine clinical practice, the prevalence of its expression in various populations of untreated and treated breast cancer patients should be established. Several reports have been published on the expression of *MDR*1 mRNA and its product, the Mdr1 isoform of P-glycoprotein, in normal human adult organs and in tumors, including breast carcinomas, for a relatively small series of patients (Table 1). The prevalence of *MDR*1 mRNA expression in normal and malignant breast tissue is somewhat controversial. In an early study of 57 patients using dot blot analysis, Goldstein et al. reported that *MDR*1 mRNA expression was infrequent (15%) in breast cancers and, when present, at low levels of message. Using *MDR*1 in situ hybridization, Kacinski et al. [11] found expression in 56% (9/16) of untreated breast cancer samples. Comparative studies using several analytical methods on aliquots of the same samples are needed to resolve these discrepancies.

P-glycoprotein has been detected by immunohistochemistry in breast surgical pathology specimens. There is a consensus that the majority of normal breast surgical specimens immunostain positively with anti-P-glycoprotein monoclonal antibodies. P-glycoprotein is also expressed in breast carcinomas although somewhat less frequently than in normal breast tissue (Table 2). It is noteworthy that nearly identical results have been obtained using monoclonal antibodies that are specific for the Mdr1 isoform of P-glycoprotein (i.e., HYB-241 and HYB-612) and monoclonal antibodies that recognize both the human Mdr1 and Mdr2 isoforms (i.e., C219) [12].

Several additional research topics are relevant to the development of laboratory tests for cancer chemosensitivity testing. In order to establish *MDR*1 mRNA/P-glycoprotein measurements as standard laboratory tests, there is a need to understand their variability and heterogeneity of expression in both normal tissues and carcinomas. Heterogeneity of P-glycoprotein

Table 2. Detection of P-glycoprotein in normal breast and cancers by immunohistochemistry

Monoclonal antibody	Expression[a]	Reference
Normal		
C219	18/26	Ro et al. [14]
C219	19/25	Coon and Weinstein
	37/51 (Av. 73%)	(unpublished data)
Carcinoma		
C219, MRK-16, JSB-1	0/6	Van der Valk et al. [19]
C219, HYB-241 HYB-612	2/14	Cordon-Cardo and O'Brien [12]
C219, JSB-1	5/13	Salmon et al. [15]
C219	20/40	Ro et al. [14]
C219, MRK-16	21/29	Wishart et al. [20]
C219	10/23	Schneider et al. [21]
C494	17/20	Verrelle et al. [22]
C219, JSB-1	30/67	Coon and Weinstein
	105/212 (Av. 50%)	(unpublished data)

[a] Number positive/total.

expression, a pattern seen in many immunohistopathology sections, complicates efforts to establish threshold levels for the expression in surgical pathology specimens. The issue of where to sample is also crucial. Our observations of P-glycoprotein expression in lymph node metastases, in cases of colon cancer where the primary tumor was P-glycoprotein negative, raises questions concerning tissue sampling that should be resolved prior to designing clinical trials to test the value of P-glycoprotein measurements for stratifying patients [13]. The clinical significance of low levels of P-glycoprotein expression in tumors remains to be determined.

Influence of Chemotherapy on P-Glycoprotein

Expression of *MDR*1 mRNA may be increased in certain tumors by exposure to natural-product chemotherapeutic agents [3]. The extent to which this occurs in breast cancer patients remains to be established by a prospective study. In a retrospective study, Ro et al. [14] examined P-glycoprotein expression before and after chemotherapy and upon recurrence of tumor in 11 patients. They found no significant differences in P-glycoprotein expression before and after chemotherapy and suggested that intrinsic rather than acquired drug resistance may play a role in the failure of induction chemotherapy for locally advanced breast cancer.

The influence of P-glycoprotein expression on breast tumor responses to therapy is also an open question. There is evidence that P-glycoprotein expression is associated with resistance to chemotherapeutic drugs in breast cancer cells [14, 15]. This is consistent with a case report of reversal of clinical doxorubicin resistance in a 57-year-old P-glycoprotein/estrogen receptor positive breast cancer patient using verapamil or a combination of vincristine, doxorubicin, and cisplatin [16].

Additional Mechanisms of P-Glycoprotein Action

A reasonable assumption has been that P-glycoprotein influences on tumor behavior are mechanistically related to drug sensitivity per se. However, this may be an oversimplification. The possibility remains that simultaneous or sequential modulation of the expression of other proteins could contribute to the prognosis of patients with P-glycoprotein positive breast cancers. For example, Vickers et al. have shown that in MCF-7/doxorubicin cells the development of multidrug resistance is associated with alterations in the expression of both cytosolic and membrane estrogen receptors, resulting in resistance to hormonal agents and the expression of hormone-independent tumor formation [17]. Studies in another organ, colon, have suggested that P-glycoprotein expression is associated with increases in local spread of tumor to regional lymph nodes [13]. Thus, the possibility is raised that P-glycoprotein may contribute to clinical outcome by multiple mechanisms.

Acknowledgement. This work was supported in part with funds from grant CA 41183 from the National Cancer Institute.

References

1. Edicott JA, Ling V (1989) The biochemistry of P-glycoprotein mediated multidrug resistance. Annu Rev Biochem 58:137–171
2. Juranka PF, Zastawny RL, Ling V (1989) P-glycoprotein: multidrug-resistance and a superfamily of membrane-associated transport proteins. FASEB J 3:2583–2592
3. Goldstein LJ, Galski H, Fojo A, Willingham M, Lai S-L, Gazdar A, Pirker R, Green A, Crist W, Brodeur GM, Lieber M, Cossman J, Gottesman MM, Pastan I (1989) Expression of a multidrug resistance gene in human cancers. J Natl Cancer Inst 81:116–124
4. Taylor CW, Dalton WS, Parrish PP, Gleason MC, Bellamy WT, Thompson FH, Roe DJ, Trent JM (1991) Different mechanisms of decreased drug accumulation in doxorubicin and mitoxantrone resistant variants of the MCF-7 human breast cancer cell line. Br J Cancer 63:923–929
5. Roninson IB (1991) P-glycoprotein-mediated drug resistance: puzzles and perspectives. In: Roninson IB (ed) Molecular and cellular biology of multidrug resistance in tumor cells. Plenum, New York, pp 395–402
6. Juliano RL, Ling V (1976) A surface glycoprotein modulating drug permeability in Chinese hamster ovary cell mutants. Biochem Biophys Acta 455:152–162
7. Tsuruo T, Iida H, Tsukagoshi S, Sakurai Y (1981) Overcoming of vincristine resistance in P388 leukemia in vivo and in vitro through enhanced cytotoxicity of vincristine and vinblastine by verapamil. Cancer Res 41:1967–1972

8. Salmon SE, Dalton WS, Grogan TM, Plezia P, Lehnert M, Roe DJ, Miller TP (1991) Multidrug-resistant myeloma: laboratory and clinical effects of verapamil as a chemosensitizer. Blood 78:44–50
9. Miller TP, Grogan TM, Dalton WS, Spier CM, Scheper RJ, Salmon SE (1991) P-glycoprotein expression in malignant lymphoma and reversal of clinical drug resistance with chemotherapy plus high-dose verapamil. J Clin Oncol 9:17–24
10. Weinstein RS, Kuszak JR, Kluskens LF, Coon JS (1990) P-glycoproteins in pathology: the multidrug resistance gene family in humans. Hum Pathol 21: 34–48
11. Kacinski BM, Yee LD, Carter D (1989) Quantitation of tumor cell expression of the P-glycoprotein (*mdr*1) gene in human breast carcinoma clinical specimens. Cancer Bull 41:44–48
12. Cordon-Cardo C, O'Brien JP (1991) The multidrug resistance phenotype in human cancer. In: DeVita VT Jr, Hellman S, Rosenberg SA (eds) J.B. Lippincott, Philadelphia, pp 19–38
13. Weinstein RS, Jakate SM, Dominguez JM, Lebovitz MD, Koukoulis GK, Kuszak JR, Klusens LF, Grogan TM, Saclarides TJ, Roninson IB, Coon JS (1991) Relationship of the expression of the multidrug resistance gene product (P-glycoprotein) in human colon carcinoma to local tumor aggressiveness and lymph node metastasis. Cancer Res 51:2720–2726
14. Ro J, Sahin A, Ro JY, Fritsche H, Hortobagyi G, Blick M (1990) Immunohistochemical analysis of P-glycoprotein expression correlated with chemotherapy resistance in locally advanced breast cancer. Hum Pathol 21: 787–791
15. Salmon SE, Grogan TM, Miller T, Scheper WS, Dalton WS (1989) Prediction of doxorubicin resistance in vitro in myeloma, lymphoma, and breast cancer by P-glycoprotein staining. J Natl Cancer Inst 81:696–701
16. Salmon SE, Grogan TM, Miller TP, Dalton WS (1990) Multidrug resistance: relevance to adjuvant therapy? In: Salmon SE (ed) Adjuvant therapy of cancer. Saunders, Philadelphia, pp 26–32
17. Vickers PJ, Dickson RB, Shoemaker R, Cowans KH (1988) A multidrug-resistant MCF-7 human breast cancer cell line which exhibits cross-resistance to antiestrogens and hormone-independent tumor growth in vivo. Mol Endocrinol 2:888–892
18. Noonan KE, Beck C, Holzmayer TA, Chin JE, Wunder JS, Andrulis IL, Gazdar AF, Willman CL, Griffith B, von Hoff DD, Roninson IB (1990) Quantitative analysis of *mdr*1 (multidrug resistance) gene expression in human tumors by polymerase chain reaction. Proc Natl Acad Sci USA 87:7160–7164
19. Van der Valk P, Van Kalken CK, Ketelaars H, Broxterman HJ, Scheffer G, Kuiper CM, Tsuruo T, Lankelma J, Meijer CJLM, Pinedo HM, Scheper RJ (1990) Distribution of multi-drug resistance-associated P-glycoprotein in normal and neoplastic human tissues. Ann Oncol 1:56–64
20. Wishart GC, Plumb JA, Going JJ, McNicol AM, McArdle CS, Tsuruo T, Kaye SB (1990) P-glycoprotein expression in primary breast cancer detected by immunocytochemistry with two monoclonal antibodies. Br J Cancer 62:758–761
21. Schneider J, Bak M, Efferth T, Kaufmann M, Mattern J, Volm M (1989) P-glycoprotein expression in treated and untreated human breast cancer. Br J Cancer 60:815–818
22. Verrelle P, Meissonier F, Fonck Y, Feillel V, Dionet C, Kwiatkowski F, Plagne R, Chassagne J (1991) Clinical relevance of immunohistochemical detection of multidrug resistance P-glycoprotein in breast carcinoma. J Natl Cancer Inst 83:111–116

II. Prognosis and Prediction of Response

Prognosis of Breast Cancer Patients: How To Use What?

G.M. Clark and W.L. McGuire*

University of Texas Health Science Center, Department of Medicine/Oncology, 7703 Floyd Curl Drive, San Antonio, TX 78284-7884, USA

Why Do We Need Prognostic Factors for Breast Cancer?

There has been considerable debate about the utility of prognostic factors for breast cancer; yet, in one way or another they are routinely used by many physicians and patients every day to make a variety of decisions. We concentrate here on three areas in which the decision-making process could be improved by a better understanding of prognostic factors: (a) identification of women who will eventually develop breast cancer, (b) prediction of clinical outcome of patients who have been diagnosed with breast cancer, (c) prediction of benefit from adjuvant therapy for specific breast cancer patients.

It is estimated that one in nine women in the United States will develop breast cancer at some time during her life. Although a number of risk factors for breast cancer have been identified (e.g., a positive family history, early onset of menarche, nulliparity, first full-term pregnancy after age 30), the vast majority of women who develop the disease do not have any of these risk factors. Clearly, there is a need to improve our ability to identify future breast cancer patients. Some progress has been made using histopathological classifications of premalignant disease that have been correlated with increased risk of eventual breast cancer [1]. More recently, molecular biologists have provided new tools for identifying genetic abnormalities that might signal the development of breast cancer. We can expect a whole new generation of prognostic factors for the development of breast cancer in the next several years.

* William L. McGuire was a Clinical Research Professor of the American Cancer Society until his death on March 25, 1992.

Supported in part by NIH Grant CA30195.

Recent Results in Cancer Research, Vol. 127

Prognostic factors are commonly used to separate patients who already have breast cancer into subsets with differing expected clinical outcomes. The most frequently used clinical endpoints are disease recurrence or death. Patients with a high likelihood of poor clinical outcome are usually offered additional adjuvant therapy following primary surgery. An example of the use of prognostic factors is the traditional staging system that includes components for the size of the primary tumor, the involvement of axillary lymph nodes, and metastatic spread of the tumor. However, with the passage of time and a growing body of data, it is clear that this staging system is not optimal for making treatment decisions. For example, breast cancer patients with negative axillary lymph nodes are generally considered to have a relatively good prognosis following surgery. Yet a significant proportion of these patients will develop a recurrence of their breast cancer and die from their disease. It would be helpful if subsets of node-negative patients with different clinical outcomes could be identified [2, 3].

One possibility is to treat all node-negative breast cancer patients with adjuvant therapy. However, there are at least four reasons why this may not be the optimal strategy: (a) most node-negative patients are cured by primary surgery alone and could not benefit from additional adjuvant therapy, (b) the number of patients who would benefit from adjuvant therapy is modest, (c) some of the patients who would benefit will suffer toxic side effects, and a small fraction will die as a result of the treatment, and (d) the costs of treating all patients may be prohibitive. The recent Oxford overview analysis [4] (reprinted in part in this volume) provides a large body of data that can be used to address some of these issues.

What is the natural history of node-negative breast cancer? The 10-year recurrence and death rates for node-negative patients in untreated control arms of randomized clinical trials of tamoxifen were 37.9% and 29.0%, respectively. Thus, more than 60% of these patients were disease-free after 10 years and could not have benefited from additional adjuvant therapy. However, these absolute rates cannot be generalized to the population as a whole since many low-risk patients with small tumors are not entered into clinical trials. In addition, the use of mammography has resulted in the detection of many more smaller tumors whose clinical outcome would be expected to be better than that described in the overview analysis. The 10-year recurrence rate of all node-negative patients is probably less than 30%, indicating that more than 70% of patients could not benefit from adjuvant therapy.

What is the expected benefit from adjuvant tamoxifen? The 10-year recurrence rate in tamoxifen-treated patients was 32.9%, a decrease of 5% from the control patients. The difference in 10-year mortality rates was only 3.5%. Applying these rates to the 116 000 women in the United States who were diagnosed with node-negative breast cancer during 1991, we would expect 82 360 of these women to be alive at 10 years without adjuvant therapy and 33 640 to have died (Fig. 1). However, only 4060 of these

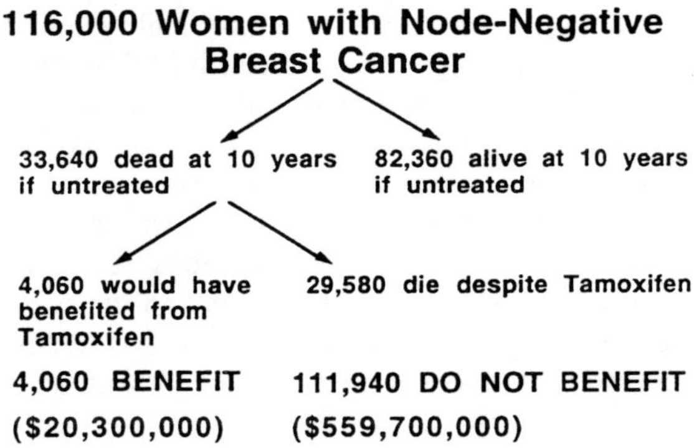

Fig. 1. Costs and benefits of treating all node-negative patients with tamoxifen. Based on mortality rates and benefits from [4], assuming U.S. $5000 for 5 years of tamoxifen

deaths could have been avoided if the patients had received tamoxifen. If we had treated all of these node-negative patients with 5 years of tamoxifen at a total cost of U.S. $5000, we would have expended $559.7 million on patients whose 10-year survival was not altered by this treatment ($411.8 million on patients alive without tamoxifen and $147.9 million on patients who died despite tamoxifen).

The alternative is to find prognostic factors that identify patients who not only have a high probability of disease recurrence, but who would also be likely to benefit from a particular therapy. For example, tumors with high proliferative rates might be more responsive to cell-cycle specific chemotherapy, or toxic agents might be linked to antibodies against the products of specific genetic alterations. Both of these strategies are currently being explored in clinical trials.

What Prognostic Factors Are Available Now?

The traditional prognostic factors in clinical use today for patients with node-negative breast cancer are (a) tumor size, (b) histopathology (ductal carcinoma in situ, pure tubular, papillary, typical medullary carcinoma), (c) histological and nuclear grade, (d) estrogen receptors (ER) and progesterone receptors (PgR), (e) DNA ploidy, and (f) proliferative rate. Tumor size is one of the most important factors in the decision-making process. Histopathology is taking on added significance. Ductal carcinoma in situ, pure tubular carcinoma, papillary carcinoma, and typical medullary carcinoma are histopathological breast cancer subtypes with an excellent prognosis when axillary nodes are negative. Nuclear and histological grade have been recommended for a long time but have fallen into disfavor because of reports of poor reproducibility. ER and PgR are routinely measured for predicting both recurrence probability and the likelihood of response to endocrine therapy. More recently, DNA ploidy and proliferative rate (e.g., S phase by flow cytometry, thymidine labeling index) have become widely available and have been shown to be useful in predicting the clinical outcome of node-negative breast cancer.

The latest generation of prognostic factors is still undergoing evaluation and includes oncogene aberrations (e.g., HER-2/neu), tumor suppressor genes (e.g., p53), growth factors and their receptors (e.g., epidermal growth factor receptor), and other factors including cathepsin D, a lysosomal enzyme that has been associated with the metastatic process.

How Can We Combine These Factors into a Prognostic Index?

Ideally, we would have a large population of breast cancer patients with long-term follow-up on whom we could measure a panel of potential prognostic factors. Then, multivariate statistical procedures such as Cox's proportional hazards model could be used to identify and validate an index or a series of indices that could be used to accurately predict the clinical outcome of future patients. Research is now underway to compare newer multivariate approaches, including decision trees constructed by recursive partitioning and neural networks, a form of artificial intelligence [5].

We have previously published guidelines for the evaluation of new prognostic factors [6, 7]. Among the minimal criteria that we listed were the necessity for multivariate analyses and procedures to validate that the results are reproducible and generalizable to other groups of patients. It is very important to analyze new factors in combination with traditional factors in multivariate analyses. Without this step, it is impossible to rule out the possibility that the new factors might be so correlated with other factors that they do not contribute any additional prognostic information beyond what can already be obtained by the standard factors. Validation of results is an often overlooked step, but one that must be taken before new factors can be recommended for routine use. All statistical techniques suffer from the problem of "overfitting" the data set being analyzed, and the results are usually worse when applied to a new set of patients. One validation procedure divides the population into a "training" set and a "validation" set to test the model's generalizability to another group of patients. Other statistical procedures to cross-validate results include jackknife and bootstrap techniques. In addition to internal validation, it is still necessary to validate the results on a truly independent, external population of patients.

Unfortunately, we do not yet have the ideal population with long-term follow-up and a complete panel of potential prognostic factors. Nevertheless, we can use available information to identify subsets of patients with different probabilities of disease recurrence. The decision to treat or not to treat should be relatively straightforward for up to one-half of the axillary node-negative breast cancer patients if we use just two factors, tumor size

Table 1. Adjuvant therapy decisions for node-negative breast cancer

	25% of patients	50% of patients	25% of patients
Number of patients per year	29 000	58 000	29 000
Tumor size	<1 cm	1–3 cm	>3 cm
Tumor subtype	DCIS Pure tubular Papillary Typical medullary		
Eventual recurrence	1%–10%	~30%	>50%
Adjuvant treatment	Few	?	Most/all

DCIS, Ductal carcinoma in situ.

and histopathology (Table 1). Approximately 25% of patients with tumors less than 1 cm in diameter, or of special histological subtypes (ductal carcinoma in situ, pure tubular carcinoma, papillary carcinoma, or typical medullary carcinoma) have an excellent prognosis, with recurrence rates ranging between 1% and 10%. The NIH Breast Cancer Consensus Conference of 1990 recommended that few of these patients should be treated with systemic therapy. Another 25% of patients have tumor size greater than 3 cm, and these tumors are also frequently associated with high-risk prognostic features. The recurrence rate in this group is greater than 50%, and most if not all of these patients should and will receive adjuvant therapy. This leaves approximately 50% of patients with intermediate-sized tumors in which the long-term recurrence rate is appreciable at 30%. This is where prognostic factors could be of greatest clinical utility.

Additional subsets of low-risk and high-risk patients based on available prognostic factors include the following: low risk – (a) ductal carcinoma in situ, pure tubular papillary, typical medullary, (b) tumor size under 1.0 cm, (c) diploid, low S phase, (d) nuclear grade I; high risk – (a) tumor size over 3 cm, (b) high S phase, (c) aneuploid/high cathepsin D. We have shown that patients with diploid, low S phase tumors have a very good prognosis, with only a 10% 4-year recurrence rate [8]. In addition, in our San Antonio series, although only 10% of our node-negative patients had nuclear grade I tumors, 92% were ER-positive, 76% were PgR-positive, 62% were small tumors, 73% were diploid, and, most importantly, as a group their 5-year disease-free survival was better than 90% [9]. On the other hand, patients with high S phase tumors [8], or aneuploid, high cathepsin D tumors [10] had particularly poor clinical outcomes.

Conclusions

In 1992, the adjuvant therapy treatment decision for patients with node-negative breast cancer is fairly straightforward for about one-half of the patients. Those with small tumors or favorable histological subtypes have such a sufficiently low recurrence rate that few should be treated. Patients with large tumors that are usually associated with poor prognostic features have such a sufficiently high recurrence rate that they should be considered candidates for adjuvant therapy. For the remaining 50% of patients with intermediate-sized tumors and a worrisome 30% overall recurrence rate we recommend the use of prognostic factors to help estimate the risk of recurrence for the individual patient so that our treatment efforts can be focused on those node-negative patients most likely to benefit from the therapy. In the near future we should be able to more accurately estimate the probabilities of clinical outcomes for all patients with node-negative breast cancer.

References

1. Page DL, Dupont WD (1990) Premalignant conditions and markers of elevated risk in the breast and their management. Surg Clin North Am 70:831–851
2. McGuire WL (1988) Adjuvant therapy of node-negative breast cancer: another point of view. J Natl Cancer Inst 80:1075–1076
3. McGuire WL (1989) Adjuvant therapy of node-negative breast cancer. N Engl J Med 320:525–527
4. Early Breast Cancer Trialists' Collaborative Group (1992) Systemic treatment of early breast cancer by hormonal, cytotoxic, or immune therapy: 133 randomised trials involving 31 000 recurrences and 24 000 deaths among 75 000 women. Lancet:1–15, 71–85
5. Ravdin PM, Hilsenbeck SG, Clark GM et al. (1991) Comparison of neural network analysis and Cox modeling for predicting relapse of axillary node positive breast cancer patients (Abstr). Proc Am Soc Clin Oncol 10:47
6. McGuire WL, Tandon AK, Allred DC et al. (1990) How to use prognostic factors in axillary node-negative breast cancer patients. J Natl Cancer Inst 82:1006–1015
7. McGuire WL (1991) Guidelines for evaluating new prognostic factors. J Natl Cancer Inst 83:154–155
8. Clark GM, Dressler LG, Owens MA et al. (1989) Prediction of relapse or survival in patients with node-negative breast cancer by DNA flow cytometry. N Engl J Med 320:627–633
9. Bustamante-Montes MA, Clark G, Langone G et al. (1989) Histopathological grading of breast specimens correlates with disease-free survival in node-negative breast cancer patients (Abstr). Proc Am Assoc Cancer Res 30:252
10. Tandon AK, Clark GM, Chamness GC et al. (1990) Cathepsin D and prognosis in breast cancer. N Engl J Med 322:297–301

DNA Flow Cytometry Measurements and Their Clinical Relevance in Node-Negative Breast Cancer Patients

L.G. Dressler

University of New Mexico School of Medicine, UNM Cancer Center, Center for Molecular and Cellular Diagnostics, Albuquerque, NM, USA

Introduction

There are at least two measurements of tumor aggressiveness that we can obtain using DNA flow cytometry techniques. One is the estimate of ploidy status or DNA content of a patient's tumor, usually referred to as DNA diploid, if the tumor contains a normal amount of DNA, or DNA aneuploid, if the tumor contains an abnormal amount of DNA (hypo or hyperdiploid). The other prognostic factor is an estimate of a tumor's proliferative capacity, obtained by measuring the percentage of nuclei in the DNA synthetic phase (S phase) of the cell cycle. The S phase is usually referred to as "high" or "low" (and sometimes intermediate), often based on a mean or median value obtained from a large database.

DNA flow cytometry measurements of DNA ploidy and proliferative capacity have had significant clinical impact in predicting relapse-free survival in early- and late-stage breast cancer [1–12]. As these studies mature, we are also observing their importance in predicting overall survival as well [2, 4–6, 13]. Most recently, we have begun to evaluate and observe that these measurements may be useful in predicting response to therapy [14–18]. This chapter summarizes data from those studies focusing on the node-negative breast cancer patient, which have evaluated the ability of DNA flow cytometry measurements to predict for patient prognosis.

Quality Control and Biologic Accuracy

In June 1990 the National Cancer Institute's Consensus Panel on Treatment of Early-Stage Breast Cancer raised concern that "due to the complexity of the technique, quality control is especially critical" when estimating proliferative capacity using DNA flow cytometry [19]. This concern has been shared by others and has stimulated the development and further progress

Recent Results in Cancer Research, Vol. 127

of several large quality-control programs in the United States and Europe to try to standardize the technique used in the clinical laboratory [20].

Preliminary results from a multicenter study conducted by Becton Dickinson Immunocytometry Systems in the United States shows very promising results [21]. In this study similar reagents are used, along with a standardized preparation and staining procedure. All samples are run on the same instrument and analyzed with the same software program. At each of the four sites in the study, similar S phase fraction was obtained for diploid and for aneuploid tumors [21]. A similar study is ongoing in Europe. Several other quality-control programs have now incorporated estimation of S phase fraction as a parameter for study (M. Waxdall and C. Hitchock, personal communication). With the availability of at least two commercial analysis programs which give similar and reproducible results, cell cycle analysis should soon be a standardized, quality-controlled parameter. It is important to keep in mind, however, that the absolute value of the S phase obtained by one laboratory compared to that from another laboratory may not be as useful in the clinical setting as the prognostic subgroup into which the value places a patient. It may be more clinically revelant that two laboratories similarly assign a tumor as "low," "high," or "intermediate" S phase, than the actual value obtained in each laboratory [20].

Another concern that has been raised is the relationship between DNA content or DNA index obtained using flow cytometry and its biologic accuracy. Although conflicting reports exist, most studies have shown that DNA index values obtained from fresh, frozen, or formalin-fixed paraffin-embedded samples of solid tumors are an accurate estimation of total chromosome number, when compared to karyotypic analysis [22–28]. Therefore, although we cannot detect structural abnormalities or indicate which chromosome(s) is duplicated and/or deleted using DNA flow cytometry, we can obtain a good estimate of the total chromosome number (DNA index X 46), reflecting total DNA content.

Relationship Between Ploidy Status and Patient Prognosis

Table 1 summarizes the results of nine published studies that have evaluated ploidy status (DNA diploid versus DNA aneuploid) as a prognostic factor in node-negative breast cancer. These studies range in patient number from 100 to nearly 400, with 4–10 years of median follow-up time. Let us first look at the ability of ploidy status to predict relapse-free survival. Three of the studies report a significant [5, 7, 29] ability of ploidy status to discriminate for relapse-free survival, i.e., patients with diploid tumors have a longer relapse-free survival compared to patients with aneuploid tumors. The other six studies, however, show conflicting results: none of these studies found that ploidy status could significantly predict relapse-free survival [6, 8, 10, 11, 30, 31]. When overall survival was reported, only Sigurdsson et al. [5]

Table 1. Ploidy (diploid/aneuploid) as a predictor of relapse-free survival (RFS) and overall survival (OS) in node-negative breast cancer patients: univariate analyses

Reference	Patients (n)	Follow-up (median years)	p value	
			RFS	OS
O'Reilly et al. [10]	169	8.00	0.60	–
Clark et al. [7]	345	6.00	0.02	–
Sigurdsson et al. [5]	286	4.00	0.03	0.005
Lewis [29]	155	10.00	0.0001	0.0001
Dressler [11]	391	4.55	0.33	–
Winchester et al. [8]	198	6.67	NS[a]	NS
Muss et al. [6]	101	4.25	0.23	–
Keyhani-rofagha	165	8.00	–	0.3
Fisher et al. [31]	243	10.00	0.7	0.9

[a] p value not given, but text indicates nonsignificant.

and Lewis [29] found a significant relationship with aneuploid tumors showing a worse survival compared to diploid tumors. Therefore, we observe inconsistent results with respect to the ability of ploidy status to predict relapse-free survival and overall survival. These inconsistencies may be due in part to different definitions of ploidy status and different interpretations of histograms, an issue that should soon be resolved when recommendations for standard definitions are employed by all investigators [32].

Relationship Between Proliferative Activity and Patient Prognosis

Now let us focus on those studies which have measured proliferative activity (S phase or S + G_2M) by DNA flow cytometry. Table 2 summarizes the results of these studies. Patient populations ranged from 100 to nearly 400 and median follow-up time was 4–10 years. In contrast to the conflicting results obtained for ploidy status, we observe uniform agreement that proliferature capacity is a significant prognostic factor. All seven studies show that S or S + G_2M consistently and significantly predict relapse-free survival [5–8, 10, 11, 31]. In the four studies which also report overall survival [5, 6, 8, 31] all but one [8] show S phase or S + G_2M to predict for overall survival. In each of these studies, patients whose tumors had a high S phase had a shortened disease-free survival compared to those with low S phase tumors. In both Clark et al.'s [7] and Dressler et al.'s [11] studies, S phase was reported to discriminate among both diploid and aneuploid tumors. Clark et al.'s [33] data represents an update of a node-negative study previously published.

Perhaps a more relevant way of summarizing this data is to look at the relationship of S phase and disease-free survival in terms of percentage of

Table 2. Proliferative capacity (High versus Low SPF) as a predictor of relapse-free survival (RFS) and overall survival (OS) in node-negative breast cancer patients: univariate analysis

Reference	Patients (n)	Follow-up (median years)	p value	
			RFS	OS
O'Reilly et al. [10]	169	8.00	$p = 0.006$	–
Clark et al. [7]	345	6.00	$p = 0.03$ (D) $p = 0.01$ (A)	–
Siguurdson et al. [5]	286	4.00	$p = 0.007$	$p = 0.005$
Fisher et al. [31]	243	10.00	$p = 0.003$	$p = 0.005$
Winchester et al. [8]	198	6.67	$p = 0.03$	NS
Dressler et al. [11]	391	4.55	$p = 0.03$ $p = 0.01$ (D) $p = 0.03$ (A)	–
Muss et al. [6]	101	4.25	$p = 0.055$ (S + G2M)	$p = 0.006$ (S + G2M)

Table 3. Five-year % disease-free survival by S phase[a]

Reference	Low S	High S	Difference
O'Rielly 1990 [10]	77%	54%	23%
Siguurdson 1990 [5][b]	89%	69%	20%
Muss 1989 [6]	82%	65%	17%
Winchester 1990 [8]	92% (D)	75% (D)	19% (D)
Clark 1991 [7]	93% (D) 81% (A)	73% (D) 64% (A)	20% (D) 17% (A)
Fisher 1991[c]	46%	27%	19%

[a] Estimated from actuarial disease-free survival curve.
[b] Estimated at 4-year follow-up.
[c] Ten-year disease-free survival figures reported only.

patients remaining free of disease. Table 3 shows the estimated 5-year disease-free survival for low S phase tumors compared to high S phase tumors. These estimates are obtained from Kaplan-Meier plots if the data were not provided in the text. We observe a striking difference in percentage of patients remaining free of disease between the low and high S phase groups; an average difference of 21% was reported among all the studies. In Winchester et al.'s [8] study, S phase predicted disease-free survival only in the diploid tumors. Clark et al.'s [7] update shows that low S phase in both diploid and aneuploid tumors correspond to a significant disease-free survival advantage compared to the high S phase group. Data from the NSABP trial show 10-year disease-free survival of 46% for low S phase patients and 27% for high S phase patients in a group of clinically node-negative patients [31]. Information was incomplete for estimating 5-year disease-free survival in this paper.

Thus far, by univariate analyses, we have observed that: (a) studies measuring proliferative capacity by flow cytometry consistently show S phase fraction to be a significant predictor of disease-free survival; (b) there is a substantial difference in the percentage of patients remaining free of disease between the low and high S phase groups; (c) ploidy status shows inconsistent results in predicting relapse-free survival and, when measured, overall survival; and (d) most studies report a significant relationship for a high S phase to predict shortened survival.

However, at least two questions continue to be asked: (1) Are DNA flow cytometry measurements providing new and useful information? (2) How can this information be used in treating a patient with breast cancer? One approach to answering the first question is to evaluate how these measurements predict patient outcome in a multivariate setting.

Multivariate Analyses of Proliferative Activity and Ploidy as Predictors of Prognosis

Table 4 shows a summary of multivariate results by five investigators evaluating DNA flow measurements as predictors of prognosis in node-negative breast cancer patients [5–8, 10]. Although different factors were included in each analysis, common to all studies were the variables of tumor size and estrogen receptor status. In Table 4, p values for proliferative capacity (high versus low S phase or S + G_2M) are listed for relapse-free survival and overall survival. Other factors in the analysis are also listed;

Table 4. Proliferative capacity (high versus low SPF) as a predictor for relapse-free survival (RFS) and overall suvivial (OS) in node-negative breast cancer patients: multivariate analysis

Reference	FU	p value		Factors
		RFS	OS	
O'Reilly et al. [10]	8.00	$p = 0.005$	–	Size[a], ER, histo
Winchester et al. [8]	6.67	$p = 0.03$ (D) $p = 0.41$ (A)	–	Size, ER, histo
Clark et al. [7]	6.00	$p < 0.03$ (D) $p < 0.01$ (A)	–	Size[a], ER[a], PgR[a], age, ploidy
Muss et al. [6]	4.25	NS	$p = 0.038$ (S + G2M)	Size, ER, age, ploidy
Siguurdson et al. [5]	4.00	$p = 0.03$	$p = 0.0001$	Size, ER, PgR, age, ploidy

[a] Significant factor.

those which remained significant are noted. We observe in O'Reilly et al.'s [10] study that S phase remains a strong independent predictor of relapse-free survival. In Winchester et al.'s [8] study, S phase maintained its significance only in the diploid group of patients whereas in Clark et al.'s [7] update it significantly predicted relapse-free survival in both diploid and aneuploid tumors. Two additional studies measured the ability of proliferative capacity to predict both disease-free survival and overall survival. In Muss et al.'s [6] study, at 4.25 years of follow-up, S + G_2M was an independent predictor of overall survival but not of relapse-free survival. Sigurdsson et al.'s [5] study, at a similar time of follow-up (4.25 years) reported S phase to maintain its significance to predict both relapse-free survival and overall survival.

Therefore, four of the five studies reporting multivariate analysis results have shown S phase or S + G_2M to be significant in the presence of other known prognostic factors and thus to represent an independent predictor of relapse-free survival. In the two studies reporting multivariate results for overall survival, there is agreement that high proliferative capacity is an independent predictor of shortened survival [5, 6].

Response to Treatment

At this time, it is difficult to make any generalizations regarding the ability of these measurements to predict response to treatment. We are just beginning to evaluate ploidy and S phase in this setting. There are at least two clinical trials in the United States currently incorporating DNA flow cytometry measurements in their clinical protocols. The current Intergroup Study 0102 uses S phase fraction to determine eligibility for randomization to one of two arms of chemotherapy in an otherwise good prognosis, node-negative population (estrogen receptor [ER] positive; tumor size <2 cm). Patients with ER-positive, small tumors who have a high S phase fraction are eligible for randomization. The patients with ER-positive, small tumors with a low S phase are observed, and no adjuvant therapy is given. The current node-negative NSABP trial B-18 is measuring S phase and ploidy in samples taken from patients undergoing pre- and postsurgical chemotherapy. This study will allow comparison of S phase and ploidy before and after chemotherapy in the presurgically treated patients. Other studies in advanced breast cancer indicate that DNA flow cytometry measurements may help to identify which cell populations of a patient's tumor respond to the chemotherapy given [14–18]. Obviously, results from these trials and others will need to be carefully evaluated to fully answer how these measurements may predict response to therapy.

In summary: (a) measurement of proliferative capacity using DNA flow cytometry is a significant, independent marker of relapse-free survival in the node-negative breast cancer patient, (b) more than 75% of patients whose tumors have a low S phase are estimated to be free of disease at 5 years, and (c) ploidy status and proliferative activity may help to identify response to therapy.

Measurements of proliferative capacity, whether by DNA flow cytometry [5–8, 10, 11, 31] or thymidine labeling index [34–38] are strong indicators of patient prognosis. Estimates of proliferative potential form the basis of our strategy for effective chemotherapy and for understanding progression of disease. It seems apparent that these markers are a critical component in the management of any breast cancer patient, particularly those with early-stage, node-negative disease.

Acknowledgements. The author gratefully acknowledges all coauthors on the Intergroup Study (0076): Robert Gray, Lynn Eudey (ECOG, Boston), Douglass Tormey, Kennedy Gilchrist (ECOG, Madison), William McGuire, Gary Clark, CK Osborne (SWOG, San Antonio), Edward Mansour (ECOG, Cleveland), Martin Abeloff (ECOG, Baltimore), and all the participating pathologists and institutions. I am indebted to Linda Richardson and Sheryl Curtin for the preparation of this manuscript.

References

1. Dressler LG, Bartow SA (1989) DNA flow cytometry in solid tumors: practical aspects and clinical applications. Semin Diagn Pathol 6:55–82
2. Coulson PB, Thornthwaite JR, Wooley TW et al. (1984) Prognostic indicators including DNA histogram type, receptor content, and staging related to human breast cancer survival. Cancer Res 44:4187–4196
3. Kallioniemi OP, Hietanen T, Mattila J et al. (1987) Aneuploid DNA content and high S phase fraction of tumor cells are related to poor prognosis in patients with primary breast cancer. Eur J Clin Oncol 23:277–282
4. Kallioniemi OP, Blanco G, Alavaikko M et al. (1988) Improving the prognostic value of DNA flow cytometry in breast cancer by combining DNA index and S phase fraction: a proposed classification. Cancer 62:2183–2190
5. Sigurdsson H, Baldetorp B, Borg A et al. (1990) Indicators of prognosis in node negative breast cancer. N Engl J Med 322:1045–1053
6. Muss HB, Kute TE, Case LD et al. (1989) The relationship of flow cytometry to clinical and biologic characteristics in women with node negative primary breast cancer. Cancer 64:1894–1990
7. Clark GM, Owens MA, McGuire WL (1991) A new S phase model predicts for recurrence for aneuploid as well as diploid node-negative breast cancer (Abstr). Proc Am Soc Clin Oncol 10:44
8. Winchester DJ, Duda RB, August CZ et al. (1990) The importance of DNA flow cytometry in node negative breast cancer. Arch Surg 125:886–889
9. Klintenberg C, Stal O, Nordenskjold B et al. (1986) Proliferative index, cytosolic estrogen receptors and axillary node status as prognostic predictors in human mammary carcinoma. Breast Cancer Res Treat 7 Suppl:99–106
10. O'Reilly SM, Camplejohn RS, Barnes DM et al. (1990) Node negative breast cancer: prognostic subgroups defined by tumor size and DNA flow cytometry. J Clin Oncol 8:2040–2046

11. Dressler LG, Eudey L, Gray R et al. (1992) Prognostic potential of DNA flow cytometry measurements in node-negative breast cancer patients: preliminary analysis of an intergroup study (INT0076). J Natl Cancer Inst 11:167–172
12. Ewers SB, Langstrom E, Baldetorp B et al. (1984) Flow cytometric DNA analysis in primary breast carcinomas and clinicopathological correlations. Cytometry 5:408–419
13. Beerman H, Klein PM, Hermans J, Van de Velde CTH, Cornelissa CJ (1990) Prognostic significance of DNA-ploidy in a series of 690 primary breast cancer patients. Int J Cancer 45:34–39
14. Brifford M, Spyratos F, Tubiana-Hulin M et al. (1989) Sequential cytopunctures during pre-operative chemotherapy for breast cancer. Cytomorphologic changes, initial tumor ploidy and tumor regression. Cancer 63:631–637
15. Spyratas F, Brifford M, Tubiana-Hulin M et al. (1992) Sequential cytopunctures during pre-operative chemotherapy for primary breast carcinoma. II. DNA flow cytometry changes during chemotherapy, tumor regression and short-term follow-up. Cancer 69:470–475
16. Remvikos Y, Beuzeboc P, Zadjela A et al. (1989) Correlation of pretreatment proliferative activity with response to cytotoxic chemotherapy. J Natl Cancer Inst 81:1383–1387
17. Seymour L, Bezwoda WR, Meyer K (1990) Response to second line hormone treatment for advanced breast cancer. Predictive value of ploidy determination. Cancer 65:2720–2724
18. Osborne CK (1989) DNA flow cytometry in early breast cancer. A step in the right direction. J Natl Concer Inst 81:1344–1345
19. National Institutes of Health (1990) Consensus Development Conference statement. Treatment of early stage breast cancer. NIM, Washington
20. Dressler LG (1990) Controls, standards and histogram interpretation in DNA flow cytometry. Methods Cell Biol 33:157–171
21. Bach BA, Knape WA, Edinger MG et al. (1991) Improved sensitivity and resolution in the flow cytometric DNA analysis of human solid tumor specimens. Use of in-vitro fine needle aspiration and uniform staining reagents. Am J Clin Pathol 96:615–627
22. Peterson SE, Friedrich V (1986) A comparison between flow cytometric ploidy investigation and chromosome analysis of 32 human colorectal tumors. Cytometry 7:307–312
23. Remvikos Y, Muleris M, Vielh PH et al. (1988) DNA content and genetic evaluation of human colorectal adenocarcinoma. A study by flow cytometry and cytogenetic analysis. Int J Cancer 42:539–543
24. Siegfried TM, Ellison DT, Resau TH (1991) Correlation of modal chromosome number of cultured non-small cell lung carcinomas with DNA index of solid tumor tissue. Cancer Res 51:3257–3273
25. Remvikos Y, Gerbault-Seurreau M, Vielh P et al. (1988) Relevance of DNA ploidy as a measure of genetic deviation: a comparison of flow cytometry and cytogenetics in 25 cases of human breast cancer. Cytometry 9:612–618
26. Dressler LG, Varsa E, Duncan M et al. (1990) Archival DNA flow cytometry is a sensitive and accurate measurement of DNA content in solid tumors. A comparison with cytogenetic analysis in 88 solid tumors (Abstr). Proc Am Assoc Cancer Res 32:159
27. Smeets AWBG, Pauwels RPE, Beck TLM et al. (1987) Tissue specific markers in flow cytometry of urological cancers. Comparing chromosomal and flow cytometric DNA analysis of bladder tumors. Int J Cancer 39:304–310
28. Tribukait B, Granberg-Ohman I, Wijkstrom H (1986) Flow cytometric DNA and cytogenetic studies in human tumors: a comparison and discussion of the differences in modal values obtained by the two methods. Cytometry 7:194–199

29. Lewis WE (1990) Prognostic significance of flow cytometric DNA analysis in node negative breast patients. Cancer 65:2315–2320
30. Keyhani-Rofagha S, O'Toole RV, Farrar WB et al. (1990) Is DNA ploidy an independent prognostic indicator in infiltrative node-negative breast adenocarcinoma? Cancer 65:1577–1582
31. Fisher B, Gunduz N, Costantino J et al. (1991) DNA flow cytometric analysis of primary operable breast cancer. Relation of ploidy and S phase fraction to prognosis of patients in NSABP B-04. Cancer 68:1465–1475
32. Hiddeman W, Schuman J, Andrey G et al. (1984) Convention on nomenclature for DNA flow cytometry. Cytometry 5:445–446
33. Clark GM, Dressler LG, Owens MA et al. (1989) DNA flow cytometry predicts for relapse and survival in node negative breast cancer patients. N Engl J Med 320:627–633
34. Meyer JS, Friedman E, McCrate MM, Bauer WC (1983) Prediction of early course of breast carcinoma by thymidine labelling. Cancer 51:1879–1886
35. Silvestrini R, Diadone MG, Gasparini G (1985) Cell kinetics as a persistent prognostic marker in node negative breast cancer. Cancer 56:1982–1987
36. Silvestrini R, Diadone MG, DiFronzo G et al. (1986) Prognostic implication of labelling index versus estrogen receptors and tumor size in node negative breast cancer. Breast Cancer Res Treat 7:161–169
37. Tubiana M, Pejovic MH, Chavaudra N, Contesso G, Malaise EP (1984) The long-term prognostic significance of thymidine labelling index in breast cancer. Int J Cancer 33:441–445
38. Courdi A, Henry M, Dahan E et al. (1989) Factors affecting relapse in node negative breast cancer. A multivariate analysis including the labelling index. Eur J Cancer Clin Oncol 25:351–356

Review of Proliferative Variables and Their Predictive Value

R. Silvestrini and M.G. Daidone

Istituto Nazionale per lo Studio e la Cura dei Tumori, Milan, Italy

The growing interest in breast cancer biology and the development of sophisticated techniques have greatly contributed to the knowledge of cellular and molecular aspects of disease progression. Markers indicative of biological aggressiveness have been identified [1], and some of these have already passed from the laboratory to clinical application as valid prognostic indicators.

Among the biological factors that have provided reliable prognostic information in breast cancer, cell kinetics has gained a prominent role. The concordant and promising results obtained in the early 1980s by three different groups on patients with early and advanced diseases [2–4] have raised interest and prompted investigation of cell proliferation for speculative and applicative purposes. Several approaches have been proposed and set up. These are based on different rationales and addressed to quantifying DNA synthesizing cells, i.e., the S phase cell fraction, or all proliferating cells, i.e., the growth fraction. The different proliferation markers have different degrees of specificity and sensitivity for target cells [5], and further research is needed on some of them to better define their functional role and relationship to biological aggressiveness.

The cell kinetic variables most throughly investigated and traditionally used for basic or clinical studies on breast cancer are [^{3}H]thymidine labeling index ([^{3}H]dT LI), flow-cytometric S phase cell fraction (FCM-S), and Ki67 immunoreactivity. These proliferation indices have already been submitted to ([^{3}H]dT LI, FCM-S) or are still completing (Ki67) the validation process for prognostic assessment [6]. The validation requires as a first step the investigation of substantial series of patients with adequate follow-up and submitted to local-regional treatment alone, to avoid any interference by systemic treatments on specific cell kinetic subsets. The prognostic relevance demonstrated in such a way must be confirmed by other groups to definitively attribute a prognostic relevance, to allow a comparison among results from different groups, and to activate multicenter clinical studies.

Recent Results in Cancer Research, Vol. 127

Ki67 is a monoclonal antibody which should recognize an antigen related to the proliferation process and provide an estimation of all proliferating cells. This methodology requires frozen tumor sections appropriately fixed in acetone and submitted to a simple immunoperoxidase procedure. Positive cells are scored and quantified at the microscope. The follow-up studies available deal with a relatively small number of patients with a short follow-up and provide controversial results for patients with node-negative or -positive tumors [7–11]. This disagreement could be the consequence of a lack of methodological standardization and quality control of the proliferation index determination, as reflected by the wide range in median values reported by different authors [7–18].

In the past few years efforts have been made to assess and improve the reliability of FCM-S determination from DNA plots obtained from paraffin-embedded specimens and generally to increase determination feasibility in aneuploid tumors, which represent about 70% of breast cancers. However, the role of FCM-S as a predictor of relapse in patients with stage I tumors has not been unequivocally demonstrated. In fact, available results show a prognostic contribution of FCM-S only in diploid [19] or in aneuploid tumors [20], or in both diploid and aneuploid tumors [21, 22]. However, in the study from the Swedish group [21], about 20% of cases had been treated with adjuvant and mostly hormonal therapy, which could have benefited patients with slowly proliferating, estrogen receptor positive tumors, thereby reducing the risk of relapse and death for this subgroup. In our experience [23], as well as in others' [24], no prognostic relevance was found even using both planimetric models and optimization procedures to increase the feasibility of FCM-S to over 85% of cases.

For some decades we have been engaged in [^{3}H]dT LI determination and in the assessment of its prognostic relevance. The consistency of the results, which indicate [^{3}H]dT LI as a prognostic marker independent of other clinical, pathological, and biological prognostic factors in all tumor types investigated, has prompted many groups to adopt this methodology. For simplification, a kit has been made available for the first methodological step. Multicenter clinical therapeutic protocols based on cell kinetics have led to activation of a quality-control program. This program, operative since 1989 [25], has demonstrated a high intra- and interlaboratory reproducibility for [^{3}H]dT LI determination.

In a recent analysis on a series of 9000 patients recruited at the Istituto Nazionale Tumori in Milan since 1972, we assessed the consistency of [^{3}H]dT LI values of primary breast cancer and their relationship to other clinical, pathological, and biological factors. The only slightly, and not significantly, higher median [^{3}H]dT LI in larger than in smaller tumors as well as the similar median values for node-negative and node-positive breast cancers observed on initially limited case series [2] were maintained in this larger series over the 20-year observation period. Similarly, we confirmed the persistence of a higher proliferative rate in estrogen receptor negative

Table 1. Prognostic relevance of [^{3}H]dT LI in breast cancer patients given local-regional therapy

Stage	Follow-up (years)	Relapse			Death		
		Low LI (%)	High LI (%)	*p*	Low LI (%)	High LI (%)	*p*
Node-negative, -positive; locally advanced [27]	14	25	70	<0.01	30	65	<0.01
Node-negative [28]	8	17	44	0.02	0	64	<0.001
Node-negative [29]	6	22	40	<0.0001	5	18	<0.0001
Node-negative [30]	5	20	40	<0.001	11	35	0.001
Node-negative [31]	3.5	6	33	0.05			

than in estrogen receptor positive tumors. Conversely, as also observed by other authors [26], the significantly different proliferative rate initially observed between tumors from pre- and postmenopausal patients was no longer observed after the 1980s due to the increase in [^{3}H]dT LI of tumors from postmenopausal patients.

Several studies [27–31] have reported the prognostic relevance of [^{3}H]dT LI in patients with early or advanced disease subjected to only local-regional treatment and followed for 3.5–14 years. In all the studies the probability of developing local-regional or distant metastases in patients with rapidly proliferating tumors was about twice as high as that of patients with slowly proliferating tumors (Table 1). Additionally, the 14-year relapse-free curves provide evidence for proliferative activity as an indicator of metastatic potential and not only of tumor growth rate [27].

[^{3}H]dT LI retains its predictive role even in the presence of prognostic information provided by tumor size, histological grade, or hormone receptors [27–31]. This finding was recently confirmed in a series of about 900 node-negative tumours, with a median follow-up of 5 years. Moreover, in this up-dated case series, [^{3}H]dT LI was a further prognostic discriminant among patients with small (<2 cm in diameter) or hormone receptor positive tumours. Such findings support the hypothesis that in breast cancer the prognostic contribution of a predictive marker could be further potentiated by considering it in association with other biological or pathological aspects that are independent or only partially related. In fact, the risk of relapse gradually increases from tumors which presented at diagnosis with two favorable prognostic factors (low proliferative rate and small tumor size or

Table 2. Four-year relapse as a function of [^{3}H]dT LI and ploidy in node-negative breast cancer patients

	Low LI (%)	High LI (%)	p
Diploid	4	24	0.05
Aneuploid	16	31	0.05

estrogen receptor positive) to tumors with two unfavorable factors (high proliferative rate and large tumor size or estrogen receptor negative).

The search for new biological markers in an attempt to increase prognostic accuracy has led to the consideration of ploidy, which is highly related to FCM-S but only weakly to [^{3}H]dT LI. In a recent series of 340 node-negative tumors, for which the determination of DNA ploidy was available (Table 2), the prognostic power of the two markers was synergistically greater than that of only one marker, mainly for defining low-risk subsets. In fact, the 4-year relapse rate was eight times lower for patients with diploid, slowly proliferating tumors than for those with aneuploid, rapidly proliferating tumors. Future efforts will be addressed to implementing, in substantial case series with adequate treatment and follow-up, the basic biological characterization. Analyses will include proliferative rate, DNA ploidy, and hormone receptors with the determination of additional promising prognostic factors such as cathepsin D, p53, nm23, and invasiveness markers [32].

Prospective studies are needed to better define the feasibility and the cost-benefit ratio of the use of biological information, as an alternative or complement to clinical and pathological factors in breast cancer patient management. Available information supports the use of proliferation markers as a complement to traditional prognostic factors to identify low- and high-risk patients. However, such encouraging findings should not be translated into a widespread use of any proliferation index proposed in the literature. All the newly proposed proliferation markers should undergo the validation process already completed for consolidated variables and which consists of biological and methodological assessments and optimization of cutoff values. In the absence of clinical validation, new proliferation markers that are inexpensive, simple, and time saving could be introduced in clinical practice once they have shown a high agreement with other established parameters.

References

1. Merkel DE, Osborne K (1989) Prognostic factors in breast cancer. Hematol Oncol Clin North Am 3:641–652
2. Tubiana M, Pejovic MH, Chavaudra G, Contesso G, Malaise EP (1984) The long-term prognostic significance of the thymidine labeling index in breast cancer. Int J Cancer 33:441–445
3. Gentili C, Sanfilippo O, Silvestrini R (1981) Cell proliferation and its relationship to clinical features and relapse in breast cancer. Cancer 48:974–979
4. Meyer JS, Friedman E, McCrate MM, Bauer WC (1983) Prediction of early course of breast carcinoma by thimidine labeling. Cancer 51:1879–1886
5. Quinn CM, Wright NA (1990) The clinical assessment of proliferation and growth in human tumours: evaluation of methods and applications as prognostic variables. J Pathol 160:93–102
6. McGuire WL (1991) Breast cancer prognostic factors: evaluation guidelines. J Natl Cancer Inst 83:154–155
7. Sahin AA et al. (1991) Ki-67 immunostaining in node-negative stage I/II breast carcinoma. Cancer 68:549–557
8. Bouzubar N, Walker KJ, Griffiths K et al. (1989) Ki67 immunostaining in primary breast cancer: pathological and clinical associations. Br J Cancer 59:943–947
9. Wintzer HO, Zipfel I, Schulte-Monting J, Hellerich U, von Keist S (1991) Ki-67 immunostaining in human breast cancer tumors and its relationship to prognosis. Cancer 67:421–428
10. Stauch G, Lelle RJ, Broermann L, Gerogii A (1988) Comparison of prognosis factors in breast cancer: grading of malignancy according to Bloom and Richardson versus determination of Ki67 growth fraction. Verh Dtsch Ges Pathol 72:256–259
11. Weilken W, Beck T, Mitze M, Knapstein PG (1991) Immunohistochemical evaluation of growth fractions in human breast cancers using monoclonal antibody Ki-67. Breast Cancer Res Treat 18:149–154
12. Brown RW, Allred DC, Clark GM, Tandon AK, McGuire WL (1990) Prognostic significance and clinical-pathological correlations of cell-cycle kinetics measured by Ki-67 immunohistochemistry in axillary node-negative carcinoma of the breast. Breast Cancer Res Treat 16:192
13. Gasparini G, Dal Fior S, Pozza F, Bevilacqua P (1989) Correlation of growth fraction by Ki-67 immunohistochemistry with histologic factors and hormone receptors in operable breast carcinoma. Breast Cancer Res Treat 14:329–336
14. Gerdes J, Lelle RJ, Pickartz H et al. (1986) Growth fractions in breast cancers determined in situ with a monoclonal antibody Ki67. J Clin Pathol 39:977–980
15. Isola J, Helin HJ, Helle MJ, Kallioniemi OP (1990) Evaluation of cell proliferation in breast carcinoma: comparison of Ki67 immunohistochemical study, DNA flow cytometric analysis, and mitotic count. Cancer 65: 1180–1185
16. McGurrin JF, Doria MI Jr, Dawson PJ, Karrison T, Stein HO, Franklin WA (1987) Assessment of tumor cell kinetics by immunohistochemistry in carcinoma of the breast. Cancer 59:1744–1750
17. Veneroni S, Silvestrini R, Costa A (1991) Relationship between ^{3}H-TdR labeling index and Ki-67 in human breast cancer. J Biol Marker 6:68
18. Veronese S, Gambacorta M (1991) Detection of Ki-67 proliferation rate in breast cancer. Correlation with clinical and pathologic features. Am J Clin Pathol 95:30–34
19. Clark GM, Dressler LG, Owens MA, Pounds G, Oldaker T, McGuire WL (1989) Prediction of relapse or survival in patients with node-negative breast cancer by DNA flow cytometry. N Engl J Med 320:627–633

20. O'Reilly SM, Camplejohn RS, Barnes DM, Millis RR, Rubens RD, Richards MA (1990) Node-negative breast cancer: prognostic subgroup defined by tumor size and flow cytometry. J Clin Oncol 8:2040–2046
21. Sigurdsson H, Baldetorp B, Borg A et al. (1990) Indicators of prognosis in node-negative breast cancer. N Engl J Med 322:1045–1053
22. Fisher B, Nurten G, Costantino J et al. (1991) DNA flow cytometric analysis of primary operable breast cancer. Cancer 68:1465–1475
23. Daidone MG, Silvestrini R, Del Bino G, Di Fronzo G (1991) Autoradiographic and flow cytometric estimations of S-phase cell fraction in node-negative (N^-) breast cancer: biologic and clinical comparison (Abstr). Proc Am Soc Clin Oncol 10:47
24. Muss H, Kute TE, Case LD et al. (1989) The relation of flow cytometry to clinical and biologic characteristics in women with node negative primary breast cancer. Cancer 64:1894–1900
25. Silvestrini R (1991) Feasibility and reproducibility of the ^{3}H-thymidine labelling index in breast cancer. Cell Prolif 24:437–445
26. Meyer JS, Prey MU, Babcock DS (1986) Breast carcinoma cell kinetics, morphology, stage, and host characteristics. Lab Invest 54:41–51
27. Tubiana M, Pejovic MH, Koscielny S, Chavaudra N, Malaise E (1989) Growth rate, kinetics of tumor cell proliferation and long-term outcome in human breast cancer. Int J Cancer 44:17–22
28. Hery M, Gioanni J, Lalanne CM, Namer M, Courdi A (1987) The DNA labeling index: a prognostic factor in node-negative breast cancer. Breast Cancer Res Treat 9:207–212
29. Silvestrini R, Daidone MG, Valagussa P, Di Fronzo G, Mezzanotte G, Bonadonna G (1989) Cell kinetics as a prognostic indicator in node-negative breast cancer. Eur J Cancer 25:1165–1171
30. Meyer JS, Province M (1988) Proliferative index of breast carcinoma by thymidine labeling: prognostic power independent of stage, estrogen and progesterone receptors. Breast Cancer Res Treat 12:191–199
31. Paradiso A, Mangia A, Picciariello M et al. (1992) Fattori prognostici nel carcinoma della mammella operabile N^-: attività proliferativa e caratteristiche clinico patologiche. Folia Oncol 13:1–13
32. Daidone MG, Silvestrini R, D'Errico A et al. (1991) Laminin receptors, collagenase IV and prognosis in node-negative breast cancer. Int J Cancer 48:529–532

Critical Review of Growth Factors as Clinical Tools in Primary and Metastatic Breast Cancer

J.G.M. Klijn[1], P.M.J.J. Berns[1], W.L.J. van Putten[2], M. Bontenbal[1], J. Alexieva-Figusch[1], and J.A. Foekens[1]

[1] Department of Medical Oncology, Division of Endocrine Oncology, Rotterdam Cancer Institute (DDHK), Groene Hilledijk 301, 3075 EA Rotterdam, The Netherlands
[2] Department of Statistics, Rotterdam Cancer Institute (DDHK), Groene Hilledijk 301, 3075 EA Rotterdam, The Netherlands

Introduction

Present research in the field of clinical breast cancer is focused on new diagnostic methods and on the development of new treatment modalities [25]. Adjuvant systemic therapy with chemotherapeutic drugs or endocrine treatment has been shown to result in a 25% reduction in annual odds of death, meaning an absolute decrease in death of 4% and 10% in node-negative and node-positive patients, respectively [13] (reprinted in part in this volume). However, it must be concluded that the majority of patients with primary breast cancer will be overtreated in cases of adjuvant therapy. Both efficacy and cost effectiveness of adjuvant systemic therapy are presently important subjects of debate [20, 27]. Identification of high-risk and low-risk patients is therefore a major issue. For patients with breast cancer a large series of classical and modern prognostic factors (Table 1) have been reported [18, 23, 28, 29]. These factors concern patient characteristics and parameters determined in blood and tumor characteristics. Most of these factors have been evaluated with respect to relapse-free survival (RFS) and overall survival (OS), but very few with respect to response to hormonal or chemotherapy in primary or metastatic disease. However, also for patients with recurrent disease (macrometastases) prognostic factors and predictors for response to treatment are clinically important for reaching decisions concerning type of therapy.

Recently a great number of modern cell biological parameters such as oncogenes/suppressor genes, growth factors, and secretory proteins appear strongly to influence the behavior of a tumor with respect to metastatic pattern, extent of cellular differentiation, growth rate, and the development of therapy resistance. Oncogenes may encode for growth factors, growth factor receptors, protein kinases, signal transducers, nuclear proteins, and transcription factors. Assessment of the value of these biological parameters as prognosticator, as predictor of response to therapy, or as possible point of

Recent Results in Cancer Research, Vol. 127

Table 1. Classification of prognostic factors in breast cancer (from [23])

- Patient characteristics
  - Race
  - Age
  - Menopausal status
  - Performance status
  - Metabolic diseases
- Variables determined in blood
  - Tumor marker levels (CEA, CA15–3)
  - Hemoglobin, alkaline phosphatase, liver function tests
  - FcτR on mononuclear cells
  - Hormone levels
- Tumor characteristics
  - Histologic features: type, grade, vascular invasion, necrosis
  - Stage (TNM), bone marrow micrometastases
  - Cytoplasmatic and nuclear steroid receptors: ER, PR, AR, vitamin D receptors
  - Membrane receptors for hormones and growth factors
    - LHRH-R
    - PRL-R
    - IGF-I-R
    - EGF-R
    - TGF-β-R
    - SS-R
  - Enzymes, proteins, and other cytoplasmatic factors
    - Human milk fat globule antigens
    - Prostaglandin levels
    - Plasminogen activator expression
    - Tyrosine kinase activities
    - Aromatase activity
    - Haptoglobin-related protein epitope expression
    - Cathepsin D
    - Heat shock proteins
    - pS2 protein
    - Growth factor content (EGF, TGF-α, -β, IGF-I)
  - Chromosomal abnormalities
    - Cytogenetic
    - Ploidy
    - Amplification, (over)expression of oncogenes (*HER2/neu*, c-*erbB*2, *int*-2, *ras*, c-*myc*)
    - Deletion or mutations of suppressor genes (Rb gene, p 53 gene)
  - Cell proliferation indices
    - Labeling index
    - S phase fraction
    - Ki-67 antigen
  - Clonogenicity
  - Immunologic phenotypes
- Response to treatment

Table 2. Incidence of positivity of various prognostic factors in primary breast cancer

Parameter	Number of series	Number of patients	Positive (%)
EGF-R	40	5 232	48
IGF-I-R	3	653	67–93
SS-R	3	470	36–60
HER2/neu amplification or (over)expression	52	11 408	20
c-*myc* amplification	18	2 493	20
Int2/bcl1 amplification	13	>1 500	13

Table 3. Relationship between EGF-R status and other prognostic factors in human primary breast cancer (number of studies with significant correlation)

ER	28/31
PR	11/18
IGF-I-R	0/3
PRL-R	0/1
LHRH-R	0/1
SS-R	1/2
Age	2/9
Menopausal status	1/7
Histologic type	3/7
Grade	10/18
Tumor size	2/17
Nodal status	5–9/20
Ploidy	1/7
Proliferation indices	3/9

action for new treatment modalities is important. Therefore characterization of individual tumors is increasingly relevant. In the present paper, we review briefly the significance of some important growth factors and oncogenes with respect to breast cancer, focusing on our own results.

Prognosis, Relapse-Free and Overall Survival

Epidermal Growth Factor

Epidermal growth factor (EGF) as well as transforming growth factor-alpha (TGF-α), both of which can activate EGF receptors (EGF-R), are probably produced locally in many tissues as local growth factors rather than as systemic hormones. EGF and TGF-α can stimulate the growth of normal mammary epithelium and human breast cancer cells in vitro. EGF-R have been demonstrated on several breast cancer cell lines, especially on estrogen receptor (ER) negative tumor cells and in human primary tumors and metastases. Recently we reviewed extensively the clinical significance of EGF-R [24]. EGF-R positivity was shown to be present in 2500 (48%) of 5232 breast tumors of 40 different series of patients (Table 2). The mean percentage of EGF-R positivity in the individual series reported by these 40 different groups of investigators is 45% (range 14%–91%). Overall there are generally no clear differences among results obtained by radioligand binding assays, immunological methods, autoradiography, and measurement of EGF-R transcripts, although the mean percentage of EGF-R positive tumors determined by immunological methods tends to be somewhat lower. Nearly all studies (Table 3) indicate a negative relationship between EGF-R and steroid receptor status (28/31 studies for ER; 12/19 for progesterone receptors, PR), showing that EGF-R positivity is twice as high in ER- or PR-negative tumors compared to ER- or PR-positive tumors (about 50%–60% versus 30%). With regard to other prognostic factors the majority of groups (10/18) also reported a significant (positive) correlation with tumor grade, but only a minority found a significant relationship between EGF-R status and patient age (2/9), menopausal status (1/7), histologic type (3/7), tumor size (2/17), nodal status (5–9/20), ploidy (1/7), or proliferation indices (3/9). No relationship was observed with tumor status regarding receptors for insulin-like growth factor-I (IGF-I-R), prolactin (PRL-R), or luteinizing hormone-releasing hormone (LHRH-R), but an inverse relationship between EGF-R and somatostatin receptor (SS-R) may be present.

However, it must be stressed that the series in which the relationship between EGF-R status and other prognostic factors were investigated contained relatively few patients (mostly less than 100). Therefore, when larger groups of patients are investigated, more significant relationships may be observed, especially with respect to nodal status, tumor ploidy, and proliferation indices. In fact, we calculated the presence of EGF-R positivity overall in 35% of 253 aneuploid tumors versus only in 15% of 114 diploid tumors ($p < 0.0001$). In addition, most studies observed a trend, if no significant correlation, between higher EGF-R levels in tumors with the highest percentages of S-phase or Ki-67 expression. With regard to RFS and OS, five of nine different groups of investigators found a significant prognostic value of EGF-R after short-term (1- to 4-year) follow-up, indicating that patients with EGF-R positive tumors have a poor prognosis. Three of five groups with a maximal follow-up of at least 6 years found only a tendency for any relationship between EGF-R status and long-term outcome. However, Nicholson et al. [31] recently reported that in a multivariate analysis at 6-year follow-up only EGF-R, out of ER, size, and grade, was significantly predictive for either RFS or OS, especially in node-negative patients. On the other hand, we found the best prognostic value of EGF-R in node-positive patients [15]. In general, with respect to subgroup analysis by nodal or ER status, there is no agreement on the best prognosticator or in which subgroup EGF-R status offers the most predictive power [24]. The differences in results and conclusions may be due partly to differences in patient number, cutoff levels for both EGF-R and ER, application of systemic adjuvant therapy, and duration of patient follow-up.

Less is known on the prognostic value of EGF itself. Previously we [14] reported a wide range of EGF-like activities in 142 breast cancers (median 86, range 26–517 ng/mg protein). A negative correlation was observed between the content of acid-ethanol extracted EGF-like activities with ER and PR. TGF-α mRNA and TGF-α protein has been found in 50%–70% of primary human breast tumors [10]. In small series of patients there appeared no association between TGF-α mRNA expression, histologic grade, nodal status, tumor cellularity, desmoplasia, and patient survival [2, 10].

Transforming Growth Factor-β

TGF-β is a growth-inhibitory factor in breast cancer. Coombes et al. [12] examined 129 primary breast carcinomas for the presence of TGF-β mRNA. Some degree of expression was observed in all patients, but high levels were inversely related to the presence of nodal metastases and were positively related to median (disease-free) survival. However, over the whole study period of 10 years, no statistical significance was observed. The presence of TGF-β transcripts in 53 out of 104 carcinomas showed no relationship with survival or other clinical features, such as tumor size and nodal or menopausal status. Thus far, there are no data on the prognostic value of receptors of TGF-β.

Insulin-like Growth Factors

IGF-I and IGF-II are potent mitogens for breast cancer cells [32]. The growth effects of both are mediated predominantly via the IGF-I receptor (IGF-I-R). IGF-I-R have been demonstrated in 50%–67% [33], 87% [35], and 93% [15] in series of 142, 297, and 214 tumors, respectively. Compared to cancer tissues, receptors for IGF-I were present less frequently in benign breast tumors (47%) and normal tissue and at lower levels. Positive relationships were observed between the levels of IGF-I-R and steroid receptors, but no associations of IGF-I-R with EGF-R, lymph node status, tumor size, differentiation grade, or menopausal status was found. However, there was a significant positive correlation with age [15]. Thus far, data of only two studies on the prognostic value of IGF-I-R have been published, showing different results. Our study [15] on 214 patients showed no relationship between IGF-I-R and RFS or OS. Recently, however, Bonneterre et al. [9] and Peyrat et al. [35] demonstrated in a study on 277 patients a significantly longer RFS and OS in patients with IGF-I-R containing tumors than in those without. The positive prognostic value of IGF-I-R on OS was confirmed by Cox analysis. The prognostic value of IGF-I-R was lower than that of ER but similar to that of PR, tumor size, lymph node status, and grade. The authors discussed that by analysis of their data comparable to our analysis, i.e., dividing the patient population into three groups of approximately equal size and with low, intermediate, and higher levels of IGF-I-R, they also found no significant prognostic value of IGF-I-R. Interestingly, the combination of IGF-I-R, tumor grade, and nodal status led to a very good evaluation of the prognosis.

Recently, we demonstrated IGF-I-R gene amplification in 2% of 975 primary breast cancers [4]. These tumors showed 35-fold higher levels of IGF-I-R than nonamplified tumors, while some other genes (three times c-*myc*, five times *int-2/blc-1*) were also amplified. Patients with tumors containing a high (≥20) IGF-I-R gene copy number tended to have a shorter median OS, but this subgroup is very small.

Previously we [14] found IGF-I-like activity in all 78 tumors investigated (median 15, range 3–131 mg/mg protein) and eightfold higher levels in acid-ethanol extracts compared to direct assays in the cytosols without prior extraction, suggesting the presence of intracellular binding proteins. Human breast cancer cell lines also express and secrete large amounts of IGF-binding proteins, which might be related to ER status [32]. With respect to tumor IGF-I content, we demonstrated a positive correlation with ER and PR levels but not with EGF-like activity [14]. In addition, plasma IGF-I concentrations appeared to be higher in patients with primary breast cancer compared to control women with the same age [35]. These findings may be important with respect to the administration of IGF-I lowering drugs such as somatostatin analogs [25, 35] and tamoxifen [36].

Somatostatin Receptors

Somatostatin is able to suppress plasma growth hormone and IGF-I concentrations and to inhibit directly human breast cancer cells in vitro [38] and SS-R positive mammary tumors in vivo (see [25]). SS-R have been found in 36%–46% of primary breast cancers (see [18, 25]), but measured in patients by receptorscintigraphy (in vivo imaging) the incidence is even 60%. These SS-R positive tumors often contain neuroendocrine histologic markers, and an inverse relationship between SS-R and EGF-R was demonstrated [37]. This latter was not confirmed in our studies [15, 16] on a larger series of patients. However, one should keep in mind that in one series only autoradiographic methods were used [37] versus autoradiography for SS-R and ligand binding for EGF-R on tissue homogenates in the other series [15, 16]. No association was found between SS-R and tumor size, nodal status, grade, or IGF-I-R levels, but SS-R was demonstrated more frequently in ER- and

PR-positive tumors. In the only reported study on the prognostic value of SS-R [15, 16] we observed that patients with SS-R positive primary tumors experienced a significantly better 5-year RFS than patients with SS-R negative tumors (82% versus 46%; $p = 0.04$).

HER2/neu

Similar to EGF-R much attention has been focussed on *HER2/neu* (c-*erbB2*) [6, 11, 18, 19, 25, 26, 29, 34]. The protein product of the *HER2/neu* oncogene is structurally homologous to the EGF-R (c-*erbB1*). In view of the close similarity between EGF-R and *HER2/neu* oncogene protein it is interesting to compare the clinical relationships and prognostic value of these two membrane markers. For the EGF-R gene a great difference has been found between the incidence of gene amplification, i.e., about 2% (range 0%–14%; Table 2) relative to protein (over) expression (48%) [24], in contrast to *HER2/neu* in which there is a strong correlation between amplification and overexpression. Amplification and/or overexpression of the *HER2/neu* gene has been described in 20% of breast tumors (range 8%–64%). In our most recent update [25] of the literature data encompassing a total of 11408 breast tumors (Table 2) we calculated a mean *HER2/neu* positivity of 20% without finding any significant difference between the incidence of amplification (953/4627, i.e., 20.6%) and overexpression (1331/6947, i.e., 19.2%). In our series of 975 tumor samples we found an incidence of *HER2/neu* amplification of 18.7% [3]. This means that EGF-R positive tumors relate to a greater proportion (45%–50%) of breast cancer patients than do *HER2/neu* positive tumors (20%), which might suggest an advantage for the measurement of EGF-R as prognostic parameter. The prognostic value of *HER2/neu* has been studied extensively since the initial report by Slamon et al. [39] showing that *HER2/neu* is an independent prognostic factor in node-positive patients. Recent reviews [6, 11, 19, 26, 34] suggest that there is no association between elevated *HER2/neu* and patient age, only a tentative relationship with tumor grade, size, or nodal involvement, and an inverse association with steroid hormone receptors. There is no consensus on the independent prognostic power of *HER2/neu* to predict either RFS or OS. In our own experience [5] *HER2/neu* amplification was not associated with RFS but weakly with shorter OS in univariate analysis ($p = 0.035$). Interestingly, however, in the small group of steroid receptor negative patients, *HER2/neu* amplification may identify patients with increased risk of relapse and death, whereas the opposite may be the case for steroid receptor positive patients. These results seem to be in contrast to the reported early recurrence of *HER2/neu* positive tumors observed in 325 patients with small (<3 cm) node-negative ER-positive breast cancers [29].

c-myc

Reviewing the data in the literature, we calculated the incidence of c-*myc* amplification (Table 2) in 20% of 2493 breast cancers [7]. However, in contrast to *HER2/neu*, the (over)expression of c-*myc* is much higher (80%–100% of tumors). In a series of 975 tumors we found c-*myc* amplification in 17.1% [3], but the incidence was higher (33%) in tumors of patients developing metastases later on [7]. The amplification of c-*myc* was more prevalent in the PR-negative subpopulation but was strongly negatively correlated with *HER2/neu* amplification. In a subgroup of 282 patients, c-*myc* amplification was observed more frequently in large tumors and in node-positive patients but was not associated with age, menopausal status, grade, or ER status [5]. In univariate analysis, amplification of c-*myc* proved to be a significant predictor of reduced RFS and OS ($p < 0.001$). In multivariate analysis for RFS, c-*myc* amplification significantly ($p = 0.001$) added to the prognostic power of tumor size, lymph node status, and ER status, with the highest relative failure rate (1.8) after lymph node status (2.2). The amplification of c-*myc* was predictive for outcome, especially among patients with node-negative disease or steroid receptor positive tumors: 51% and 46% difference in actuarial 5-year RFS compared to patients with tumors with normal c-*myc* gene copy numbers [5, 6].

Predictive Value for Response to Treatment

It appears that EGF-R positive tumors are more prone to first relapses at visceral sites, while EGF-R negative tumors recur more often in the bone [24]. Interestingly, Kallioniemi et al. [21] recently demonstrated a significant association also between *HER2/neu* overexpression and increased risk of visceral metastases. In addition, in our experience *HER2/neu* amplified tumors tended to relapse relatively frequently in liver and lung and tumors, with c-*myc* amplification especially locoregionally and in the brain, but significantly less in bone [8].

Patients with advanced disease and EGF-R positive tumors respond less well to first-line endocrine treatment as compared to those with EGF-R negative tumors, but the significance of this independence of ER status is unknown [24, 30]. There is no apparent relationship between EGF-R status and response to first-line chemotherapy, but this has not been well studied. In our experience, *HER2/neu* amplified tumors showed a poor response to endocrine therapy, but a good response to subsequent chemotherapy [8]. The c-*myc* amplified tumors, however, showed a worse response to chemotherapy, but not to endocrine therapy, compared to nonamplified tumors. Eventually, either for *HER2/neu* or c-*myc*, opposite effects on duration of response to endocrine and subsequent chemotherapy resulted in the lack of

Table 4. Difference in 5 year relapse-free survival in node-negative breast cancer according various prognosticators [23, 29]

Prognostic factor	Difference between high and low risk (%)
1 *HER2/neu*	NS
2 IGF-I-R	NS
3 ER	8
4 Tumor size	13
5 Ploidy	14
6 Grade	16
7 Labeling index	18
8 S phase	20
9 Cathepsin D	8–23
10 pS2	31
11 EGF-R	0–35
12 c-*myc*	51
Combinations	
1 S phase/diploid	20
2 Cathepsin D/aneuploid	31
3 *HER2*/ER+, <3 cm	35

a significant association between gene amplification and (overall) postrelapse survival.

Discussion

The efficacy and cost effectiveness of adjuvant systemic therapy in women with primary breast cancer are important subjects of current debate. More selective use of chemotherapy to maximize the benefit to individual patients may be possible with refinements in risk stratification and better assessment of the patient's risk preferences [20]. This concerns especially patients with primary node-negative breast cancer. Numerous prognostic factors have been reported with different prognostic values within this subgroup (Table 4) [23, 29]. There is less agreement on the value of several factors such as EGF-R and cathepsin D. The differences in results and conclusions may be due partly to differences in patient number, cutoff levels, administration of systemic adjuvant therapy, and duration of patient follow-up – generally, concerns affecting the evaluation of other prognostic factors. The discriminatory effect of EGF-R status seems to decrease with long-term follow-up compared to short-term follow-up, as previously shown and discussed by some authors for ER status [1, 22]. Interestingly, the relationships and conclusions reported for *HER2/neu* are similar and comparable to those described for EGF-R [24]. Few authors have compared the prognostic power of EGF-R and *HER2/neu* in the same study, and these show conflicting results [see 18, 24]. With respect to our own experience, especially c-*myc* [5, 7] and pS_2 protein [17] are the most powerful prognosticators, especially for node-negative breast cancer.

Especially the overall influence of adjuvant systemic treatment on the prognostic power of several prognostic factors has yet to be established. In addition, presently there are conflicting reports on the value of *HER2/neu* with respect to predictability of response to endocrine and chemotherapy, showing a poor response of *HER2/neu* positive tumors to adjuvant chemotherapy but a good response to chemotherapy in metastatic disease. However, in view of the protracted indirect endocrine effect of adjuvant chemotherapy in premenopausal patients by "chemical castration" and the observed relationship between efficacy and tumor PR levels, it can be expected that adjuvant chemotherapy may be more effective, especially in *HER2/neu* negative primary premenopausal breast cancer, because of our observation of a relatively good response of *HER2/neu* negative metastatic tumors to endocrine therapy [8].

Ultimately, further refinements in risk stratification by combined use of several prognosticators may be possible, but evaluation of these combinations by multivariate analysis in very large series is necessary. Therefore, we hope to extend our series of patients to approximately 4000–5000 in the coming years.

References

1. Alexieva-Figusch J, van Putten WLJ, Blankenstein MA, Blonk-van der Wijst J, Klijn JGM (1988) The prognostic value and relationships of patient characteristics, progestin receptor, estrogen receptor, and site of relapse in primary and metastatic human breast cancer. Cancer 61:758–768
2. Barrett-Lee P, Travers M, Luqmani Y, Coombes RC (1990) Transcripts for transforming growth factors in human breast cancer: clinical correlates. Br J Cancer 61:612–617
3. Berns PMJJ, Klijn JGM, van Staveren IL, Portengen H, Noordergraaf E, Foekens JA (1992) Prevalence of amplification of the oncogenes c-*myc*, *Her2/neu*, and *int*-2 in one thousand human breast tumours: correlation with steroid receptors. Eur J Cancer 28:697–700
4. Berns PMJJ, Klijn JGM, van Staveren IL, Portengen H, Foekens JA (1992) Sporadic amplification of the insulin-like growth factor 1 receptor gene in human breast tumors. Cancer Res 52:1036–1039
5. Berns PMJJ, Klijn JGM, van Putten WLJ, van Staveren IL, Portengen H, Foekens JA (1992) c-*myc* amplification is a better prognostic factor than *HER-2/neu* amplification in primary breast cancer. Cancer Res 52:1107–1113
6. Berns PMJJ, Klijn JGM, Foekens JA (1992) Oncogene amplification in human breast and ovarian cancer. Current Perspectives on Molecular and Cellular Oncology. 1B:81–94
7. Berns PMJJ, Foekens JA, van Putten WLJ, van Staveren IL, Portengen H, De Koning WCH, Klign JGM (1992) Prognostic factors in human primary breast

cancer: comparison of c-*myc* and *HER2/neu* amplification. J Steroid Biochem Mol Biol 43:13–19

8. Berns PMJJ, Foekens JA, van Staveren IL, Portengen H, van Putten WLJ, de Koning H, Klign JGM (1992) Amplification of the *HER2/neu* gene and not of c-*myc* is associated with a poor response to endocrine and good response to chemotherapy in recurrent breast cancer. 5th EORTC Breast Cancer Conference, Leuven, 3–6 Sept 1991, abst A213
9. Bonneterre J, Peyrat JP, Beuscart R, Demaille A (1990) Prognostic significance of IGF-I receptors in human breast cancer. Cancer Res 50:6931–6935
10. Ciardiello F, Kim N, McGeady ML, Liscia DS, Saeki T, Bianco C, Salomon DS (1991) Expression of transforming growth factor alpha (TGF α) in breast cancer. Ann Oncol 2:169–182
11. Clark GM, McGuire WL (1991) Follow-up study of *HER-2/neu* amplification in primary breast cancer. Cancer Res 51:944–948
12. Coombes RC, Barrett-Lee P, Luqmani Y (1990) Growth factor expression in breast tissue. J Steroid Biochem Mol Biol 37:833–837
13. Early Breast Cancer Trialists' Collaborative Group (1992) Systemic treatment of early breast cancer by hormonal, cytotoxic, or immune therapy: 133 randomised trials involving 31000 recurrences and 24000 deaths among 75000 women. Lancet 339:1–15, 71–85
14. Foekens JA, Portengen H, Jansen M, Klijn JGM (1989) Insulin-like growth factor I (IGF-I) receptors and IGF-I-like activity in human primary breast cancer. Cancer 63:2139–2147
15. Foekens JA, Portengen H, van Putten WLJ, Reubi JC, Trapman AMAC, Alexieva-Figusch J, Klijn JGM (1989) The prognostic significance of receptors for insulin-like growth factor-I, somatostatin, and epidermal growth factor in human primary breast cancer. Cancer Res 49:7002–7009
16. Foekens JA, van Putten WLJ, Portengen H, Rodenburg CJ, Reubi JC, Berns PMJJ, Henzen-Logmans SC, van der Burg MEL, Alexieva-Figusch J, Klijn JGM (1990) Prognostic value of pS2 protein, and receptors for epidermal growth factor (EGF-R), insulin-like growth factor-I (IGF-I-R), and somatostatin (SS-R), in patients with breast and ovarian cancer. J Steroid Biochem Mol Biol 37:815–822
17. Foekens JA, Rio M-C, Seguin P, van Putten WLJ, Fauque J, Nap M, Klijn JGM, Chambon P (1990) Prediction of relapse and survival in breast cancer patients by pS2 protein status. Cancer Res 50:3832–3837
18. Foekens JA, Peters HA, Portengen H, Noordergraaf E, Berns PMJJ, Klijn JGM (1991) Cell biological prognostic factors in breast cancer: a review. J Clin Immunoassay 14:184–196
19. Gullick WJ (1990) The role of the epidermal growth factor receptor and the c-*erbB*-2 protein in breast cancer. Int J Cancer Suppl 5:55–61
20. Hillner BE, Smith TJ (1991) Efficacy and cost effectiveness of adjuvant chemotherapy in women with node-negative breast cancer. A decision-analysis model. N Engl J Med 324:160–169
21. Kallioniemi PO, Holli K, Visakorpi T, Koivula T, Helin HH, Isola JJ (1991) Association of c-*erbB*-2 protein over-expression with high rate of cell proliferation, increased risk of visceral metastasis and poor long-term survival in breast cancer. Int J Cancer 49:650–655
22. Kinsel LB, Szabo E, Greene GL, Konrath J, Leight GS, McCarty KS Jr (1989) Immunocytochemical analysis of estrogen receptors as a predictor of prognosis in breast cancer patients: comparison with quantitative biochemical methods. Cancer Res 49:1052–1056
23. Klijn JGM, Foekens JA (1990) Prognostic factors in breast cancer. In: Goldhirsch A (ed) Endocrine therapy of breast cancer IV. Springer, Berlin Heidelberg New York, pp 17–25 (ESO monographs)

24. Klijn JGM, Berns PMJJ, Foekens JA (1992) The clinical significance of epidermal growth factor receptor (EGF-R) in human breast cancer: a review on 5232 patients. Endocr Rev 13:3–17
25. Klijn JGM, Berns PMJJ, Bontenbal M, Alexieva-Figusch J, Foekens JA (1992) Clinical breast cancer, new developments in selection and endocrine treatment of patients. J Steroid Biochem Mol Biol 43:211–221
26. MaGuire HC, Greene MI (1989) The *neu* (c-*erbB*-2) oncogene. Semin Oncol 16:148–155
27. McGuire WL (1989) Adjuvant treatment of node-negative breast cancer. N Engl J Med 320:525–527
28. McGuire WL (1989) Prognostic factors for recurrens and survival. In: Educational Booklet American Society of Clinical Oncology, 25th Annual Meeting, pp 89–92
29. McGuire WL, Tandon AK, Allred DC, Chamness GC, Clark GM (1990) How to use prognostic factors in axillary node-negative breast cancer patients. J Natl Cancer Inst 82:1006–1015
30. Nicholson S, Sainsbury JRC, Halcrow P, Chambers P, Farndon JR, Harris AL (1989) Expression of epidermal growth factor receptors associated with lack of response to endocrine therapy in recurrent breast cancer. Lancet 1:182–184
31. Nicholson S, Richard J, Sainsbury C, Halcrow P, Kelly P, Angus B, Wright C, Henry J, Farndon JR, Harris AL (1991) Epidermal growth factor (EGF-r); results of a 6 year follow-up study in operable breast cancer with emphasis on the node negative subgroup. Br J Cancer 63:146–150
32. Osborne CK, Clemmons DR, Arteaga CL (1990) Regulation of breast cancer growth by insulin-like growth factors. J Steroid Biochem Mol Biol 37:805–809
33. Pekonen F, Partanen S, Mäkinen T, Rutanen EM (1988) Receptors for epidermal growth factor and insulin-like growth factor I and their relation to steroid receptors in human breast cancer. Cancer Res 48:1343–1347
34. Perren TJ (1991) c-*erbB*-2 oncogene as a prognostic marker in breast cancer. Br J Cancer 63:328–332
35. Peyrat JP, Bonneterre J, Vermin PH, Jammes H, Beuscart R, Helquet B, Djiane J, Lefebvre J, Demaille A (1990) Insulin-like growth factor I receptors (IGF-I-R) and IGF-I in human breast tumors. J Steroid Biochem Mol Biol 37:823–827
36. Pollak M, Polychronakos C, Bauer S, Kaplan R, Guyda H, Constantino J, Redmond C, Fisher B, Margolese R (1990) Effect of tamoxifen on serum insulin-like growth factor I (IGF-I) levels of stage I breast cancer patients (Abstr). Proc Am Soc Clin Oncol 9:20
37. Reubi JC, Waser B, Foekens JA, Klijn JGM, Lamberts SWJ, Laissue J (1990) Somatostatin receptor incidence and distribution in breast cancer using receptor autoradiography. Relationship to EGF receptors. Int J Cancer 46:416–420
38. Setyono-Han B, Henkelman MS, Foekens JA, Klijn JGM (1987) Direct inhibitory effects of somatostatin (analogues) on the growth of human breast cancer cells. Cancer Res 47:1566–1570
39. Slamon DJ, Clark GM, Wong SG, Levin WJ, Ullrich A, McGuire WL (1987) Human breast cancer: correlation of relapse and survival with amplification of the Her-2/neu oncogene. Science 235:177–182

Prognosis and Prediction for Early Breast Cancer

M. Baum

Department of Surgery, The Royal Marsden Hospital, Fulham Road, London SW3 6JJ, UK

Introduction

In the United Kingdom some wit who wishes to remain anonymous has coined the expression "YAPI", which stands for "yet another prognostic indicator". I am sure that many share my irritation when reading countless papers claiming yet another prognostic indicator, whilst people have completely lost sight of the appropriate use and the frequent abuse of these tests.

In broad terms, there are two appropriate uses for "prognostic indicators", the first is to define a subgroup of patients with early breast cancer whose prognosis is so good (i.e., equivalent to an age-matched population) that there is no room for improvement, and therefore their cure by surgery alone is likely. (The possible exception for this generalisation might be the prolonged use of tamoxifen in the hope of preventing the contra-lateral breast cancer.) The second use of a prognostic indicator is in determining which subsets of breast cancer respond preferentially to either endocrine or cytotoxic chemotherapy – in other words, determining whether there are qualitative interactions between the choice of therapy and the eventual outcome of treatment.

As far as the first issue is concerned, we can already state with confidence that screen-detected duct carcinoma in situ and special types of breast cancer such as the tubular variety are almost certainly cured by adequate local therapy alone. In addition, some might argue that a 1-cm, well-differentiated, node-negative cancer also has such an excellent chance of cure that there is little additional room for improvement by a systemic option. Beyond these rare exceptions, which are now becoming more frequent thanks to the implementation of screening programmes, one could argue that there is always room for improvement.

However, I must caution that the converse is not necessarily true. There is a widespread assumption that the worse the prognosis, the more appropriate it is to use aggressive systemic chemotherapy, and yet we have already learned from the International Breast Cancer Study Group that

Recent Results in Cancer Research, Vol. 127

those cases with the worst prognosis, as judged by the over-expression of the C-*erbB2* oncogene, are the very subgroup who fail to respond to cytotoxic chemotherapy. At the same time it must be recognised that the world overview has described a fairly constant relative risk reduction across all prognostic subgroups using the conventional prognostic indicies of tumour size, nodal status and receptor status, so that in absolute terms, the greater the risk of relapse, the greater is the absolute benefit of the appropriate systemic therapy. What is meant therefore by *appropriate* systemic therapy? The plausible assumption that only those primary tumours that express the oestrogen receptor (ER) would respond to adjuvant tamoxifen has been refuted to my satisfaction. I am not arguing that ER-negative cases respond to the same extent (although I could do so if pressured) but wish merely to state that ER measurement alone does not define a subgroup of patients who are wholly unresponsive to adjuvant endocrine therapy. For example, the world overview described a relative risk reduction for relapse of 13% for ER-negative postmenopausal patients treated with adjuvant tamoxifen, and this included data from the confounded trials in which tamoxifen was added to cytotoxic chemotherapy. This benefit is of the same order as that achieved with six cycles of cyclophosphamide, methotrexate and fluorouracil (CMF) in the same subgroup of patients; this suggests that in choosing one treatment, tamoxifen because of its low toxicity would be more appropriate than a course of polychemotherapy.

What we still need, therefore, are prognostic indicies, probably better referred to as biological discriminants, that would allow a rational choice of systemic therapy for the individual patient. So far, I believe that no such test exists.

I would now like to illustrate some of the points in this introduction by referring to the four papers that were presented in this session.

Prognosis of Breast Cancer Patients: How To Use What?

G.M. Clarke and W.L. McGuire

Dr. Clarke began his presentation by drawing attention to the fact that 29% of node-negative patients are dead within 10 years despite their apparently good prognosis. This translates into 34 000 deaths per year in the United States. He then went on to describe a cost-benefit analysis for tamoxifen in an unselected group of node-negative patients, suggesting that over a 10-year period only 4000 patients would benefit, at a cost of $5000 a year.

I must take exception to this analysis, which assumes that only a small proportion of patients benefit substantially, whereas a similar difference in actuarial survival curves could also be interpreted as most patients benefitting a little.

He then described their studies on the expression of a mutant p53 tumour suppression gene. This appeared to corralate well with all other markers of proliferation apart from S phase fraction. It could be argued therefore that those node-negative patients with the over-expression of a mutated p53 have the worst prognosis and might benefit to the greastest extent by adjuvant systemic therapy. Once again, there was the assumption that the greater the risk of relapse, the better would be response to toxic therapy. I believe that this needs to be tested in prospective trials with patients stratified according to the presence or absence of the mutant p53.

DNA Flow Cytometry Measurements and Their Role in Node-Negative Breast Cancer Patients (L.G. Dressler)

Dr. Dressler introduced her paper by describing the evidence that the DNA content of a breast cancer represents the summation of all the genetic amplifications present; as such it would be a crude marker for predicting the behaviour of an individual breast cancer. In contrast, however, the S phase fraction calculated using flow cytometry measurements must be an expression of the "positive drive" of a breast cancer. She then described the data in a study following the prospective stratification of node-negative breast cancers into two groups, described as low or high S phase fraction. In a multi-variate analysis, tumour size and S phase were shown to be independent prognostic variables. In an inter-group study, node-negative patients were randomised between an observation-only arm and a group receiving chemotherapy with the CMF plus prednisone regimen. A significant improvement in relapse-free survival was observed for the whole group receiving CMF plus prednisone. On sub-dividing the patients into those with low S phase and high S phase tumours, both appeared to have achieved the same order of benefit with adjuvant systemic chemotherapy. S phase alone was not sufficient to identify qualitative interactions between improvements in relapse-free survival and the choice of chemotherapy. However, it could be argued that a much larger sample size would be needed to demonstrate a true qualitative interaction if one existed. Nevertheless, this is a valiant attempt to grapple with the needs of a predictive marker for response to adjuvant chemotherapy.

Review of Proliferative Value Variables and Their Predictive Value (R. Silvestrini)

Dr. Silvestrini pointed out that several biological indicators of clinical aggressiveness had been proposed, but that the results are inconsistent. She suggested that these disagreements could be ascribed to the lack of quality control of biological determinations and the heterogeneity of series in terms of tumour stage and type of treatment. In contrast, there is a remarkable programme of quality assurance in Italy for the use of the thymidine labelling index (TLI) as a marker of proliferation. In addition, her group studied

Ki67 as an antigen expressed by cells that are actively proliferating and showed that this is not independent as a prognostic variable when compared with the S phase fraction. The Milan group studied 985 node-negative cases and stratifed them according to high or low TLI. TLI appears to be independent of T size and N status. A study is now in progress in which patients are originally stratified according to low or high TLI. Those node-negative patients with low TLI are randomised between tamoxifen and a control group, whereas those with high TLI are randomised to CMF or a control group. Once again, an assumption has been made that patients of TLI with active proliferation are more likely to respond to chemotherapy whilst those whose tumour is less actively proliferating might better respond to adjuvant tamoxifen. I believe an opportunity has been missed here for stratifying the patients into the two TLI groups and then randomising them three ways, between tamoxifen, CMF and a control group. Using the approach described above, it will never be possible to demonstrate whether there is a true qualitative interaction between TLI and response to chemotherapy or endocrine therapy.

Critical Review of Growth Factors as Clinical Tools in Clinical and Metastatic Breast Cancer (J. Klijn et al.)

Dr. Klijn opened his discussion by describing how oncogenes and growth factors not only play an important role in the growth regulation of breast cancer cells but are also related to the prognosis of patients with primary or metastatic breast cancer. However, so far there has been no consensus on the prognostic value of these factors or their predictive value in selecting appropriate systemic therapy. Their group made a unique study of the expression of insulin-like growth factor receptor and found it ubiquitously expressed in all breast cancers and therefore of no prognostic significance. In contrast, the expression of epidermal growth factor receptor was found to be present in 48% of cancers, and its expression was associated with a poor prognosis and was inversely correlated with the expression of ER. Surprisingly, the epidermal growth factor receptor was not always related to gene amplification and was probably an example of post-transcriptional events. Amplification or over-expression of the *HER2/neu* oncogene was found in 20% of their large series and appeared only of moderate prognostic value amongst patients who were ER and progesterone receptor (PR) negative. In contrast, the c-*myc* amplification strongly indicated a poor prognosis in node-negative, node-positive and ER-, PR-positive patients. *HER2/neu* amplification in tumours appears to predict a poor response to endocrine therapy. They described a discriminant function making use of the various growth factors, together with ER and PR, which was able to define a group of patients with an excellent prognosis, in whom there was no room for improvement with adjuvant systemic therapy, and the remainder who were likely to benefit from the said treatments. However, once again, they are unable to describe or predict qualitative interactions among the growth factors, their receptors and specific treatment types.

In the general discussion that followed, most participants agreed that there are now sufficient prognostic indicators to select those rare patients who would not benefit from adjuvant systemic therapy, but that we were a long way from identifying biological variables that would usefully predict the magnitude of benefit from either a cytotoxic or a endocrine option.

Conclusion

I have one additional general concern about most of the work reported so far on prognostic variables and discriminant functions. Most groups use Cox's regression model to create prognostic indicies identifying two or three "independent prognostic variables" which account for the majority of the prognostic information within the data set. I understand that this is a mathematical expression, but I think that there is a dangerous assumption that it also tells something of biological importance. There must be truly independent biological variables which are related to genetic mutation amplifications or deletions on different arms of different chromosomes. In addition, there no doubt also exist time-dependent variables. I can understand how tumour size and perhaps the presence or absence of positive lymph nodes are time-dependent variables, and I can also accept that with time there may be a drift from a well-differentiated to a poorly differentiated malignant pheonotype. However, some of the interpretations of Cox's model produce nonsensical results in biological terms. For example, I could understand that the presence of a mutant p53 oncogene and the deletion of the retinoblastoma gene (Rb) could represent independent variables because they arise on different chromosomes; yet proliferation indicies or histological grade must be epiphenomena produced as the net effect of multiple somatic mutations. To believe, therefore, that Cox's model gives us any biological insight into the nature of breast cancer is clearly wrong.

My final concern relates to the statistical problems of demonstrating that any of these biological markers can accurately predict qualitative interactions between treatment and outcome for subsets of patients. For example, it would take 2000 patients randomised between two treatments to have sufficient statistical power to demonstrate that one treatment is, say, 10% better than another. If a variable were equally distributed, as either present or absent, amongst this group of patients, we would need 4000 patients to be able to show a qualitative interaction. However, most of the putative predictive indicies are asymmetrically distributed, with some of the more interesting ones only appearing in, say, 20% of cases. We would therefore need about 8000 patients to stand about a 90% chance of demonstrating true heterogeneity of outcome with the given treatment. I believe that so far none of the trials have had sufficient power, and that in the next decade we must devote outselves to addressing some of these fascinating biological questions, whilst at the same time gearing up our trial activity to recruit at two to three times the rate to which we have become accustomed in the previous decade.

III. Primary Therapy for Early Breast Cancer

Trials of Breast Conservation: A Critical Review of All Options

W.C. Wood

Department of Surgery, Emory University School of Medicine, Atlanta, GA, USA

Introduction

The role of breast conservation in the local management of primary breast cancer is in evolution today. The first major clinical question addressed was the adequacy of therapy that spared the breast as compared with total mastectomy. A series of trials in single institutions suggested relative equivalence of local and regional control with a combination of excisional tumor surgery, axillary dissection, and breast irradiation [1]. Many breast surgeons, who remain the primary health care providers making an initial diagnosis, continued to harbor anxiety about the systemic effects and ultimate survival of patients treated with differing local therapies.

These concerns led to marked differences in the degree to which breast conservation was used for primary therapy, at least as can be measured in the data available in the United States. Undoubtedly, local culture and conversations among regional physicians and surgeons also influenced the degree of acceptance of breast conservation therapy. As seen in Table 1, considerable differences existed among geographic regions in the United States in 1988 in the acceptance of breast conservation therapy [2]. This was prior to the National Institutes of Health Consensus Conference of 1990 [1] and its recommendations concerning the role of breast conservation treatment.

Six randomized, prospective trials have been performed to address this major question (Table 2) [1, 3]. These trials differ from one another in a variety of ways, including criteria for eligibility, the definition of excision margins, the definition of radiation to be delivered, and – in one instance – the method of randomization. These differences, particularly the difference in randomization that allows a possibility of skew among the different arms, pose a potential difficulty in interpretation of these trials. If the results of the trials differed significantly from one another, these differences in trial design would greatly complicate any attempt to draw general principles

Recent Results in Cancer Research, Vol. 127

Table 1. Breast cancer patients with breast conservation: 41 680 cases reported (from [2])

	Stage I	All
New England	53.1%	40.2%
Mid-Atlantic	35.2%	28.1%
South Atlantic	29.4%	21.0%
East north central	28.2%	23.8%
East south central	15.3%	11.5%
West north central	19.1%	13.6%
West south central	26.0%	20.9%
Mountain	30.5%	27.9%
Pacific	34.5%	29.8%
Total	31.9%	25.5%

Table 2. Randomized trials of breast conservation (see [1])

Institution	*n*	Stage	Margins	Follow-up (years)
Institut Nazionale Tumori, Milan	705	T1, N0	2–3 cm	10–17
Institut Gustave-Roussy	179	T1, N0–1	Micro clear	>10
National Surgical Adjuvant Breast Program (B-06)	1855	T1–2, N0–1	Micro clear	5–9
European Organization for Research and Treatment of Cancer (10801)	903	T1–2, N0–1	1 cm	4–10
Danish Breast Cancer Cooperative Group Trial	859	T1–3, N0–1	Grossly clear	1–7
National Cancer Institut	247	T1–2, N0–1	Grossly clear	1–11

from the trials that have already been performed. The relative uniformity of results achieved by these six trials performed in significantly different ways tends, instead, to reinforce the major lessons of these prospectively randomized trials.

What These Trials Answer

These trials have demonstrated first that the choice of breast conservation therapy or local control achieved with total mastectomy does not lead to significant differences in survival. The second conclusion that can be determined from these trials is that different levels of local control are not directly related to differences in subsequent survival. The third finding is that improved local control conserves breasts. Although this might be considered a truism, it has been overlooked in some discussions in the past.

What The Trials Have Not Answered

Individual institutional experiences compared with one another suggest that large increases in the thickness of surgical margins translate into small improvements in local control [1]. The balance of cosmesis improved by smaller margins and local control improved by larger margins has not been addressed in a prospective trial. The role of histologic type and grade of the primary tumor, the extent of intraductal component, and the size of the primary tumor in relation to the extent of surgical margin have not been addressed in any prospective manner. The balance of surgical margin and radiation dose or the use of boost radiation to the area immediately surrounding the tumor have not been addressed in a prospective fashion. The balance of the extent of surgery required after shrinkage of a primary tumor by neoadjuvant therapy has not been prospectively studied. Finally, the identity of subgroups of tumors not requiring radiation to achieve local control and, thus, ultimate breast preservation is still under active investigation. These all involve techniques of optimal local control and cosmesis.

The biological question not answered is: "Does inferior local control have any survival risk?" Local failure after the management of primary breast cancer has four possible sources, as listed in Table 3. Follow-up of patients who present with chest wall failure after mastectomy has demonstrated that in the majority this is the first manifestation of disseminated disease, and that only a small minority represent isolated disease in the chest wall. Patients undergoing breast conservation therapy also have the possibility of progression of residual breast carcinoma and, by definition, the possibility of a new primary arising in the preserved breast. A question of major biological interest is whether the progression of residual breast carcinoma presents additional risk to the woman who fails or simply serves as a marker of high risk on the basis of her tumor biology. A recent analysis of the data of the National Surgical Adjuvant Breast Program Trial B-06 has suggested that

Table 3. Causes of local failure in breast cancer

	TM	BCT
Manifestation of disseminated disease	X	X
Isolated disease in chest wall	X	X
Progression of residual breast cancer	0	X
New primary in preserved breast	0	X

TM, Total mastectomy; BCT, breast conservation therapy.

progression of residual breast carcinoma is a marker for poor prognosis but does not contribute to poor prognosis [4, 5]. Although the numbers of patients demonstrating ipsilateral breast tumor recurrence after breast conservation therapy are not sufficiently large to answer the biologic question of risk with absolute certainty, they are sufficient to address any clinical concern associated with this biologic question. There is no evidence that variation in the method of local therapy significantly impacts upon survival.

References

1. Dorr A (1992) NIH Consensus Development Conference on the management of early breast cancer. J Natl Cancer Inst Monogr 11
2. Osteen RT, Steel GD Jr, Menck HR, Winchester DP (1992) Regional differences in surgical management of breast cancer. CA 42:39–43
3. Sarrazin D, Le MG, Arrigada R et al. (1989) Ten-year results of a randomized trial comparing a conservative treatment to mastectomy in early breast cancer. Radiother Oncol 14:177–184
4. Gelman R, Gelber R, Henderson IC et al. (1990) Improved methodology for analyzing local and distant recurrence. J Clin Oncol 8:548–555
5. Fisher B, Anderson S, Fisher E et al. (1991) Significance of ipsilateral breast tumor recurrence after lumpectomy. Lancet 338:327–331

Selection and Technique for Lumpectomy

R.G. Margolese

McGill University, Department of Oncology, Jewish General Hospital, 3755 Cote Ste Catherine, Montreal, Quebec, Canada H3T 1E2

The performance of a proper lumpectomy requires balancing the features required for cancer control against those for best cosmesis. Certain caveats have been established by custom without evaluation of their true importance. These include the need for clear margins, concerns for any extensive component of duct carcinoma-in-situ (DCIS), and the size of the primary tumor. Surveys of present clinical practice indicate that lumpectomy has not replaced mastectomy as the common operation for breast cancer in most centers. This suggests an incorrect understanding of the relation of lumpectomy or mastectomy to distant treatment failures, and also of the importance of local tumor control as a factor in the selection of primary treatment.

Clinical Studies

The National Surgical Adjuvant Breast Project (NSABP) conducted two breast cancer surgical trials in the 1970s. The first compared Halsted radical mastectomy to simple mastectomy with or without radiation (Protocol B-04). The second study (Protocol B-06) compared total mastectomy and axillary dissection against lumpectomy with or without breast irradiation plus axillary dissection (Fig. 1). In both studies the primary end points compared outcomes for the various procedures but in addition, both studies were aimed at providing biologic information important for the understanding of breast cancer. Both studies compared an extensive surgical procedure against a lesser one, and both explored a third arm using radiotherapy in place of the extended surgical therapy.

In both cases there was a significant incidence of local or regional recurrence in the area not treated by surgery or radiation. Thus axillary node recurrence in B-04 patients who had no treatment of lymph nodes approached 20% [1]. Recurrence of tumor at the site of the lumpectomy in B-06 patients who did not receive radiation approaches 50% [2, 3]. How-

Recent Results in Cancer Research, Vol. 127

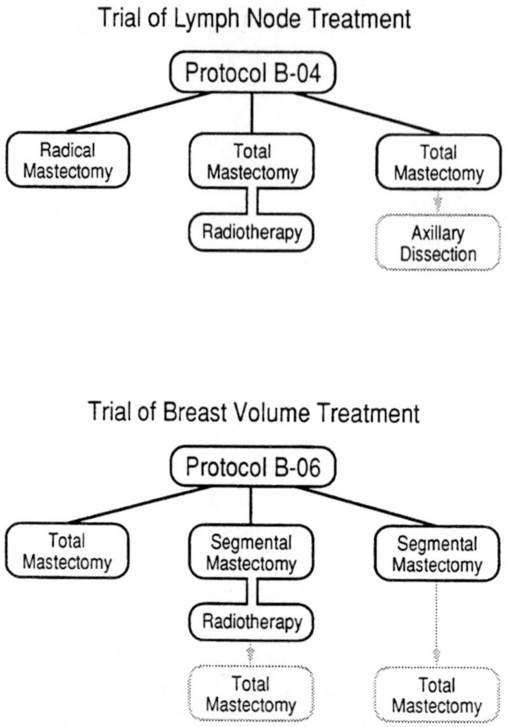

Fig. 1. *Top*, Protocol B-04. Comparison of radical mastectomy and total mastectomy with and without radiation therapy. *Bottom*, Segmental mastectomy protocol B-06. Comparison of total mastectomy and segmental mastectomy with or without radiation therapy

ever, in both studies the overall long-term rates of distant metastases and overall survival are the same in all treatment arms (Fig. 2). This means that less aggressive treatments permit local or regional recurrence but have no impact on factors allowing distant metastases to occur. These metastases must therefore occur before the primary diagnosis is made, since they are not influenced by local or regional treatment variations.

Local Recurrence

To better understand the biology of the problem, we must examine the nature of local recurrence following lumpectomy. Figure 3 shows two distinct representative patterns: Type I is a focal residual tumor, almost always at the same site as the original tumor. Type II is a diffuse process involving much or most of the breast, and perhaps the skin overlying the breast, and frequently extends off the breast onto the adjacent chest wall. The

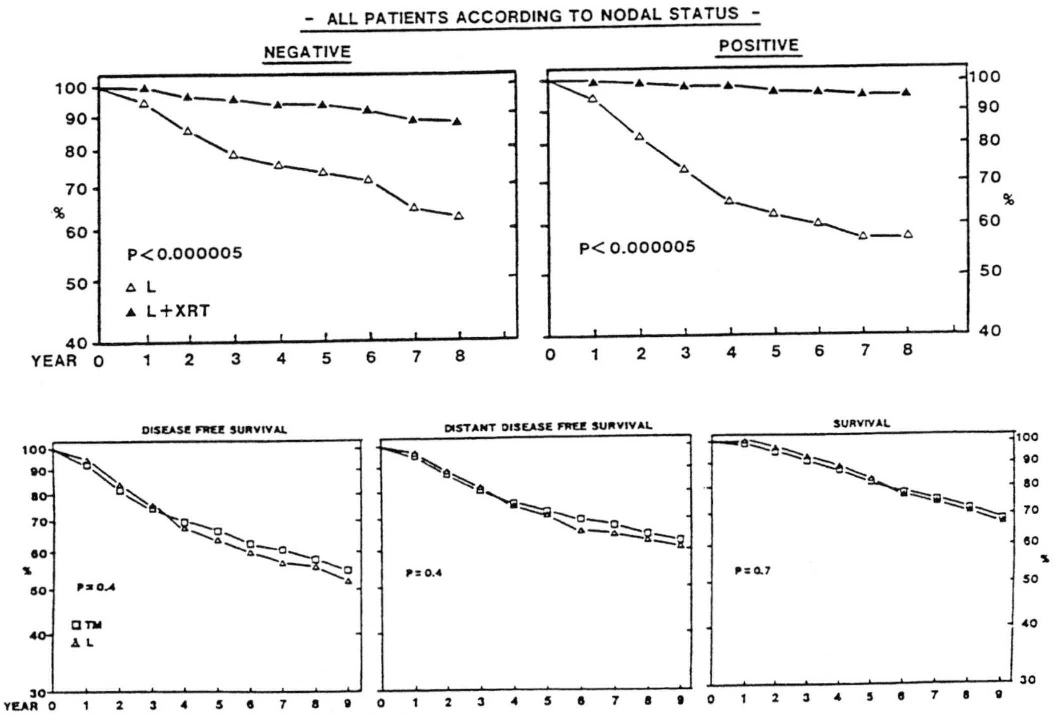

Fig. 2. Protocol B-06 results. *Top*, Local recurrence rates for negative-node (*left*) and positive-node (*right*; adjusted for number of nodes) patients. *White triangles* indicate patients who underwent lumpectomy; *black triangles* indicate patients who underwent lumopectomy and breast radiation. *Bottom*, Disease-free survival (*left*; adjusted for number of positive nodes), distant disease-free survival (*middle*), and survival (*right*) for total mastectomy patients (*squares*) compared with lumpectomy-only patients (*triangles*).

mechanisms of these two patterns are almost certainly quite different. Type I represents residual disease incompletely removed by initial lumpectomy and has a high salvage rate with secondary surgery [4]. Type II represents circulating cancer cells, and its local pattern is very similar to the type of "local recurrence" seen in the chest wall incision following the Halsted type of mastectomy.

In protocol B-06, local recurrence rates in nonirradiated patients approximate 50%, but with breast irradiation drop to less than 10% (Fig. 2). The most reasonable explanation for this difference is that minimal residual tumor at the margins is well controlled and eliminated by radiation therapy, but frequently grows to proportions of clinical manifestation in nonirradiated patients. The 10% not controlled by radiation therapy represent either those cases whose tumors are radioresistant or the cases of Type II recurrence

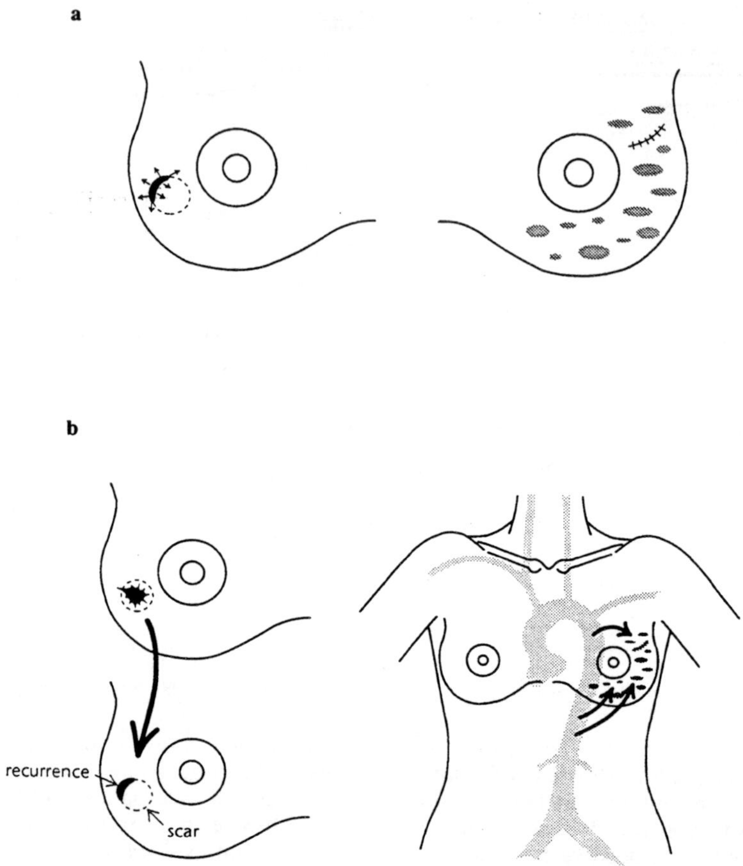

Fig. 3. a Patterns of local recurrence. *Left*, solitary mass usually near original surgery; *right*, diffuse intramammary spread with cutaneous and lymphatic involvement. **b** Mechanisms of local recurrence. *Left*, residual tumor; *right* hematogenous spread

which are associated with widespread metastases and do not reflect local phenomena.

A third type of recurrent carcinoma is represented by tumors in other quadrants of the breast which fit the definition of new primaries, but these are extremely uncommon.

Multicentricity

It has been repeatedly demonstrated over many decades that sampling of mastectomy specimens will reveal an incidence of multicentric carcinoma in

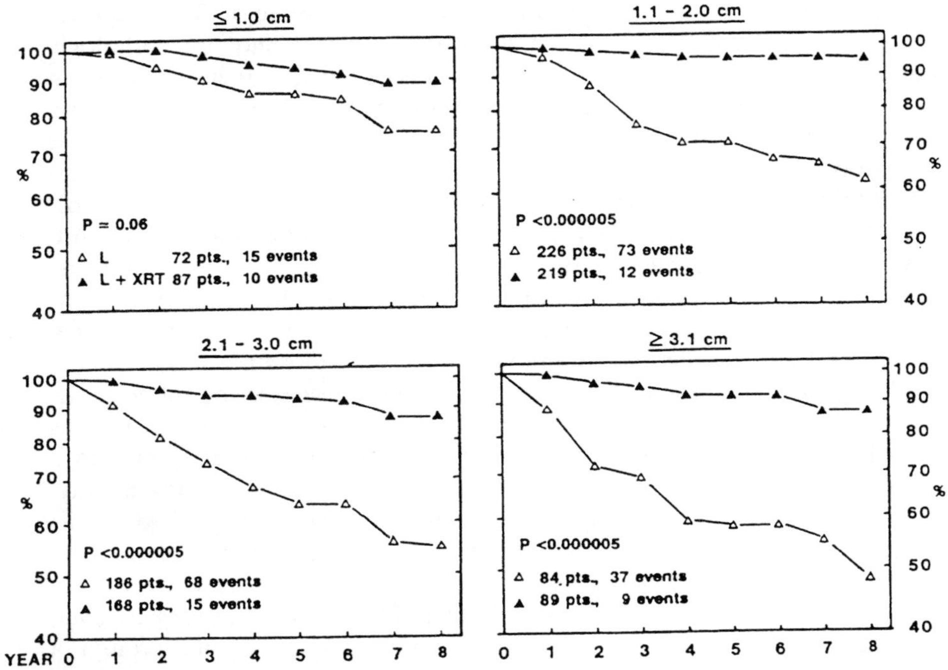

Fig. 4. NSABP Protocol B-06. Local recurrence rates according to tumor size. *White triangles* indicate lumpectomy only; *black triangles* indicate lumpectomy and breast radiation (*pts*, patients)

15%–45% of cases [5], the higher numbers being associated with more thorough practices of serial sectioning. Random biopsies of the contralateral breast reveal an incidence of 10%–25% [6, 7], which indicates that the process is bilateral and symmetrical. There is good evidence that most type I local recurrence stems from residual tumor or foci of DCIS adjacent to the original tumor within the same duct system. Multicentric neoplasia in other duct systems remote from the original primary are uncommonly associated with recurrent or future carcinoma. Holland [8], using mammographic/pathologic correlations of mastectomy specimens has shown that DCIS frequently extends several centimeters outside of the area grossly identified as tumor on the specimen. Evidence that these foci are related to local recurrence stems from the observation that local radiation therapy prevents most of these. Furthermore, the Milan Study of quadrantectomy, a more extensive surgical procedure, shows a very low rate of local recurrence, whereas patients in the study treated by lumpectomy show a 7% local recurrence rate [9]. In protocol B-06 the smallest tumors, those less than 1 cm, had a lower recurrence rate even if radiation therapy was not used, but larger tumors have higher rates (Fig. 4). We can conclude that positive margins occur frequently, since half of the patients with pathologically assessed negative margins recurred if not treated by radiation. Thus, despite the apparent control for margins that is achieved with modern pathologic practices of inking and inspecting the margins of the specimens, there is an element of residual neoplasia at the margins of many lumpectomy cases. We can speculate that radiation will probably control those patients in whom we see microscopically positive margins, just as it does in those where we do not identify the residual tumor (negative margin patients). A recent NSABP review of factors in local recurrence confirms the view that this feature may give rise to persisting or recurrent local disease, but that distant disease incidence and overall survival are not affected by either treatment option and that metastases are not facilitated through the pathway of local recurrence [10] (see Fig. 2). Therefore except for those uncommon tumors which extend visibly throughout the breast, lumpectomy is the initial treatment of choice. This conclusion is supported by statistical data as well as biologic understanding and is the position of the NIH Consensus Conference of 1990. Despite this, many surgeons continue to recommend mastectomy, often because of concerns about local recurrence. To take the logic to its extreme, many patients are advised to accept a mastectomy in order to prevent the need for a mastectomy in the future should local recurrence become a problem. Of course local control is still an important surgical goal, and the presence of extensive disease at the margins should prompt a surgical re-excision in order to improve the chances of permanent local control, but mastectomy is rarely indicated for most patients with primary breast cancer.

Influence of Adjuvant Therapy on Local Recurrence

In later NSABP protocols where adjuvant therapy was given routinely to lumpectomy and radiation therapy patients, the average annual ipsilateral breast recurrence rates are much lower than those reported in B-06. Although direct cross-protocol comparisons cannot be made because of different selection factors, it is clear that annual recurrence rates in patients receiving chemotherapy and/or tamoxifen are now in the range of 0.5%. The presence of tumor at the margins seen on histology is an anatomic event; the growth of residual tumor is a biological process. The results described the clinical trials discussed above confirm the biologic principles of the Fisher hypothesis, not the anatomic basis of the Halsted approach.

Techniques

The first objective of breast cancer surgery is control of the tumor. The second objective is to preserve the best cosmesis while keeping in mind the

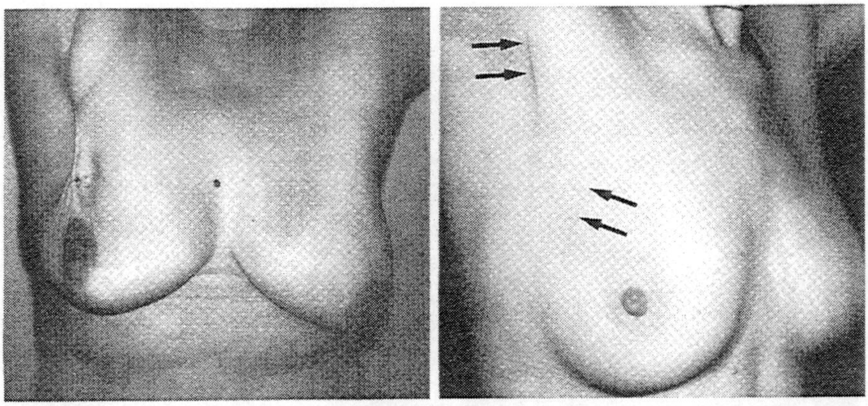

Fig. 5. **a** Patient with tumor in the upper outer quadrant of the right breast treated by segmental mastectomy and axillary dissection with one continuous incision. The result is contracture and deformity. **b** Patient with similar tumor treated by two separate incisions. No distortion or deformity

first objective. Although the first lumpectomies were done by surgeons who were uncertain of lumpectomy's place and who were not trained or experienced in the operation, this has now changed. Extensive operations which destroy the contours and symmetry should be avoided. They represent irreconcilable philosophies of aggressive and conservative surgery.

Incisions

Most tumors are in the upper outer quadrants, and many surgeons will instinctively extend a radial incision from the operative site into the axilla in order to accomplish the axillary dissection through the same incision. This incision crosses the natural elastic contour lines and because of its length will frequently produce contractions and distortion (Fig. 5a). It is preferable to do the lumpectomy through one incision and the axillary dissection through another (Fig. 5b). The en bloc concept is proven by these studies to be a false one and need not be considered.

Skin Removal

Removal of wide wedges of skin especially in the inferior part of the breast will produce significant cosmetic distortion. The distance from the areola to the inframammary fold is fairly constant, even with varying overall size of

a b

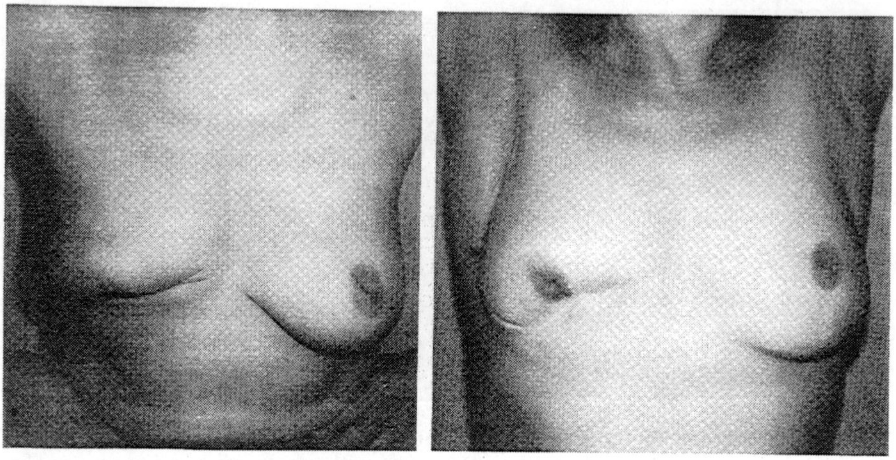

Fig. 6. Patient with extensive skin removal in lower half of breast causing loss of contour and extreme deformity

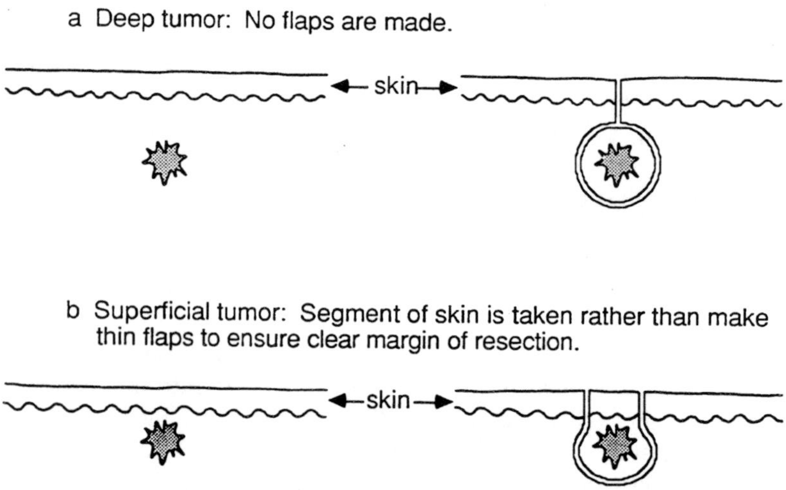

Fig. 7. Recommended treatment of skin for: **a** Deep-seated tumor. **b** Superficial tumor

the breast, and removal of too much skin and breast tissue can be very disfiguring (Fig. 6). It is best not to remove any skin at all, but in those situations where the tumor is very superficial, it is preferable to remove a wedge of skin overlying the tumor rather than undermine the flaps too thinly (Fig. 7). Thin flaps will lose their vascularity and will result in wider scar often with some collapse or saucerization.

Summary

The preoccupation with local recurrence in breast-conserving surgery represents the dominance of anatomic worries over biologic ones and is similar to the concerns that led our ancestors to devise the radical mastectomy which we now know to be an inappropriate solution to the cancer problem. Local recurrence in a conserved breast is not seen to be a cause of distant failure or death, but is often a reflection of metastases in those patients that have them. With the advent of adjuvant chemotherapy, even in node-negative cases, we have seen a conspicuous decline in local recurrence rates. The vast majority of patients with primary breast cancer can be safely and adequately treated by lumpectomy with radiation therapy and axillary dissection. Local recurrence rates are suppressed by the routine addition of adjuvant therapy. Careful attention to the principles of breast-conserving surgery will give the best cosmesis and the best rates of local control.

References

1. Fisher B, Redmond C, Fisher ER, Bauer M, Wolmark N, Wickerham L, Deutsch M, Montague E, Margolese R, Foster R (1985) Ten-year results of a randomized clinical trial comparing radical mastectomy and total mastectomy with or without radiation. N Engl J Med 312:11:674–681
2. Fisher B, Bauer M, Margolese R, Poísson R, Pilch Y, Redmond C, Fisher E, Wolmark N, Deutsch M, Montague E, Saffer E, Wickerham L, Lerner H, Glass A, Shibata H, Deckers P, Ketcham A, Oishi R, Russell I (1985) Five-year results of a randomized clinical trial comparing total mastectomy and segmental mastectomy with or without radiation in the treatment of breast cancer. N Engl J Med 312:11:665–673
3. Fisher B, Redmond C, Poisson R, Margolese R, Wolmark N, Wickerham L, Fishier E, Deutsch M, Caplan R, Pilch Y, Glass A, Shibata H, Lerner H, Terz J, Sidorovitch L (1989) Eight-year results of a randomized clinical trial comparing total mastectomy and lumpectomy with or without irradiation in the treatment of breast cancer. N Engl J Med 320:13:822–828
4. Kurtz JM, Amalric R, Brandone H, Ayme Y, Sjpitalier JM (1988) Results of wide excision for mammary recurrence after breast-conserving therapy. Cancer 61:1969–1972
5. Morgenstern L, Kaufman PA, Friedman NB (1975) The case against tylectomy for carcinoma of breast – factor of multicentricity. Am J Surg 130:251
6. Sandison AT (1975) Multicentric breast cancer: incidence of new cancers in homolateral breast after partial mastectomy. Cancer 35:475
7. Crile G (1975) Results of conservative treatment of breast cancer at 10 and 15 years. Ann Surg 181:26–30
8. Holland R, Solke H, Veling J et al. (1985) Histologic multifocality of T1, T_{1-2} breast carcinomas – implications for clinical trials of breast conserving surgery. Cancer: 979–990
9. Veronesi U, Volterrani F, Luini V, Saccozzi R, Del Vecchio M, Zucali R, Galimberti V, Rasponi A, Di Re E, Squicciarini P, Salvadori B (1990)

Quadrantectomy versus lumpectomy for small size breast cancer. Eur J Cancer 26:6:671–673

10. Fisher B, Anderson S, Fisher ER, Redmond C, Wickerham DL, Wolmark N, Mamounas EP, Deutsch M, Margolese RG (1991) Significance of ipsilateral breast tumour recurrence after lumpectomy. Lancet 338:8763:327–331

Salvage Treatment After Local Breast Cancer Relapse

F. Harder, R. Hünig, U. Laffer, N. Lüscher, R. de Roche, and J. Torhorst

University Hospital, Kantonsspital, 4031 Basel, Switzerland

Local recurrence after mastectomy as primary treatment of breast cancer has been associated with poor prognosis. In a Swiss study analyzing prospectively the outcome of 225 local recurrences after mastectomy, Brunner et al. [1] observed in 1988 a somewhat better prognosis than generally published, partly as a consequence of a strict search for distant metastases at the time of treatment of the recurrence and as an ineligibility criterion for this study. Under these conditions, disease-free survival was 47% at 5 years. The strongest factors in the multivariate analysis determining disease-free survival were the initial axillary lymph node status and the time elapsed between mastectomy and appearance of the local recurrence.

After conservative treatment of breast cancer, ipsilateral breast recurrence carries a distinctly better prognosis. An estimated 10% of patients have clinically apparent distant metastases or are technically inoperable [2, 7]. Published 5-year survival rates after treatment of local recurrence are between 50% and 80%. Locoregional control at 5 years is higher after salvage mastectomy (88%) than after further breast-conserving procedures (64%), according to Kurtz et al. [5]. The surgical principles and possibilities after salvage mastectomy for local recurrence are the same as for recurrence after mastectomy as primary treatment. One decisive difference between the two situations, however, is the fact that in one case the area to be reoperated has already been irradiated. Adjuvant radiation in addition to salvage mastectomy is therefore no longer possible. The conditions of the tissues are different. Systemic treatments are possible in both situations, however.

Our considerations are limited to surgical treatment of local failure after breast conservation, and two main questions are addressed: (a) the rate of ipsilateral breast recurrence in a relatively large series of one center and (b) the surgical solutions for salvage treatments.

Between January 1977 and December 1990, 832 breasts in 814 patients were treated by lumpectomy, axillary clearance, and radiotherapy following

Recent Results in Cancer Research, Vol. 127

a defined treatment protocol (not described here) that has been modified in details over time. Two thirds of the patients were operated at the two Basel University clinics of general surgery or of gynecology in equal numbers and one third in near-by hospitals. All had their radiotherapy at one single unit. Due to a low patient accrual of 20–40 patients per year between 1977 and 1984, the median time of follow-up was 3.9 years, but 97.5% complete. Overall ipsilateral breast recurrence as first tumor manifestation was 5.2% and regional failure 1.9%. Distant disease was seen in 9.4%.

The rate of recurrence depended, as expected, on nodal status. Limiting the analysis to the 163 patients of the first 7 years (1977–1983), the median follow-up was 8.8 years, the difference between patients with and those without nodal involvement was clearly evident: 9% in 100 node-negative patients (1% per year) and 27% in 63 node-positive patients (2.3% per year). This amounts to 15.5% in all 174 patients (1.7% per year). The local failure rate for all 832 breasts treated up to the end of 1990 (node-negative and -positive together) was 5.2% (median follow-up 3.9 years).

An important determinant of local outcome in the whole series was age [6]: 140 patients under the age of 40 years had a 11.4% incidence of breast recurrence and 85 patients aged between 65 and 75 years one of 1.7% (equal follow-up time). The 355 premenopausal patients had a higher recurrence rate (9.1%) than peri- (2.3%) and postmenopausal (3.5%) patients. Clear margins on frozen section were associated with less recurrence than involved margins (4.4% versus 10.6%; $p = 0.012$, X^2 test); when the margins were classified as doubtful by the pathologist, the rate was of 6.2%. Concerning histological grade of differentiation or type, none of the 66 tubular or 19 mucinous carcinomas had a recurrence. High-grade malignancies had a 6% and low-grade lesions a 3% recurrence rate, in situ lesions being excluded. The actuarial survival of patients free of local recurrence was of 90% and 80% at 5 and 10 years, and for patients developing local recurrence of 85% and 57% at 5 and 10 years. In our series, young age, resection margins, nodal status, and histology determined ipsilateral breast recurrence [3].

The second part of this presentation deals with the surgical treatment of local failure after initial breast conservation. While primary treatment has been clearly defined in our protocol, treatment options for local failure have not. The total number of 43 isolated ipsilateral recurrences in 832 treated breasts (or 47 local failures altogether) is too small to allow any analysis of subgroups.

Ten patients were offered wide local excisions, with variable success. Five were free of disease between 1.2 and 6.2 years after excision, two of whom needed a subsequent amputation for a second local failure. Three patients died after 0.9, 5.2, and 7 years. One is alive with local recurrence at 1.6 years and one with distant metastases at 1.0 year. Local excision offers a shorter local control [5]. Fowble [2] mentions age under 35 years, positive nodes, recurrences in a new quadrant, lobular carcinoma, vascular invasion, and extensive intraductal component as contraindications to wide local excision for local failure. Most importantly, excision must be accompanied by multiple frozen section analyses.

Generally, the diagnosis of local failure is followed by amputation of the breast. The condition of the tissues in this irradiated area needs very special attention. The skin is generally less expandable, wound healing can be disturbed, and ongoing tissue retraction is observed. This means that some reconstructive techniques applicable to mastectomy without radiation must be avoided as they put too much strain on the tissues. This does not imply that reconstruction cannot be immediate. However, it excludes some options. Submuscular implantation of tissue expanders or other implants carry a very high risk of necrosis and infection if used primarily after amptuation of the irradiated breast. The best choice is the transposition of healthy, well vascularized, unirradiated tissue into the created defect. Even then, an immediate implant in a submuscular position is not without risk. Flaps based on the rectus abdominis, such as the transverse rectus abdominis musculocutaneus (TRAM) [4], the vertical rectus abdominis musculocutaneous (VRAM), or the thoracoepigastric flap are the best choices. These may bring enough tissue into the defect to guarantee tension-free closure and often also an adequate contour. For symmetry, however, contralateral reduction mammoplasty is usually necessary. The main possibilities are the following.

1. The use of the omentum to cover wide problematic tissue defects is obsolete today; it can represent a last salvage procedure when other methods have failed. The omentum itself is covered with split-thickness skin grafts.

2. A safe and relatively simple musculocutaneous flap is the latissimus dorsi flap. Its volume is limited but often suffices to cover the defect. In the presence of expandable, relatively healthy skin in the irradiated area, even an expander prothesis may be implanted at a later time with intermittent overexpansion to allow for a definitive adequate shape. A correction of ptosis on the contralateral side to achieve symmetry is usually necessary.

3. Technically more demanding, but also more suitable for the coverage of large defects and for obtaining a satisfactory contour, rectus abdominis-based musculocutaneous flaps are the best choice. A large skin island with a sufficient subcutaneous fat pad based on one or eventually both rectus muscles and on their perforators is transposed to the defect created by amputation. In bilateral mastectomy, it can be performed bilaterally. However, this creates a very extensive wound surface and may be a rather burdening operation even for younger patients. The silhouette obtained by this technique can be remarkable, without any implant. The VRAM flap is safer than the TRAM flap, as it is based directly on the rectus abdominis muscle on its whole extension. Cosmetically it is inferior and smaller than the TRAM flap. A combination of the TRAM and VRAM flaps may be necessary to cover huge defects. Such a procedure may be rather risky, as flap necrosis may occur (7% in our series).

Today the most adequate means of covering even large areas of irradiated terrain after amputation for local recurrence in conservatively treated breast cancer is a musculocutaneous flap based on the rectus abdominis muscle. Other tissue transfers are reserved for salvage procedures. Surgery must be extensive and with clean margins, as additional radiotherapy is not possible. The role and mode of chemotherapy needs to be defined and probably has a place in inflammatory, rapidly evolving lesions. Wound healing is affected in some delicate flaps, and the necessary extension of amputation may be difficult to determine when multiple inflammatory lesions temporarily disappear to the naked eye under induction chemotherapy.

References

1. Brunner KW, Harder F, Greiner R, Frost M, Cavalli F, Senn HJ, Schatzmann E (1988) Das loko-regionale Rezidiv nach operiertem Mammakarzinom: prognostische Faktoren und therapeutische Konsequenzen. Schweiz Med Wochenschr 118:1976–1981
2. Fowble B, Solin LJ, Schultz DJ, Rubenstein J, Goodman RL (1990) Breast recurrence following conservative surgery and radiation: patterns of failure, prognosis and pathologic findings for mastectomy specimens with implications for treatment. Int J Radiat Oncol Biol Phys 19:833–842
3. Harder F, Laffer U, Lüscher N, Torhorst J, Almendral A, Herrmann R, Hünig R (1992) Vorgehen beim Rezidiv nach limitierter Chirurgie des Mammacarcinoms. Chirurg 63:483–490
4. Hartrampf CR, Scheflan M, Black PW (1982) Breast reconstruction with a transverse abdominal island flap. Plast Reconstr Surg 69:216
5. Kurtz JM, Amalric R, Brandone H, Ayme Y, Jacquemier J, Pietra J-C et al. (1989) Local recurrence after breast-conserving surgery and radiotherapy. Cancer 63:1912–1917
6. Kurtz JM, Jacquemier J, Amalric R, Brandone H, Ayme Y, Hans D, Bressac C, Roth J, Spitalier JM (1990) Why are local recurrences after breast conserving therapy more frequent in younger patients? J Clin Oncol 8:1–8
7. Recht A, Schnitt SJ, Connolly JL, Rose MA et al. (1989) Prognosis following local or regional recurrence after conservative surgey and radiotherapy for early stage breast carcinoma. Int J Radiat Oncol Biol Phys 16:3–9

Primary Chemotherapy for Resectable Breast Cancer

G. Bonadonna, U. Veronesi, C. Brambilla, L. Ferrari, P. Passoni, G.F. Coopmans de Yoldi, A. Luini, M. Greco, and P. Valagussa

Istituto Nazionale Tumori, Milan, Italy

Introduction

Primary (neoadjuvant, preoperative) chemotherapy for surgically curative breast cancer is a novel treatment approach. The sequentially combined strategy derives from prior experience achieved with locally advanced (stage III) disease in which primary chemotherapy including a regimen containing doxorubicin (Adriamycin) was delivered to achieve prompt tumor shrinkage and thus facilitate subsequent mastectomy and/or irradiation [1–4]. In recent years primary chemotherapy has been tested in resectable breast cancer with multifold clinical aims: (a) to increase the frequency of breast-saving procedures in tumors whose size would require mastectomy, (b) to decrease the frequency of local recurrence, and (c) to further improve relapse-free and total survival rates over those recently achieved with systemic adjuvant treatments [2, 5, 6] (the latter of these is reprinted in part in this volume). This paper summarizes and updates the clinical results of the prospective trial started in 1988 at the Milan Cancer Institute [7].

Patients and Treatments

The patient population was enrolled in this pilot study from January 1988 to October 1990; the main characteristics of women selected are shown in Table 1. Patients had a primary tumor that was at least 3 cm in largest diameter, as determined by palpation and mammography. The only criteria for exclusion was tumor fixation to underlying pectoral fascia and/or muscle, or direct tumor extention to chest wall or skin. Patients with central or retroareolar tumors and those presenting with more than one nodule at mammography were included in the study. Four patients were not evaluable; three refused to continue drug treatment after starting primary chemotherapy and preferred to have immediate mastectomy in spite of decreasing

Recent Results in Cancer Research, Vol. 127

Table 1. Main patient characteristics ($n = 227$)

Primary tumor size	
3.0–4.0 cm	50%
4.1–5.0 cm	32%
>5.0 cm	18%
Menopause status	
Premenopausal	65%
Postmenopausal	35%
Median age	49 years
Progression during primary chemotherapy	7 (3.0%)
Conservative surgery	201/220[a] (91.4%)
Mastectomy	19/220 (8.6%)
Median follow-up time from primary chemotherapy	30 months

[a] Subjected to surgery.

tumor size, and a fourth died of fulminant viral hepatitis in another hospital after three cycles of chemotherapy. Clinical staging followed morphological diagnosis, which was established in all patients by fine needle aspiration cytology. In addition, either Tru-cut biopsy (48 women) or small surgical incisional biopsy (173 women) was performed.

Five drug regimens were used, and all agents were administered by intravenous bolus injection [1, 5]. Seven consecutive groups of 33 patients each were treated as follows: (a) three or four courses of cyclophosphamide, methotrexate, and fluorouracil (CMF), (b) three or four courses of fluorouracil, doxorubicin (Adriamycin), and cyclophosphamide (FAC), (c) three courses of fluorouracil, epirubicin and cyclophosphamide (FEC), (d) three courses of fluorouracil, mitoxantrone (Novantrone), and cyclophosphamide (FNC), and (e) three courses of doxorubicin alone at the dose of 75 mg/m^2 every 3 weeks.

Surgery was performed within 3 weeks from the last dose of chemotherapy. The surgical technique was that of quadrantectomy [7] except in patients whose tumors did not regress sufficiently for this. The incision was related mainly to postchemotherapy dimensions, with specimen margins grossly free of tumors. The specimen was then cut and measured by a ruler, and when the size of residual tumor was less than 3 cm in largest diameter, the operation was completed with full axillary dissection. Modified radical mastectomy was performed when a single or bifocal tumor measuring 3 cm or more in diameter was present at surgery. Postoperative radiotherapy was delivered to all patients subjected to breast-conserving surgery.

Further (adjuvant) chemotherapy was administered to patients with node-positive tumors and to those with node-negative and receptor-negative tumors. The number of adjuvant cycles was two or three.

Table 2. Operable breast cancer candidates for mastectomy: clinical versus surgical diameters following three or four cycles of primary chemotherapy

Initial tumor size	Patients subjected to surgery	Tumor size at surgery			Conservative surgery
		<3 cm	0	pCR	
3.0–4.0 cm	110	93%	11	5	97%
4.1–5.0 cm	73	79%	10	3	92%
>5.0 cm	37	62%	5	0	73%

pCR, Pathological complete remission.

Table 3. Pathological axillary node involvement following primary chemotherapy

	n	%
Negative	87/220	40
Positive	133	60
1–3	78/133	59
4–10	33	25
>10	22	16

Results

Objective clinical response by palpation was as follows: progressive disease 3%, objective improvement 15%, partial response 57%, complete remission 21%. There was no difference in the response rate among the five regimens utilized nor between three and four treatment cycles of either CMF or FAC. Thus, in this study, only a full dose of doxorubicin yielded a response rate (79%) equivalent to any of the triple-drug combinations tested. Dose intensity for the regimens ranged from 0.88 to 0.99.

The surgical findings are summarized in Table 2. As can be seen, tumor shrinkage to less than 3 cm (the main initial objective of this study) was inversely related to the initial tumor diameter. Histological complete remission occurred in 4% of the 201 patients subjected to quadrantectomy. It should be mentioned that breast-conserving surgery was carried out in 15 patients in whom the residual tumor burden was greater than 3 cm. Although this was a deviation from protocol, the surgeon felt that a conservative procedure was feasible and justified because of a large breast size. Thus, in the present series, conservative surgery was performed in a total of 201 of 220 patients (91%). Table 3 reports the pathological involvement of axillary lymph nodes following primary chemotherapy.

Toxicity from primary chemotherapy was modest and reversible [7]. The lowest frequency of vomiting (13%) and hair loss (6%) was produced by

Table 4. Treatment outcome following primary chemotherapy (PC)

	%	SE
Freedom from progression at 30 months from PC (*n* = 227)	69	3
Total survival at 30 months from PC (*n* = 227)	93	2
Relapse-free survival at 24 months from surgery (*n* = 220)	73	3
Causes of death (*n* = 227)		
Disease progression	7.5	
Second cancer (gastric)	0.4	
Thromboembolism (lung)	0.4	
Local recurrence	2	

the FNC regimen followed by CMF regimen (17% and 11%, respectively). The highest incidence of transient grade 3 leukopenia (27%) was associated with the administration of mitoxantrone.

Table 4 shows some preliminary data on treatment outcome. Although the 2-year results are premature, we can also add that tumor size and nodal extent remain prognostically important. Local recurrence is 2%.

Conclusions

Our experience indicates that the delivery of several drug regimens as primary chemotherapy can down-stage a large but resectable breast cancer to less than 3 cm in most patients (initial tumor size 3–5 cm, 91%; greater than 5 cm, 73%). Three cycles of full-dose primary chemotherapy can safely induce prompt tumor shrinkage and allow substitution of conservative for mutilating surgery, thus improving the patients' quality of life. It is important to stress that the response rate was unrelated to age, menopause, tumor cell proliferative activity, or type of drug regimen.

These findings, as well as those of other investigators [8–11], add to our experience and emphasize the important role of medicine also in the primary management of mammary carcinoma.

References

1. Bonadonna G (1989) Conceptual and practical advances in the management of breast cancer. Karnofsky Memorial Lecture. J Clin Oncol 7:1380–1397
2. Bonadonna G (1992) Evolving concepts in the systemic adjuvant treatment of breast cancer. Cancer Res 52:2127–2137

3. Valagussa P, Zambetti M, Bonadonna G et al. (1990) Prognostic factors in locally advanced noninflammatory breast cancer. Long-term results following primary chemotherapy. Breast Cancer Res Treat 15:137–147
4. Hortobagyi GN (1990) Comprehensive management of locally advanced breast cancer. Cancer 66:1387–1391
5. Bonadonna G, Valagussa P, Brambilla C et al. (1991) Adjuvant and neoadjuvant treatment of breast cancer with chemotherapy and/or endocrine therapy. Semin Oncol 18:515–524
6. Early Breast Cancer Trialists' Collaborative Group (1992) Systemic treatment of early breast cancer by hormonal, cytotoxic or immune therapy: 133 randomised trials involving 31 000 recurrences and 24 000 deaths among 75 000 women. Lancet 339:1–15, 71–85
7. Bonadonna G, Veronesi U, Brambilla C et al. (1990) Primary chemotherapy to avoid mastectomy in tumors with diameters of three centimeters or more. J Natl Cancer Inst 82:1539–1545
8. Forrest APM, Levack PA, Chetty U et al. (1986) A human tumour model. Lancet 2:840–842
9. Mansi JL, Smith IE, Walsh G et al. (1989) Primary medical therapy for operable breast cancer. Eur J Cancer Clin Oncol 25:1623–1627
10. Jacquillat C, Weil M, Baillet F et al. (1990) Results of neoadjuvant chemotherapy and radiation therapy in the breast-conserving treatment of 250 patients with all stages of infiltrative breast cancer. Cancer 66:119–129
11. Banzet P, Holland JF, Khayat D, Weil M (eds) (1991) Neoadjuvant chemotherapy. Springer, Berlin Heidelberg New York

IV. Radiation Therapy as Part of Primary Treatment

Radiation Therapies for Breast Cancer: Current Knowledge on Advantages and Disadvantages

L.E. Rutqvist

Oncologic Centre, Karolinska Hospital, 104 01 Stockholm, Sweden

Introduction

In the middle of the 1970s both American and European research groups reported significant benefits with adjuvant chemotherapy in terms of the recurrence-free survival of patients with early-stage breast cancer. Since then there has been a continued emphasis on the use of adjuvant systemic therapy in the primary management of breast cancer. The fact that many radiation therapy studies have failed to show an overall survival benefit has often been used as an argument against radiation therapy. However, local control of the disease through the use of adjuvant radiation should not be underrated because locoregional recurrences decrease the patient's quality of life and shorten disease-free survival. Recent information also suggests that failure to control the disease locally may compromise overall survival. An unbiased assessment of the role of adjuvant radiation in the primary management of breast cancer should acknowledge the fact that many of the radiation trials reported in the literature used out-dated orthovoltage treatment techniques that are not relevant to current medical practice.

Prevention of Locoregional Recurrence with Radiation Therapy

Postmastectomy Radiation Therapy. Several randomized trials have established that postmastectomy radiation prevents locoregional recurrences [1–4]. This effects contributes to the sustained improvement of recurrence-free survival observed with radiation therapy. Trials directly comparing adjuvant chemotherapy or adjuvant tamoxifen with radiation therapy have consistently demonstrated that radiation is the currently most effective treatment modality to control the disease locally [5, 6].

Radiation Therapy Following Breast-Conserving Surgery. At present there are only two unconfounded randomized studies evaluating the role of radia-

Recent Results in Cancer Research, Vol. 127

Table 1. Breast recurrence rates by allocated treatment in two unconfounded randomized trials of radiation therapy (RT) after breast-conserving surgery: the NSABP B-06 [7] and the Uppsala-Örebro trial [8]

Trial, tumor stage	Breast recurrence rate		*p*
	Surgery alone	Surgery + RT	
NSABP B-06[a]			
Node-negative	37%	12%	<0.001
Node-positive[b]	43%	6%	<0.001
Uppsala-Örebro[c]	8%	3%	0.06

[a] Eight-year results; all patients were required to have tumors not larger than 4 cm.
[b] All patients had chemotherapy.
[c] Three-year results; and patients were required to have node-negative tumors not larger than 2 cm.

tion therapy to the breast after breast conserving surgery: the National Surgery Adjuvant Breast Program (NSABP B-06) trial [7] and the Swedish Uppsala-Örebro trial [8]. Both studies showed that radiation decreased the number of breast recurrences (Table 1). The incidence of such recurrences in the control group appeared to be different in the two studies: 37% of node-negative cases in NSABP B-06 and 8% in the Swedish trial (which only included stage I cases). It is possible that more extensive surgery, the exclusion of patients with tumors larger than 2 cm, a higher percentage of mammography screening cases, and the short median follow-up in the Swedish trial may help to explain this difference. However, the authors of that study suggested that radiation therapy after breast-conserving surgery possibly need not be given to patients with a very low risk of breast recurrence, particularly since such recurrences have not been shown to compromise overall survival. It seems reasonable to interpret the results of the Swedish trial cautiously until longer follow-up is available, and breast-conserving surgery without postoperative radiation therapy remains experimental in most institutions. It is possible that an improved understanding of factors predicting the risk of breast recurrences in the future will permit identification of subgroups of patients who have such a low risk that the potential benefit with radiation therapy may not be considered clinically worthwhile. However, at present there is no consensus on how to define such subgroups.

Radiation Therapy Combined with Systemic Treatment

The 5- and 10-year results of the Oxford overview of adjuvant cytotoxic and tamoxifen trials showed significant survival benefits with both types of treatment [9] (reprinted in part in this volume). Adjuvant systemic treatment is therefore generally considered standard therapy in selected subgroups of patients. The role of postoperative radiation therapy should thus be considered in such a setting.

Two large Scandinavian trials have evaluated the role of radiation therapy in postmenopausal, high-risk patients treated with adjuvant tamoxifen: the South Swedish Trial and the Danish Breast Cancer Cooperative Group (DBCG-82c) trial [4, 6]. Both studies showed significant decreases in locoregional recurrences among those who received both radiation and tamoxifen compared to those treated with tamoxifen alone. The Danish DBCG-82b trial – which included nearly 1500 patients – evaluated the addition of radiation therapy to adjuvant chemotherapy in pre- or perimenopausal, high-risk patients. Patients treated with chemotherapy (cyclophosphamide, methotrexate, fluorouracil) plus radiation therapy had significantly fewer locoregional recurrences as well as a significant improvement in both recurrence-free and overall survival.

The results of these Scandinavian studies illustrate that in patients with high-risk tumors there is a significant benefit in terms of local control of the disease with the addition of radiation therapy to adjuvant cytotoxic treatment or adjuvant tamoxifen. The question of whether there is also a survival benefit with radiation – as suggested by the DBCG-82b trial – is addressed below in the context of the overviews of radiation therapy trials.

Is Deferred Treatment Equally Effective?

It has been suggested that postmastectomy radiation therapy should be deferred until a locoregional relapse is diagnosed so that patients who do not develop such a recurrence are spared the inconvenience and potential hazards of radiation therapy. However, such a treatment policy is based on the assumption that the eventual local control rate – that is, after salvage treatment – is the same as that of a policy of giving adjuvant radiation treatment. This hypothesis was studied in the first Stockholm trial [10]. Among those patients who developed a locoregional recurrence the response to salvage treatment was evaluated using UICC/WHO criteria. Treatment after recurrence was decided individually by the responsible clinician. This implied that the patients received a wide variety of treatments, including different types of surgery and radiation therapy as well as various endocrine agents and cytotoxic chemotherapy.

There was no significant difference in the distribution of best response to salvage treatment between the two radiation therapy groups compared to the surgery alone group (Table 2). About 70% in the radiation therapy groups achieved an objective response (complete or partial remission) or disease stabilization, compared to 78% in the surgery alone group. Similarly, there was no significant difference in the proportion who developed progressive disease after an initial response to treatment. The total proportion

Table 2. Long-term local tumor control according to allocated adjuvant treatment among patients with a locoregional recurrence in the Stockholm trial of pre- or postoperative radiation therapy (RT) [10]

	Pre- and postoperative RT (n = 639)		Surgery alone (n = 321)	
	n	%	n	%
No. of patients with a locoregional recurrence	64	10	105	33
Best response to salvage treatment[a]				
Complete remission	32/63	51	67/101	66
Partial remission or disease stabilization	12/63	19	12/101	12
Progressive disease	19/63	31	22/101	22
No. with progressive disease after an initial objective response or disease stabilization	16/44	36	36/79	46
No. with uncontrolled local disease at death or at last follow-up[b]	39/639	6	50/314	16[c]

[a] One irradiated and four surgery alone patients were unevaluable.
[b] Seven surgery alone patients were unevaluable.
[c] Irradiated versus surgery alone patients: $p < 0.01$.

of patients who eventually showed progressive disease was high in both the irradiated group and the surgery alone group: 66% compared to 68%. The long-term outcome of salvage treatment was thus poor irrespective of the initially allocated adjuvant therapy. However, since the total number of locoregional failures was greater in the surgery alone group, the overall proportion of patients with uncontrolled locoregional disease present at death or at last follow-up was significantly greater in that group compared to the irradiated groups (16% versus 6%; $p < 0.01$).

These results indicate that a policy of deferred treatment only for those who actually develop a locoregional recurrence eventually results in a higher incidence of patients with uncontrolled local disease compared to a policy of prevention of locoregional recurrences by the use of adjuvant radiation therapy.

Overall Survival Benefit with Radiation Therapy

In 1987 Cuzick et al. published two overviews ("meta-analyses"), including selected radiation therapy studies [11, 12]. No overall survival benefit with radiation was observed during the first 10 years of follow-up. The radiation therapy used in the trials was even suggested to have had an adverse effect on survival in subgroups of patients after 10 years. These results were interpreted to support the view that adjuvant radiation therapy is unable to prevent distant dissemination, and that a survival benefit only can be achieved with systemic treatment. However, the overviews have been criticized because they included several trials with inadequate treatment techniques, for example, orthovoltage radiation [13]. This circumstance may have obscured a clinically worthwhile benefit with radiation in the more recent trials using modern, megavoltage techniques. The overviews also included several studies with methodological flaws, such as biased methods of treatment allocation.

These circumstances were the main reason for a joint analysis of two of the trials included in the overviews: the Stockholm and Oslo-II trial. These studies differed from the other trials in the overviews in several important respects: they both used modern, megavoltage radiation techniques, the treatment included the regional nodal areas, the tumor dose was appropriate (45–50 Gy/4–5 weeks), and the design of trials permitted an unconfounded, unbiased evaluation of the effect of treatment by histological nodal status.

The results showed a significant benefit with radiation for all patients in terms of distant metastasis-free survival ($p < 0.01$) [14]. The relative risk (RR) of distant metastasis for irradiated versus control patients was 0.75 (95% confidence interval: 0.61–0.92). However, there was no significant overall survival benefit with radiation: the RR of death for the irradiated patients was 0.92 (0.77–1.10). There was a significant interaction between treatment and nodal status ($p < 0.05$); the irradiated node-positive patients had an RR of distant metastasis of 0.63 (0.48–0.83; $p < 0.001$) versus 0.97 (0.70–1.33; n.s.) for the irradiated node-negative patients. There was also an overall survival difference in favor of the irradiated patients in the node-positive subgroup ($p = 0.06$) with an RR of death of 0.78 (0.61–1.00). This corresponds to a 22% relative reduction of deaths. In contrast, there was no survival benefit with radiation among the node-negatives; the RR of death was 1.10 (0.85–1.43).

One aim of overviews is to obtain a more stable estimate of the effect of a certain therapy by increasing the number of patients available for analysis. An overview may also aim at avoiding selection bias by including all available trials of a particular treatment modality. In practice this implies that the included trials are dissimilar, for instance, in regard to the performance of the therapy used. Because of this, a "negative" overview result does not imply that the tested treatment modality invariably is ineffective. For instance, the mentioned overviews of radiation therapy trials included large, older trials using orthovoltage X-rays. This may have obscured a clinically worthwhile benefit in the more recent radiation therapy trials using adequate, megavoltage treatment techniques. The results of the joint analysis of the Stockholm and Oslo-II trial suggests such an interpretation. In fact, an updated overview of all available unbiased, unconfounded radiation therapy trials is currently underway which will include an in-depth analysis of the significance of treatment technique.

Side Effects of Radiation Therapy

Cardiovascular Side Effects. One concern with radiation therapy is that it may be associated with cardiovascular side effects. Analyses of cause-specific mortality in individual radiation trials [2, 15] and one population-based cohort study [16] have shown an increase in mortality due to ischemic heart disease associated with radiation, but the effect in quantitative terms, dose-effect relationships, and the significance of treatment technique were not evaluated in these studies.

To assess the potential cardiovascular effects of the radiation therapy used in the first Stockholm trial, radiation dose-volumes in the myocardium were estimated for each of the techniques used in the study since it seemed reasonable to assume that any adverse cardiac effect of radiation should be correlated with both the dose and the irradiated cardiac volume [17]. The randomization in the trial was between pre- or postoperative radiation therapy or surgery alone. The internal mammary nodes, chest wall and breast in the preoperative cases were generally treated with tangential cobalt-60 beams. The chest wall among the postoperative cases was treated with electrons. The consistently highest radiation dose and the largest irradiated volume was obtained with left-sided tangential cobalt-60 fields. The consistently smallest dose-volume was obtained with right-sided tangential cobalt-60 fields. Irrespective of the laterality of the tumor, the electron techniques resulted in intermediate dose-volumes.

An analysis of cause-specific mortality by estimated radiation dose-volume showed that there was no significant trend with increasing dose-volume in mortality due to breast cancer, other types of cancer, cardiovascular diseases other than ischemic heart disease, miscellaneous causes, or all causes [17]. However, mortality due to ischemic heart disease was significantly higher in the highest dose-volume group (that is, patients with left-sided tumors treated with tangential cobalt-60 fields) compared to the surgical controls ($p < 0.01$). The difference between the groups emerged after 4–5 years and appeared to increase with longer follow-up. In the intermediate and low dose-volume group the mortality due to ischemic heart disease was similar to that among the surgical controls.

The study thus indicated that an increased cardiovascular mortality related to radiation therapy probably can be avoided by the use of appropriate treatment techniques and avoidance of excessive treatment.

Second Cancers. Radiation is potentially carcinogenic. An increased number of second malignancies may therefore theoretically offset the benefit with adjuvant radiation therapy. In the Cancer Research Campaign trial

Table 3. Total number of new primary malignancies in the first Stockholm trial of pre- and postoperative radiation therapy (RT) versus surgery alone [1]

Allocated treatment	Observed no. of cancers	Expected no. of cancers	Rate per 1000 WYR[a]	Relative risk[b] (95% C.I.)
Preoperative RT	48	30.9	13.0	1.03 (0.68–1.54)
Postoperative RT	35	31.4	9.3	0.73 (0.47–1.14)
Surgery alone	45	29.7	12.7	1.00

The follow-up ranged from 13 to 19 years, with a mean of 16 years. The data on second cancers were obtained from the Swedish Cancer Registry. The expected number of tumors was calculated for an age-matched general population.
[a] WYR, woman-years at risk.
[b] Relative to the surgery alone group.

Table 4. Analysis of second, contralateral breast cancers in the Stockholm trial of pre- and postoperative radiation therapy versus surgery alone [1]

Allocated treatment	Observed no. of cancers	Expected no. of cancers	Rate per 1000 WYR	Relative risk[a] (95% C.I.)
Preoperative RT	24	7.7	6.5	1.16 (0.64–2.09)
Postoperative RT	20	7.8	5.3	0.94 (0.51–1.75)
Surgery alone	20	7.3	5.6	1.00

[a] Relative to the surgery alone group.

there was, in fact, an increased number of deaths due to second malignancies among the irradiated patients [15]. However, this increase concerned mainly abdominal malignancies, that is, tumors outside the radiation fields. This observation makes it likely that the increase was related to distant metastases from breast cancer that were incorrectly diagnosed as new primary malignancies. In the Stockholm trial of adjuvant radiation there was no increase in second primary cancer associated with radiation during a follow-up of 13–19 years (Table 3). In particular, there was no increase in second, contralateral breast cancer (Table 4). The absence of an increased frequency of second malignancies with radiation therapy may be related to the fact that cell death predominates over sublethal injury at the radiation doses commonly used in therapeutic radiology.

Other Side Effects. Radiation therapy that includes the regional nodes may cause arm edema, decreased shoulder mobility, radiation pneumonitis, and brachial plexus neuropathy [18–20]. Radiation therapy to the breast after breast-conserving surgery may compromise the cosmetic results through breast edema, fibrosis, and nipple retraction [21]. These effects are related to the biological dose and appear to be enhanced by the concomitant use of chemotherapy, particularly if the chemotherapy is given concurrently with the radiation. Single doses in excess of 2 Gy should probably also be avoided since large single fractions have been shown to increase late side effects.

Summary

Radiation therapy continues to be the most effective adjunct to surgery to achieve long-term local control of breast cancer. In this respect it is more effective than both adjuvant cytotoxic therapy and adjuvant tamoxifen. Radiation therapy therefore plays an important role in the primary management of selected groups of breast cancer patients. However, radiation therapy may be related to potentially serious side effects, including ischemic heart disease and pneumonitis. After breast-conserving surgery radiation therapy may also compromise the cosmetic outcome. An appropriate treatment technique and avoidance of excessive treatment is essential to decrease the risk of adverse side effects. Concomitant administration of chemotherapy should probably be avoided, as well as treatment schedules with single fractions in excess of 2 Gy.

References

1. Retqvist LE, Cedermark B, Glas U et al. (1989) Radiotherapy, chemotherapy and tamoxifen as adjuncts to surgery in early breast cancer: a summary of three randomized trials. Int J Radiat Oncol Biol Phys 16:629–639
2. Höst H, Brennhovd I, Loeb M (1986) Postoperative radiotherapy in breast cancer – long-term results from the Oslo study. Int J Radiat Oncol Biol Phys 12:727–732
3. Griem KL, Henderson IC, Gelman R, Ascoli D, Silver B, Recht A, Goodman R, Hellman S, Harris JR (1987) The five-year results of a randomized trial of adjuvant irradiation therapy after chemotherapy in breast cancer patients treated with mastectomy. J Clin Oncol 5:1546–1555
4. Overgaard M, Juul Christensen J, Johansen H et al. (1990) Evaluation of radiotherapy in high-risk breast cancer patients: report from the Danish Breast Cancer Cooperative Group (DBCG 82) Trial. Int J Radiat Oncol Biol Phys 19:1121–1124
5. Rutqvist LE, Cedermark B, Glas U et al. (1990) Randomized trial of adjuvant tamoxifen combined with postoperative radiation therapy or adjuvant chemotherapy in postmewnopausal breast cancer. Cancer 66:89–96
6. Rydén S, Fernö M, Möller T et al. (1992) Long-term effects of adjuvant tamoxifen and/or radiotherapy. The South Sweden Trial. Acta Oncol (in press)
7. Fisher B, Redmond C, Poisson R, Margolese R, Wolmark N, Wickerham L, Fisher E, Deutsch M, Caplan R, Pilch Y, Glass A, Shibata H, Lerner H, Terz J,

Sidorovich L (1989) Eight-year results of a randomized clinical trial comparing total mastectomy and lumpectomy with or without irradiation in the treatment of breast cancer. N Engl J Med 320:822–828

8. Uppsala-Örebro Breast Cancer Study Group (1990) Sector resection with or without postoperative radiotherapy for stage I breast cancer: a randomized trial. J Natl Cancer Inst 82:277–282
9. Early Breast Cancer Trialists' Collaborative Group (1992) Systemic treatment of early breast cancer by hormonal, cytotoxic, or immune therapy, 133 randomised trials involving 31 000 recurrences and 24 000 deaths among 75 000 women. Lancet 339:1–15, 71–85
10. Rutqvist LE, Pettersson D, Johansson H (1992) Adjuvant radiation therapy versus surgery alone in operable breast cancer: long-term follow-up of a randomized trial. Radiother Oncol (submitted)
11. Cuzick J, Stewart H, Peto R, Baum M, Fisher B, Höst H, Lythgoe JP, Ribeiro G, Scheurlen H, Wallgren A (1987) Over-view of randomised trials of post-operative adjuvant radiotherapy in breast cancer. Cancer Treat Rep 71:15–29
12. Cuzick J, Stewart H, Peto R, Fisher B, Kaae S, Johansen H, Lythgoe JP, Prescott RJ (1987) Over-view of randomised trials comparing radical mastectomy against simple mastectomy with radiotherapy in breast cancer. Cancer Treat Rep 71:7–14
13. Levitt S (1988) Is there a role for post-operative adjuvant radiation in breast cancer? Beautiful hypothesis versus ugly facts: 1987 Gilbert H. Fletcher Lecture. Int J Radiat Oncol Biol Phys 14:787–796
14. Auquier A, Rutqvist LE, Höst H, Arriagada R, Rotstein S (1992) Postmastectomy megavoltage radiation: the Oslo and Stockholm trials. Eur J Cancer (in press)
15. Haybittle JL, Brinkley D, Houghton J, A'Hern RP, Baum M (1989) Postoperative radiotherapy and late mortality: evidence from the Cancer Research Campaign trial for early breast cancer. Mr Med J 298:1611–1614
16. Rutqvist LE, Johansson H (1990) Mortality by laterality of the primary tumour among 55 000 breast cancer patients from the Swedish Cancer Registry. Br J Cancer 61:866–868
17. Rutqvist LE, Lax I, Fornander T, Johansson H (1992) Cardiovascular mortality in a randomized trial of adjuvant radiation therapy versus surgery alone in primary breast cancer. Int J Rad Oncol Biol Phys (in press)
18. Swedborg I, Wallgren A (1981) The effect of pre- and postmastectomy radiotherapy on the degree of edema, shoulder-joint mobility and gripping force. Cancer 47:877–881
19. Lingos TI, Recht A, Vicini F et al. (1991) Radiation pneumonitis in breast cancer patients treated with conservative surgery and radiation therapy. Int J Rad Oncol Biol Phys 21:355–360
20. Olsen NK, Pfeiffer P, Mondrup K, Rose C (1990) Radiation-induced brachial plexus neuropathy in breast cancer patients. Acta Oncol 29:885–890
21. Abner AL, Recht A, Vicini FA et al. (1991) Cosmetic results after surgery, chemotherapy, and radiation therapy for early breast cancer. Int J Radiat Oncol Biol Phys 21:331–338

How To Combine Adjuvant Chemotherapy and Radiation Therapy

J.R. Harris and A. Recht

Departments of Radiation Oncology, Beth Israel Hospital and Dana-Farber Cancer Institute; Joint Center for Radiation Therapy; Harvard Medical School, Boston, MA USA

The use of breast-conserving treatment (combining breast-conserving surgery and irradiation, RT) had been well established based on the results of clinical trials demonstrating equivalent survival for patients with early-stage breast cancer treated by this approach or by mastectomy [1–5]. Breast-conserving treatment results in important gains in body image and sexuality for many patients and is now widely used in both the United States and Europe. Over a similar time frame, clinical trials have also demonstrated the effectiveness of adjuvant systemic therapies in prolonging survival [6] (reprinted in part in this volume). Therefore clinicians are now commonly faced with the necessity of combining RT and systemic therapy in patients following conservative surgery. In this chapter we review the available information regarding the integration of RT and chemotherapy (CT) following conservative surgery. We do not address issues related to the combination of RT and tamoxifen or the use of initial CT (discussed elsewhere in this volume).

It is useful at the start to state the goals, options, and issues in combining RT and CT. The chief goal for nearly all patients is to obtain the highest rate of survival; additional important goals are to maintain a low rate of local recurrence, a low rate of complications, and a high rate of satisfactory cosmetic results. The options for combining RT and CT are to give the RT first followed by CT, the CT first followed by RT, or to give both simultaneously or to start with some number of cycles of CT, then give RT, and the finish CT (commonly referred to as 'sandwich' therapy). In considering this issue of combining RT and CT it would be useful to know the answers to a number of questions: Does a delay in CT decrease its effect? Does a delay in RT decrease its effect? Can RT and CT be given simultaneously without a large increase in complications and a decrease in the cosmetic outcome? Does prior RT affect CT doses? In addressing these questions, it is also important to bear in mind that there are differences in the implementation of breast-conserving surgery, RT, and CT from center

Recent Results in Cancer Research, Vol. 127

to center; therefore, the optimal combination of RT and CT may differ among centers.

It seems intuitively logical that delays in the initiation of CT may decrease its effectiveness; however, firm data demonstrating this are not available. Efforts to address this have focused on the possible benefit of perioperative CT and on the results obtained in patients treated with mastectomy. In the International Breast Cancer Study Group trial testing the value of perioperative treatment with cyclophosphamide, methotrexate, and fluorouracil (CMF) [7], node-positive patients were randomized to one cycle of perioperative CMF (within 36 h of surgery), this treatment followed by (six cycles of conventionally timed CT, or six cycles of conventionally timed CT alone. With a median follow-up of 42 months, disease-free survival was equivalent for patients treated with conventionally timed CT with or without one cycle of perioperative CT, and both of these groups had improved disease-free survival compared with patients treated with one cycle of perioperative CT alone. These results suggest that very prompt initiation of CT is not required. Similar results have been reported in studies from Austria [8], and from Italy [9] using perioperative epidoxorubicin. Other studies testing the value of perioperative CT are underway or have been completed but have not published results.

There are results from a randomized clinical trial in which patients treated with mastectomy were randomized to RT followed by CT (six cycles of CMF), CT followed by RT, or a sandwich approach using three cycles of CT initially, RT, then completion of the CT. With a relatively small number of patients in each arm (about 80), the best results were observed in patients treated with the sandwich approach [10]. Retrospective reviews examining the influence of the delay of CT on outcome have demonstrated conflicting results [11–15].

It is also possible that delays in the initiation of RT to give CT first may decrease its effectiveness. The information available on this issue is also not definitive. Among a group of patients treated *without* adjuvant chemotherapy, local recurrence was greater among patients treated with RT which was started more than 7 weeks following conservative surgery compared with patients treated within 7 weeks ($p = 0.01$ on univariate analysis, but nonsignificant in a mutlivariate analysis). We have previously reported a retrospective analysis on 295 node-positive patients treated with RT and CT using a variety of sequences which were not randomly assigned. Of note, in this series of patients treated between 1976 and 1985, careful mammographic and pathologic evaluation was not performed routinely and the extent of breast resection was typically limited to a gross excision of the tumor with a small rim of adjacent breast tissue. These results have been updated, and there is now a median follow-up time of 99 months among surviving patients. As shown in Fig. 1, among the 34 patients who received RT more than 16 weeks after surgery, the 5-year actuarial local recurrence rate was 28% compared with only 5% for the 252 patients who received RT

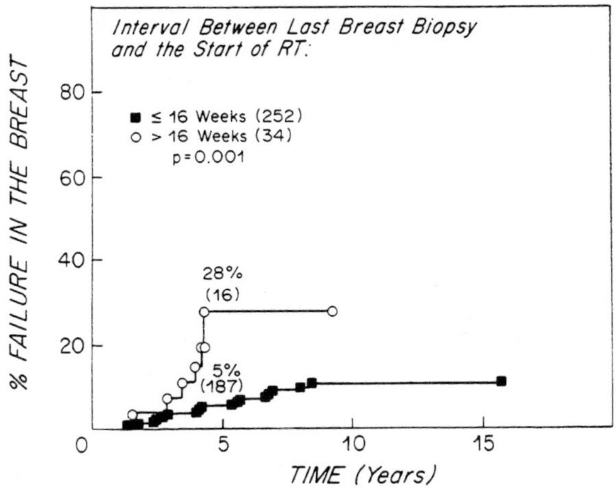

Fig. 1. Actuarial rate of local recurrence in the treated breast comparing patients irradiated within 16 weeks of surgery and patients irradiated after 16 weeks to allow the use of initial chemotherapy

within 16 weeks of surgery ($p < 0.05$; in nine patients the time to the initiation of RT could not be determined precisely). It should be noted in Fig. 1 that this apparent difference in local recurrence was not seen until after the first 3 years following treatment.

Table 1 shows the distribution of clinical and pathologic features comparing the groups treated within 16 weeks and those treated after 16 weeks. The two groups were balanced with regard to patient age, percentage infiltrating duct, tumor size, percentage of patients whose tumor contained an extensive intraductal component, and the frequency of reexcision of the primary site prior to RT. These groups were not balanced with regard to the frequency of lymphatic vessel invasion associated with the tumor and the number of positive nodes; patients with four or more positive nodes were more likely to have received delayed RT. However, the 5-year actuarial rate of local recurrence among patients with four or more positive nodes was 26% for patients who received RT more than 16 weeks after surgery and 10% for patients who received RT within 16 weeks. The corresponding figures for patients with one to three positive nodes were 28% and 4%. These results suggest that a delay in the initiation of RT beyond 16 weeks in order to give CT first may result in an increased rate of local recurrence. There are a number of caveats regarding this finding: (a) the study is based on a retrospective analysis involving small numbers of patients, especially those with long delays; (b) the study does not evaluate the most important endpoint (namely, survival) in relation to sequencing; and (c) even if these results were to be confirmed in randomized clinical trials, they may not apply to patients undergoing wider resections as opposed to the limited ones

Table 1. Clinical and pathologic features of patients treated with RT within 16 weeks and those treated after 16 weeks from last breast resection

	Patients (n)	Mean age (years)	Mean tumor size (cm)	Infiltrating duct	EIC+	LVI+	Reexc	1–3 N+	≥4 N+
>16 weeks	34	44.5	2.2	79%	23%	73%	29%	50%	50%
≤16 weeks	252	45	2.1	87%	31%	51%	22%	79%	21%
p value		NS	NS	NS	NS	0.06	NS	0.001	0.001

EIC+, Infiltrating duct carcinomas with an extensive intraductal component; LVI+, lymphatic vessel invasion present; Reexc, patient underwent a reexcision of the primary site prior to RT; N+, positive nodes.

performed here. Of note in this regard, among a series of patients treated with quadrantectomy and presented in a poster at this conference, no effect was seen with delays greater than 16 weeks [16].

More recently, at our institution, we have been conducting a prospective randomized trial to test more formally the effect of sequencing of RT and CT on outcome. In this trial, patients at moderate or high risk for relapse (typically node-positive) are randomized to receive irradiation followed by four cycles of cyclophosphamide, doxorubicin, methotrexate, fluorouracil, and prednisone or this CT followed by RT. Approximately 250 patients have been randomized on this protocol, but results are not yet available.

Another important question regarding sequencing is whether RT and CT can be given simultaneously without a large increase in complications and a decrease in the cosmetic outcome? The use of simultaneous RT and CT has the advantage that it would eliminate the necessity for delaying one of the modalities, and it may also provide an additive or synergistic interaction between the RT and CT. The available information on the effects of simultaneous treatment is conflicting, and this is likely due to differences in the details of the RT and CT protocols used (e.g., the number, types, and doses of drugs, the daily and total doses of RT, the machine energy, the use of two compared with three fields, and the specific details by which RT and CT are given simultaneously). In some studies, patients treated with simultaneous treatment have had greater skin reactions compared with patients treated sequentially [17–21], but this has not been seen in other studies [22–26]. In our experience at the Joint Center for Radiation Therapy, acute skin reactions were more pronounced with simultaneous treatment compared with sequential treatment, particularly in patients who received full doses of RT and four injections of methotrexate during RT [17]. We have also found that patients treated with simultaneous treatment have an increased rate of radiation pneumonitis (particularly when a third field was used to treat the axillary and/or supraclavicular nodal areas) [27] and a decrease in the long-term cosmetic result [28]. In contrast, the University of Pennsylvannia group reported in this meeing that neither an increase in radiation pneumonitis nor a decrease in the cosmetic outcome was seen when patients were treated with simultaneous RT and CMF where methotrexate was omitted during the RT [29]. An increase in cardiac complications has been reported by the Milan group for patients treated with simultaneous RT and doxorubicin-containing CT [23]; this is described in greater detail elsewhere in this volume. Others have not found an increase in cardiac complications when RT and doxorubicin-containing CT are given sequentially [30], and this has been our experience in the randomized trial described above. Thus, the use of simultaneous RT and CT has potential advantages, but the precise details of the administration of these two modalities is important to insure its safety. We are currently investigating the use of simultaneous full-dose CMF and RT (restricted to the breast alone and given at 180 cGy per day to a total dose which is approximately 10% lower than used with sequential treatment) in patients with up to three positive nodes.

A final question regarding sequencing is whether prior RT affects the ability to give full doses of CT. The available information on this question is also conflicting, and here too this is likely due to differences in the specifics of the RT (areas treated and technique) and CT (types and doses of drugs including the rules for CT dose modifications). Two randomized trials comparing breast-conserving treatment with mastectomy are useful to assess the impact of prior irradiation on CT doses. In the study from the United States National Cancer Institute [31], no significant difference was found in CT doses between the patients treated with breast-conserving treatment and those with mastectomy, while in the Guy's Hospital trial [32] patients treated with mastectomy were able to receive greater amounts of CT. In the Guy's Hospital trial, however, at least some patients received irradiation of the internal mammary nodes through a separate direct anterior field, and drug dose reductions were made using the total white cell count and were not reescalated if counts improved. Experience has shown that dose reductions should be made based on the granulocyte count since RT can result in a large reduction in the lymphocyte count, and that reescalation of CT doses is possible. The results from other randomized studies have found that CT doses are only slightly lower when RT is added [33–35].

In summary, given the more widespread use of breast-conserving treatment (using breast-conserving surgery and RT) and adjuvant CT, clinicians are now commonly faced with the necessity of combining RT and CT in patients following conservative surgery. The chief goal in designing the optimal sequence of CT and RT is to obtain the highest rate of survival; additional important goals are to maintain a low rate of local recurrence, a low rate of complications, and a high rate of satisfactory cosmetic results. The available information regarding the optimal sequencing of CT and RT is limited and is often conflicting. Differences in the details of the treatment (surgery, RT, and CT) may explain some of the conflicting results. At this time, there are concerns regarding delaying the initiation of CT, and retrospective data from our institution on a limited number of patients suggest that a delay in the initiation of RT may be associated with an increase in the rate of local recurrence. It may be possible to deliver RT and CT simultaneously in a safe and effective manner, but the precise details for this have not been established. Additional data from randomized clinical trials addressing this important issue are required and will be available over the next couple of years.

References

1. Fisher B, Redmond C, Poisson R, Margolese R, Wolmark N, Wickerham L (1989) Eight-year results of a randomized clinical trial comparing total mastectomy and lumpectomy with or without irradiation in the treatment of breast cancer. N Engl J Med 320:822–828
2. Lichter A, Lippman M, Danforth D, d'Angelo T, Steinberg S (1992) Mastectomy versus breast-conserving therapy in the treatment of stage I and II carcinoma of the breast: a randomized trial at the National Cancer Institute. J Clin Oncol 10:976–983
3. Sarrazin D, Le M, Arriagada R (1989) Ten-year results of a randomized trial comparing a conservative treatment to mastectomy in early breast cancer. Radiother Oncol 14:177–184
4. Versonesi U, Banfi A, Salvadori B, Luini A, Saccozzi R, Zucali R (1990) Breast conservation is the treatment of choice in small breast cancer: long-term results of a randomized trial. Eur J Cancer 26:668–670
5. Von Dongen J (1990) Randomized clinical trial to assess the value of breast conserving therapy in stage I and II breast cancer: EORTC trial 10801 (Abstr). Proc NIH Consensus Development Conf: 25–27
6. Early Breast Cancer Trialist's Collaborative Group (1992) Systemic therapy of early breast cancer by hormonal, cytotoxic, or immune therapy: 133 randomized trials involving 31,000 recurrences and 24,000 deaths among 75,000 women. Lancet 339:1–15, 71–84
7. Ludwig Breast Cancer Study Group (1989) Prolonged disease-free survival after one course of perioperative adjuvant chemotherapy for node-negative breast cancer. N Engl J Med 320:491
8. Kraniner M, Sevelda P, Salzer H et al. (1991) Comparison between the application of intra- versus 3-week postoperative adjuvant chemotherapy in breast cancer (Abstr). Eur J Cancer 27 Suppl 2:39
9. Sertoli M, Pronzato P, Querolo P et al. (1992) Perioperative polichemotherapy for primary breast cancer. Recent Results Cancer Res 115:57
10. Lara Jimenez P, Garcia Puche J, Pedraza V (1991) Adjuvant combined modality treatment in high risk breast cancer patients: ten years results (Abstr). Proc 5th EORTC Breast Cancer Working Conf. A293
11. Recht A, Come S, Gelman RS et al. (1991) Integration of conservative surgery, radiotherapy, and chemotherapy for the treatment of early-stage node-positive breast cancer: sequencing, timing, and outcome. J Clin Oncol 9:1662
12. Glucksber H, Rivkin S, Rasmussen S et al. (1982) Combination chemotherapy (CMFVP) versus i-phenylalanine mustard (L-PAM) for operable breast cancer with positive axillary nodes: a Southwest Oncology Group study. Cancer 50:423
13. Buzdar A, Smith T, Powell KC et al. (1982) Effect of timing of initiation of adjuvant chemotherapy on disease-free survival in breast cancer. Breast Cancer Res Treat 2:163

14. Dalton W, Brooks R, Jones SE et al. (1987) Breast cancer adjuvant therapy trials at the Arizona Cancer Center using Adriamycin and cyclophosphamide. In: Salmon SE (ed) Adjuvant therapy of cancer, vol 5. Grune and Stratton, Orlando, p 263
15. Brufman G, Sulkes A (1991) A retrospective analysis of adjuvant chemotherapy with and without radiotherapy for stage II breast cancer: a 10-year update (Abstr). Proc 5th Europ Conf Clin Oncol P-0882
16. Pacini P, Cappeline M, Cardona G et al. (1992) Conservative treatment of breast cancer: influence of boost dose and interval between surgery and radiotherapy on breast relapses. Recent Results Cancer Res 115:65
17. Botnick L, Come S, Rose CM et al. (1983) Primary breast irradiation and concomitant adjuvant chemotherapy. In: Harris JR, Hellman S, Silen W (eds) Conservative management of breast cancer. Lippincott, Philadelphia, p 321
18. Hahn P, Hallberg O, Vikterlof K (1978) Acute skin reactions in postoperative breast cancer patients receiving radiotherapy plus adjuvant chemotherapy. AJR 130:137
19. Hansen R, Erickson B, Komaki R et al. (1990) Concomitant adjuvant chemotherapy and radiotherapy for high risk breast cancer patients. Breast Cancer Res Treat 17:171
20. Meek A, Order S, Abeloff MD et al. (1983) Concurrent radiochemotherapy in advanced breast cancer. Cancer 51:1001
21. Sponzo R, Cunningham T, Caradonna R (1979) Management of non-resectable (stage III) breast cancer. Int J Radiat Oncol Biol Phys 5:1475
22. Bontenbal M, Sieuwerts A, Foekens JA et al. (1991) Enhanced antitumor effects of combination chemo- and radiotherapy on the cytotoxicity in human breast cancer cells in vitro (Abstr). Proc 5th EORTC Breast Cancer Working Conf A196
23. Buzzoni R, Bonadonna G, Valagussa P et al. (1991) Adjuvant chemotherapy with doxorubicin plus cyclophosphamide, methotrexate, and fluorouracil in the treatment of resectable breast cancer with more than three positive axillary nodes. J Clin Oncol 9:2134
24. Moliterni A, Bonadonna G, Valagussa P et al. (1991) Cyclophosphamide, methotrexate, and fluorouracil with and without doxorubicin in the adjuvant treatment of resectable breast cancer with one to three positive axillary nodes. J Clin Oncol 9:1124
25. Perez C, Presant C, Philpott G (1979) Phase I–II study of concurrent irradiation and multi-drug chemotherapy in advanced carcinoma of the breast: a pilot study by the Southeastern Cancer Study Group. Int J Radiat Oncol Biol Phys 5:1329
26. Piccart M, de Valeriola D, Pardiaens R et al. (1988) Six-year results of a multimodality treatment strategy for locally advanced breast cancer. Cancer 62:2501
27. Lingos T, Recht A, Vicini F et al. (1991) Radiation pneumonitis in breast cancer patients treated with conservative surgery and radiation therapy. Int J Radiat Oncol Biol Phys 21:355
28. Abner A, Recht A, Vicini FA et al. (1991) Cosmetic results after conservative surgery, chemotherapy, and radiation therapy for early breast cancer. Int J Radiat Oncol Biol Phys 21:331
29. Overmeyer B, Fowble B, Solin L, Goldstein L, Glick J (1992) The long-term results of conservative surgery and radiation with concurrent chemotherapy for early breast cancer. Recent Results Cancer Res 115:61
30. Pandya K, Olson J, Neuberg D et al. (1989) Observations on caridac toxicity in a treatment program containing Adriamycin and radiation therapy for stage III breast cancer: an Eastern Cooperative Oncology Group Study (Abstr). Breast Cancer Res Treat 14:148

31. Lippman M, Lichter A, Edwards BK et al. (1984) The impact of primary irradiation treatment of localized breast cancer on the ability to administer systemic adjuvant chemotherapy. J Clin Oncol 2:21–27
32. Habibollahi F, Fentiman I, Chaudary M (1989) Influence of radiotherapy on the dose of adjuvant chemotherapy in early breast cancer. Breast Cancer Res Treat 13:237
33. Ahmann D, O'Fallon J, Scanlon PW et al. (1982) A preliminary assessment of factors associated with recurrent disease in a surgical adjuvant clinical trial for patients with breast cancer with special emphasis on the aggressiveness of therapy. Am J Clin Oncol 5:371
34. Cooper M, Rhyne A, Muss HB et al. (1981) Randomized comparative trial of chemotherapy and irradiation therapy for stage II breast cancer. Cancer 47:2833
35. Ragaz J, Ng V (1988) Correlation of dose intensity (DI) of individual chemotherapy agents (CA) in CMF combined with survival – a review of a randomized adjuvant study (Abstr). Proc Am Assoc Cancer Res 29:A788

Factors Which Predict Breast Relapse

J.M. Kurtz

Radiation Oncology, Division, University Hospital, Geneva, Switzerland

Introduction

The clinical and pathologic characteristics of recurrent cancer in the conservatively operated and radically irradiated breast have only begun to be investigated and defined during the past decade. Compared with local failure in the skin flaps after total mastectomy, intramammary recurrences are generally considered to have a more protracted time course and a more favorable prognosis [13, 22, 35]. Furthermore, since the mechanism of failure presumably differs in the two cases, the factors influencing the incidence of relapse in the breast are not necessarily the same as those which correlate with the risk of local failure following primary radical surgery.

This chapter summarizes what is currently known regarding possible factors influencing the risk of intramammary recurrence after conservative surgery and irradiation for clinical stages I and II breast cancer. No consideration is given to the question of breast conservation in more advanced stages, nor are the results of radiotherapy alone, without tumor excision, discussed. As data concerning patients treated by conservative surgery alone are limited, only series including treatment with megavoltage radiotherapy are analyzed.

Most local failures occur at or near the site of primary tumor excision. Less frequently, and more often as a late event, tumor formation is observed at a clear distance from the primary tumor bed and is considered a "new" cancer [13, 22, 35]. More difficult to classify precisely are recurrences involving the skin of the breast or diffuse recurrences with extensive parenchymal and cutaneous involvement. Such unfavorable events represent about 10% of local failures and are usually considered recurrences of the primary tumor [27]. To distinguish between "true" recurrences and new tumors is to some extent arbitrary, and any calculation of local recurrence rates should include both types. In any event, the rate of recurrent cancer elsewhere in the breast is rather invariable (3%–4% at 10 years) and is not influenced by known

Recent Results in Cancer Research, Vol. 127

risk factors, provided that standard radiotherapy is administered [24, 35, 44]. Therefore, the risk factors outlined in the subsequent discussion can be thought of as relating principally to recurrences within the immediate vicinity of the primary tumor area.

Patient-Related and Tumor-Related Factors

Age and Menopausal Status

An association of young age with increased risk of failure in the breast has been found by almost all investigators who have analyzed this factor [3, 5, 12, 16, 25, 42, 44]. Representative data, presented in Table 1 from three large series, suggest that there is a continuously increasing risk of local failure with decreasing age. Although age subdivisions are arbitrary, it is clear that patients in the oldest age groups have a very low risk of local failure with standard therapy, and that the youngest patients are exposed to a risk which is considerably greater.

The age dependence of local recurrence risk is not well understood. It may reflect a tendency for younger patients either to have a greater residual tumor burden after local excision or to respond differently to radiation therapy, or alternatively it may stand in relation to the effects of circulating estrogens on residual cancer foci or premalignant changes in the treated breast. It is not known whether the risk of local recurrence in premenopausal patients can be reduced by hormonal manipulation. It is possible that this age effect is related to the age dependence of certain histologic features associated with local recurrence risk (see below).

Table 1. Rate of recurrence in the breast after conservative surgery and irradiation in three large series, as a function of patient age

	Patients (*n*)	Age cohort (years)	Breast recurrence (%)
Vicini et al. [46]	1382	<35	17
		35–50	12
		>51	6
Kurtz et al. [25]	1683	<40	21
		40–54	11
		>54	7
Veronesi et al. [44]	1232	<36	10
		36–45	7
		>45	3

Breast Size

Recent data suggest that recurrence risk may be influenced by the size of the patient's breast [4]. In a series of 324 breast cancers 2 cm or smaller treated in a standard fashion, local failure was observed in 2% of patients with large breasts, 8% of patients with medium-sized breasts, and 14% of patients with small breasts. Although this is probably related to the facility of obtaining wide resection margins in voluminous breasts, a hormonal effect related to obesity cannot be excluded.

Tumor Location

There are no striking relationships between the location of the primary tumor and the risk of local failure, at least when tumors are subclassified as medial, lateral, or central (Table 2). Conservative excisions of subareolar tumors are frequently considered unwise because of the risk of nipple involvement and the necessity in some instances of resecting the nipple-areolar complex. Most series presumably contain few patients with subareolar tumors, but there is no convincing evidence that such lesions are at higher risk of local recurrence.

Skin Dimpling, Nipple Retraction

While deep tumor fixation and gross skin infiltration are considered contraindications for classical breast-conserving techniques, neither nipple retraction nor skin dimpling appear to be associated with a higher risk of local failure. Among 385 stage I and II patients noted preoperatively to have skin dimpling or nipple retraction, 41 (11%) local recurrences were observed, identical to the rate observed in patients without these changes (101/930, 10.9%) [21].

Table 2. Rate of recurrence in the breast after conservative surgery and irradiation in three large series, as a function of tumor location

	Patients (*n*)	Location (%)			
		Outer	Inner	Central[a]	Subareolar
Boyages et al. [3]	783	11	9	–	9
Kurtz [21]	1219	11	13	13	11
Fowble et al. [15]	886	8	5	5	9

None of the differences were significant.
[a] 6 or 12 o'clock.

Table 3. Rate of recurrence in the breast after conservative surgery and irradiation in three large series, as a function of clinical tumor size (T1 versus T2)

	Patients (n)	Tumor size (%)	
		<2 cm	2.1–5 cm
Boyages et al. [3]	783	10	10
Kurtz [21]	1350	11	11
Fowble et al. [14]	697	8	8

Tumor Size

Contrary to a widely held belief, within the range of tumor sizes generally considered for breast-conserving surgery, the clinical diameter of the primary tumor has little influence on local recurrence risk, provided that a macroscopically complete resection had been performed and standard radiotherapy administered (Table 3). This is consistent with pathologic studies of mastectomy specimens, indicating that the likelihood of residual cancer after simulated tumorectomy for tumors less than 5 cm in diameter is independent of tumor size [18, 31]. Although an adequate local excision may be more difficult to perform in larger tumors, depending on the volume of the breast, data from virtually all large series confirm that local failure is not more frequent in larger than in smaller tumors [1, 3, 5, 14, 16, 21, 42]. Data from the National Surgical Adjuvant Breast Project (NSABP), however, suggest that tumor size may influence local recurrence risk in patients not receiving radiotherapy [10, 11].

Axillary Lymph Node Status

There are virtually no series in which the independent influence of nodal status can be adequately evaluated, as in most older series axillary dissections were not routinely performed, and in most contemporary series adjuvant systemic therapy was given preferentially to node-positive patients. Although there is some suggestion from small series that node-positive patients have a greater inherent tendency to recurrence in the breast [33], most series (Table 4) tend to show fewer local failures in these patients than in those without nodal involvement [3, 8, 14, 16, 44]. This is attributed to the use of adjuvant systemic treatment in node-positive patients (see below).

Table 4. Rate of recurrence in the breast after conservative surgery and irradiation in four large modern series, as a function of histologic lymph node status

	Patients (n)	Lymph node status (%)	
		Node-negative	Node-positive
Boyages et al. [3]	470	14	9
Veronesi et al. [44]	1232	5	3
Fisher et al. [8]	569	12	6
Fowble et al. [14]	697	8	7

Almost all node-positive patients received adjuvant chemotherapy. In the series of Veronesi and Fisher, the differences were significant.

Macroscopic Multiplicity

Patients with diffuse mammographic malignant calcifications or multiple gross tumor masses are seldom treated with conservative surgery and radiotherapy. However, two series report the results of breast-conserving treatment in a small number of patients with clinically or mammographically multifocal tumors or tumors which consisted of more than one separate nodule on gross pathologic examination [28, 30]. The local recurrence rates in these patients were approximately twice as high as in patients with unifocal tumors, confirming the greater risk associated with macroscopically multiple cancers. It remains open to debate under what circumstances such tumors can be safely treated with breast conservation.

Hormone Receptors and Other Biologic Factors

Evaluation of receptor data with regard to local failure is difficult since the frequency of observed recurrences can be confounded by interrelated factors such as menopausal status and hormonal manipulations. In a series from Marseille Cancer Institute, estrogen receptor negative patients failed more frequently in the breast than did patients with positive or unknown receptors, but this effect was not significant in multivariate analysis. There was no effect of progesterone receptor status [26]. In the experience of the Joint Center for Radiation Therapy, breast failure at 5 years was 14% for estrogen receptor negative tumors, compared with 9% for those with postive or unknown receptors, a nonsignificant difference [3]. Moreover, in a report from a large prospective study, hormone receptors had no relation to the risk of local failure [10]. Thus, at present there is no evidence that hormone receptor status is useful as a risk factor for local recurrence.

A host of other biologic features are under investigation as prognostic factors in breast cancer, including markers of cell proliferation, measures of tumor cell DNA content, growth factors, and oncogene amplification. To date there are no published studies on the possible influence of such factors on local failure risk.

Histologic Type

Although 80%–90% of breast cancers are classified as invasive ductal carcinomas, the limited data available suggest that standard breast-conserving therapy achieves local control rates with the less common histologic types which are similar to those observed after treatment of infiltrating duct cancers [23]. Single institutional series of in situ carcinomas are generally small, and reliable information on long-term results has only recently been gained from the pooling of data from multiple centers. In a combined series of 261 noninvasive intraductal carcinomas selected for breast-conserving therapy, 5- and 10-year local control rates were comparable to those commonly reported for invasive breast cancers [40].

For the usual classification of infiltrating carcinomas, local control after breast-conserving treatment appears to be little affected by histologic subtype (Table 5). Certainly there is no reason to exclude medullary or colloid cancers from such treatment. Similarly, the treatment results for lobular carcinomas, despite their predilection for multicentricity, appear to be adequate, at least with 5-year follow-up, reflecting the effectiveness of whole-breast irradiation [37].

Extensive Intraductal Component

Morphologic risk factors for invasive ductal cancers have been most extensively studied, particularly the extent of intraductal carcinoma and its

Table 5. Rate of recurrence in the breast after conservative surgery and irradiation in four series, as a function of histologic types of invasive carcinoma

	Patients (*n*)	Histologic type (%)			
		Ductal	Lobular	Medullary	Colloid
Schnitt et al. [39]	610	11	12	–	–
Kurtz et al. [23]	861	9	14	4	0
Weiss et al. [48]	879	8	9	4	18
Ribeiro et al. [37]	316	3	5	–	0

None of the differences were significant.

Table 6. Rate of recurrence in the breast after conservative surgery and irradiation, as a function of the extent of intraductal carcinoma within the primary tumor

	Extent of intraductal carcinoma			
	<25%		>25%	
	n	%	*n*	%
Boyages et al. [2]	16/279	5.7	37/166	22.3
Jacquemier et al. [20]	39/382	10.2	22/114	19.3
Fourquet et al. [12]	33/361	9.1	12/63	19.0
Lindley et al. [32]	21/213	9.9	13/59	22.0

The differences were significant in each series.

influence on local failure. Extensive intraductal component (EIC) was defined by investigators at Harvard University Medical School as being present when at least 25% of an invasive tumor mass was composed of intraductal cancer, provided that intraductal cancer could also be identified outside the limits of the main mass. The definition also includes tumors which are predominantly intraductal with foci of invasion [3]. Although varying definitions have been employed by different investigators, the original observation that tumors having a prominent in situ component are at high risk of failure in the breast has been since confirmed by several groups (Table 6).

Subsequent pathologic studies have shed light on the likely mechanism of the importance of EIC as a risk factor. Patients undergoing reexcision of the primary tumor area following excisional biopsy showed a high likelihood of positive reexcision specimens for EIC+ tumors, particularly with regard to the presence of extensive residual intraductal cancer [34, 38]. In addition, in a study of mastectomy specimens after simulated tumorectomy, breasts with EIC+ tumors had a much higher likelihood than those with EIC− tumors to have residual carcinoma, predominantly intraductal, at any given distance from the edge of the primary tumor mass. Furthermore, the amount of residual intraductal cancer tended to be much more extensive in breasts with EIC+ tumors [19]. It thus appears that EIC can be considered a marker for both the presence of residual tumor as well as for the quantity of residual cancer present, at least after a narrow local excision. The value of EIC as a risk factor may be less important in patients treated with very wide excisions such as quadrantectomy.

Other Morphologic Features

None of the other morphologic features studied have proven to be as consistently reliable as EIC, nor are the gradations of risk associated with other factors generally as striking as those between EIC+ and EIC− tumors. In a large cooperative study comparing lumpectomy with or without irradiation, lymphatic vascular invasion was an important risk factor for local failure in unirradiated patients, but this effect became insignificant when radiotherapy was added [11]. In most other studies, however, patients with lymphatic vessel invasion were at higher risk of local failure [3, 12, 26, 32, 33]. As lymphatic invasion potentially represents a significant mechanism of local tumor extension, this remains a plausible risk factor for further study.

The evaluation of tumor grade as a risk factor is made difficult by the variety of grading systems used. With one exception [12], groups employing histologic grading based on the Bloom-Richardson system show a clear correlation between increasing grade and local failure in the breast [6, 26, 32, 33]. Other features suggested as possible adverse risk factors include necrosis within the invasive cancer [25], the degree of intraductal necrosis [32], and the presence of a moderate to marked lymphocytic stromal reaction [25, 32].

An age dependence in the prevalence of certain morphologic risk factors has been shown by some authors. For example, the proportion of ductal cancers demonstrating EIC is greater in premenopausal patients [17, 25]. In the Marseille study, a particularly marked form of EIC was more frequently observed in patients younger than 40 years, who also had a higher incidence of high-grade tumors and marked lymphocytic stromal reactions [25]. This age dependence of risk factors may reflect the well-established correlation between age and local recurrence and may allow identification of young patients at particularly high risk.

Treatment-Related Factors

Adequacy of Surgical Excision

The adequacy of surgical resection can be influenced by the type of primary excision technique employed, by the histopathologic evaluation of the margins of excision, and by the use of reexcision. If no microscopic control of resection margins is carried out, and reexcision is not performed, a reduction in the rate of recurrences within or immediately around the tumor bed can be expected from the routine use of quadrantectomy rather than excisional biopsy or lumpectomy. The 10-year cumulative risk of "true" or "marginal" recurrence was 4% in the Milan quadrantectomy series [44], compared to 10% in two large series using more limited excision techniques [24, 35]. These long-term results have been confirmed by preliminary data from a randomized clinical trial [45].

However, the value of very wide excisions such as quadrantectomy presumably relates to greater reliability in achieving microscopically negative resection margins, which can probably be obtained in small tumors with less generous, and cosmetically more acceptable, excisions. Although criteria for assessing what constitutes "inadequate" margins are often arbitrary, most studies indicate that positive or close resection margins are correlated with a higher risk of local failure [1, 12, 26, 45]. In one large study in which no correlation between local recurrence and margin status was found, the dose of radiotherapy had been individualized as a function of the closeness of resection margins [41].

Given the adequate local control provided by gross macroscopic excision and radiotherapy, even in older series, it is likely that microscopic margins represent an important element only for a minority of patients, depending on the presence of other tumor-related risk factors. In a study of local recurrence related to volume of excised tissue, Vicini et al. [47] found local control in excess of 90% for both T1 and T2 tumors, independently of the resected volume, provided that EIC was not present. For EIC+ tumors, however, only excisions in excess of 48 cm^3 for T1 tumors and 75 cm^3 for T2 tumors resulted in a comparable level of local control.

Concern about resection margins has given rise to the increased use of local reexcision, which is positive for residual cancer in 32%–62% of patients suspected of having inadequate margins at initial resection [41]. It is likely that the examination of reexcision specimens can be used to assess risk, as this procedure may provide additional information regarding the amount of residual disease remaining in the conserved breast. It is unclear whether or not the use of reexcision results in a reduction of local failure rates.

Adequacy of Radiotherapy

Factors potentially influencing the effectiveness of radiation therapy include the delay between surgery and the beginning of treatment, the technique of whole breast irradiation, and the use of supplemental irradiation to the tumor bed ("boost"). The interval between surgery and radiotherapy is of increasing concern, as radiation treatment is frequently deferred several months until completion of adjuvant chemotherapy. A retrospective study suggests a markedly increased local risk for patients whose radiation treatment was delayed longer than 16 weeks, but unbiased data on the question of timing of radiotherapy and chemotherapy await completion of a randomized trial [36].

Because the dose and fractionation utilized in external-beam whole-breast irradiation is quite standardized in most Western countries, variations in technique are not likely to be responsible for significant differences in recurrence rates among various series. The application of 50 Gy in standard fractionation reduces local recurrence risk by a factor of four or five compared to microscopically complete tumor excision alone [10]. A significant increase in the total dose of whole-breast irradiation above this level is generally not advised because of the risk of unacceptable cosmetic results.

Although it is unknown to what extent the total dose may be reduced or other fractionation programs employed without compromising treatment results, there is evidence suggesting that undue protraction of radiotherapy may be associated with poorer local control [29].

The use of a "boost" to the primary tumor area provides an opportunity to reduce recurrence risk without significantly jeopardizing the cosmetic result. Two retrospective analyses concluded that significantly higher local control was achieved if a total dose equivalent to 60–65 Gy in standard fractionation had been applied to the tumor bed [6, 43], and a large Canadian series suggested a significant reduction in local failure associated with boost irradiation [5]. It is customary to use either external beam irradiation (either electrons or photons) or interstitial iridium-192 implantation for boost treatment, and at present no comparative data exist which convincingly demonstrate a clear advantage for either method over the other. The precise effect of a boost on the results of breast-conserving therapy is currently being evaluated in a prospective randomized trial by the EORTC Radiotherapy Cooperative Group.

In order to abbreviate and simplify treatment, some groups have proposed limiting radiation therapy to the area of the tumor bed, without whole-breast irradiation [7]. This option, a legitimate research question, is currently under study in a prospective randomized trial. Preliminary results, however, already indicate significantly increased recurrence rates without whole-breast irradiation, at least for certain subgroups of patients [37].

Effect of Systemic Therapies

Assessment of the effect of chemotherapy or hormone therapy on the risk of local failure is made difficult by differences in tumor-related characteristics between patients traditionally offered adjuvant systemic treatment and those treated with local-regional modalities alone. The first convincing evidence of a significant local effect of combination chemotherapy in conjunction with breast irradiation was provided by data from a large cooperative American study [8]. Patients treated by lumpectomy and breast irradiation had a significantly lower local failure rate when adjuvant chemotherapy was administered (node-positive patients), compared with patients receiving no chemotherapy (node-negative patients), despite the inherently higher local failure risk of node-positive patients compared with node-negative patients when only chemotherapy but no radiotherapy was administered. These observations are supported by retrospective data [16, 17]. In addition, preliminary data from a randomized trial suggest that the administration of tamoxifen to estrogen receptor positive patients results in a lower rate of local failure in patients treated with standard breast-conserving therapy [9]. It is unknown whether an interaction between radiotherapy and systemic agents is operative in this setting, or whether the observed effects are simply additive, nor is it clear whether the sequencing of treatments is important.

Conclusions

For grossly unifocal cancers less than 5 cm in clinical diameter, macroscopically complete excision followed by standard megavoltage radiotherapy produces highly satisfactory long-term control in most patients. Considerable progress has been made during the last decade in defining patient-related, tumor-related, and treatment-related factors which may help to identify the small minority of patients destined to fail locally. It is clear that recurrence risk is a decreasing function of age, and that premenopausal patients comprise the group at greatest risk (Table 1). The only tumor-related feature thus far identified that reproducibly correlates with a higher probability of local failure is extensive intraductal component (Table 6), which has been shown to be a marker for the extent of residual cancer after limited local excision. However, in most series EIC does not explain the majority of local recurrences, and reliable risk factors for the definition of other high-risk subgroups have not been clearly identified.

If whole-breast radiotherapy is given according to current standards, treatment-related factors are likely to have modest effect on the overall risk of local failure. Quadrantectomy studies have shown that local control can be improved by very wide excision, but it is possible that equivalent results can be obtained by lumpectomy in most patients if particular attention is paid to microscopic resection margins. Wider reexcision can be selectively employed, especially in cases with tumor-related risk factors, particularly EIC. It is likely that supplemental irradiation to the tumor bed will also reduce risk, and modest reductions in local failure have been demonstrated with effective systemic therapies.

References

1. Bartelink H, Borger JH, van Dongen JA, Peterse JL (1988) The impact of tumor size and histology on local control after breast-conserving therapy. Radiother Oncol 11:297–303
2. Boyages J, Recht A, Connolly J et al. (1989) Factors associated with local recurrence as a first site of failure following the conservative treatment of early breast cancer. Recent Results Cancer Res 115:2–102
3. Boyages J, Recht A, Connolly JL et al. (1990) Early breast cancer: predictors of breast recurrence for patients treated with conservative surgery and radiation therapy. Radiother Oncol 19:29–41
4. Chauvet B, Simon JM, Reynaud-Bougnoux A et al. (1990) Récidives mammaires après traitement conservateur des cancers du sein: facteurs prédictifs et signification pronostique. Bull Cancer 77:1193–1205

5. Clark RM, Wilkinson RH, Miceli PN, MacDonald WD (1987) Breast cancer. Experiences with conservation therapy. Am J Clin Oncol 10:461–468
6. Clarke DH, Lê MG, Sarrazin D et al. (1985) Analysis of local-regional relapses in patients with early breast cancers treated by excision and radiotherapy: experience of the Institut Gustave-Roussy. Int J Radiat Oncol Biol Phys 11:137–145
7. Fentiman IS, Poole C, Tong D et al. (1991) Iridium implant treatment without external radiotherapy for operable breast cancer: a pilot study. Eur J Cancer 27:447–450
8. Fisher B, Redmond C, Poisson R et al. (1989) Eight-year results of a randomized trial comparing total mastectomy and lumpectomy with or without irradiation in the treatment of breast cancer. N Engl J Med 320:822–828
9. Fisher B, Constantino J, Redmond C et al. (1989) A randomized clinical trial evaluating tamoxifen in the treatment of patients with node-negative breast cancer who have estrogen receptor-positive tumors. N Engl J Med 320:479–484
10. Fisher B, Anderson S, Fisher ER et al. (1991) Significance of ipsilateral breast tumor recurrence after lumpectomy. Lancet 338:327–331
11. Fisher ER, Sass R, Fisher B et al. (1986) Pathologic findings from the National Surgical Adjuvant Breast Project (protocol 6). II. Relation of local breast recurrence to multicentricity. Cancer 57:1717–1724
12. Fourquet A, Campana F, Zafrani B et al. (1989) Prognostic factors of breast recurrence in the conservative management of early breast cancer: a 25-year follow-up. Int J Radiat Oncol Biol Phys 17:719–725
13. Fowble B, Solin LJ, Schultz DJ, Rubenstein J, Goodman RL (1990) Breast recurrence following conservative surgery and radiation: patterns of failure, prognosis, and pathologic findings from mastectomy specimens with implications for treatment. Int J Radiat Oncol Biol Phys 19:833–842
14. Fowble BL, Solin LJ, Schultz DJ, Goodman RL (1991) Ten-year results of conservative surgery and irradiation for stage I and II breast cancer. Int J Radiat Oncol Biol Phys 21:269–277
15. Fowble B, Solin LJ, Schultz DJ et al. (1991) Breast recurrence and survival related to primary tumor location in patients undergoing conservative surgery and radiation for early breast cancer. Int J Radiat Oncol Biol Phys 23:933–939
16. Haffty BG, Fischer D, Rose M, Beinfield M, McKhann C (1991) Prognostic factors for local recurrence in the conservatively treated breast cancer patient: a cautious interpretation of the data. J Clin Oncol 9:997–1003
17. Harris JR, Recht A (1991) Conservative surgery and radiotherapy. In: Harris JR, Hellman S, Henderson IC, Kinne DW (eds) Breast diseases, 2nd edn. Lippincott, Philadelphia, pp 388–419
18. Holland R, Veling SHJ, Mravunac M, Hendriks JHCL (1985) Histologic multifocality of Tis, T1–2 breast carcinomas. Implications for clinical trials of breast-conserving surgery. Cancer 56:979–990
19. Holland R, Connolly JC, Gelman R et al. (1990) The presence of an extensive intraductal component (EIC) following a limited excision correlates with prominent residual disease in the remainder of the breast. J Clin Oncol 8: 113–118
20. Jacquemier J, Kurtz JM, Amalric R, Brandone H, Ayme Y, Spitalier J-M (1990) An assessment of extensive intraductal component as a risk factor for local recurrence after breast-conserving therapy. Br J Cancer 61:873–876
21. Kurtz JM (1988) The problem of mammary recurrence after breast-conserving therapy. Thesis, University of Basel
22. Kurtz JM, Amalric R, Brandone H et al. (1989) Local recurrence after breast-conserving surgery and radiotherapy. Frequency, time course and prognosis. Cancer 63:1912–1917

23. Kurtz JM, Jacquemier J, Torhorst J et al. (1989) Conservation therapy for breast cancers other than infiltrating ductal carcinoma. Cancer 63:1630–1635
24. Kurtz JM, Spitalier JM, Amalric R et al. (1990) The prognostic significance of late local recurrence after breast-conserving therapy. Int J Radiat Oncol Biol Phys 18:87–93
25. Kurtz JM, Jacquemier J, Amalric R et al. (1990) Why are local recurrences after breast conserving therapy more frequent in young patients? J Clin Oncol 8: 591–598
26. Kurtz JM, Jacquemier J, Amalric R et al. (1990) Risk factors for breast recurrence in premenopausal and postmenopausal patients with ductal cancers treated by conservation therapy. Cancer 65:1867–1878
27. Kurtz JM, Jacquemier J, Brandone H et al. (1991) Inoperable recurrence after breast-conserving surgical treatment and radiotherapy. Surg Gynecol Obstet 172:357–361
28. Kurtz JM, Jacquemier J, Amalric R et al. (1991) Breast-conserving therapy for macroscopically multiple cancers. Ann Surg 212:38–44
29. Kurtz JM, Amalric R, Brandone H, Ayme Y, Spitalier JM (1991) How important is adequate radiotherapy for the long-term results of breast-conserving treatment? Radiother Oncol 20:84–90
30. Leopold KA, Recht A, Schnitt SJ et al. (1989) Results of conservative surgery and radiation for multiple synchronous cancers of one breast. Int J Radiat Oncol Biol Phys 16:11–16
31. Lesser ML, Rosen PP, Kinne DW (1982) Multicentricity and bilaterality in invasive breast cancer. Surgery 91:234–240
32. Lindley R, Bulman A, Parsons P, Phillips R, Henry K, Ellis H (1989) Histologic features predictive of an increased risk of early local recurrence after treatment of breast cancer by local tumor excision and radical radiotherapy. Surgery 105:13–20
33. Locker AP, Ellis IO, Morgan DAL, Elston CW, Mitchell A, Blamey RW (1989) Factors influencing local recurrence after excision and radiotherapy for primary breast cancer. Br J Surg 76:890–894
34. Peterse JL (1991) The predictive value of an extensive intraductal component for residual tumor. Findings in 168 cases of reexcision after tumorectomy. Proc Fifth Breast Cancer Working Conference, EORTC Breast Cancer Cooperative Group, Abstract A-12
35. Recht A, Silen W, Schnitt SJ et al. (1988) Time course of local recurrence following conservative surgery and radiotherapy for early stage breast cancer. Int J Radiat Oncol Biol Phys 15:55–266
36. Recht A, Come SE, Gelman RS et al. (1991) Integration of conservative surgery, radiotherapy, and chemotherapy for the treatment of early-stage node-positive breast cancer: sequencing, timing, and outcome. J Clin Oncol 9: 1662–1667
37. Ribeiro GG, Dunn G, Swinell R, Harris M, Banerjee SS (1990) Conservation of the breast using two different radiotherapy techniques: interim report of a clinical trial. Clin Oncol 2:27–34
38. Schnitt SJ, Connolly JL, Khettry U et al. (1987) Pathologic findings on re-excision of the primary site in breast cancer patients considered for treatment by primary radiation therapy. Cancer 59:675–681
39. Schnitt SJ, Connolly JL, Recht A et al. (1989) The influence of lobular histology on local tumor control in patients treated with conservative surgery and radiotherapy. Cancer 64:448–454
40. Solin LJ, Recht A, Fourquet A et al. (1991) Ten year results of breast-conserving surgery and definitive irradiation for intraductal carcinoma of the breast. Cancer 68:2337–2344

41. Solin LJ, Fowble BL, Schultz DJ, Goodman RL (1991) The significance of the pathology margins of the tumor excision on the outcome of patients treated with definitive irradiation for early stage breast cancer. Int J Radiat Oncol Biol Phys 21:279–287
42. Stotter AT, McNeese MD, Ames FC, Oswald MJ, Ellerbroek NA (1989) Predicting the rate and extent of locoregional failure after breast conservation therapy for early breast cancer. Cancer 64:2217–2225
43. Van Limbergen E, van den Bogaert W, van der Schueren E, Rijnders A (1987) Tumor excision and radiotherapy as primary treatment of breast cancer. Analysis of patient and treatment parameters and local control. Radiother Oncol 8:1–9
44. Veronesi U, Salvadori B, Luini A et al. (1990) Conservative treatment of early breast cancer. Long-term results of 1232 cases treated with quadrantectomy, axillary dissection, and radiotherapy. Ann Surg 211:250–259
45. Veronesi U, Volterrani F, Luini A et al. (1990) Quadrantectomy versus lumpectomy for small size breast cancer. Eur J Cancer 26:671–673
46. Vicini F, Recht A, Abner A et al. (1990) The association between very young age and recurrence in the breast in patients treated with conservative surgery (CS) and radiation therapy (RT) (Abstr). Int J Radiat Oncol Biol Phys 19 Suppl 1:132
47. Vicini FA, Eberlein TJ, Connolly JL et al. (1991) The optimal extent of resection for patients with stages I or II breast cancer treated with conservative surgery and radiotherapy. Ann Surg 214:200–205
48. Weiss MC, Fowble B, Solin LJ et al. (1991) The results of conservative therapy for histologic subtypes of invasive breast cancer. Int J Radiat Oncol Biol Phys 23:941–947

Summary Report: Radiation Therapy as Part of Primary Treatment

S. Hellman

It is important to recognize that for many women the primary tumor contains the only malignant cells, and thus its control determines whether or not the cancer is cured, while even for others who have occult micrometastatic disease, improper treatment may result in local recurrence or a poor cosmetic result. This session therefore focused on issues which influence the use of radiation therapy in the treatment of the primary tumor. Overview analyses give clear evidence of the advantages of radiation therapy in improving local control but also provide an important cautionary note concerning the need for satisfactory technique if complications which result in significant irradiation of the heart may be responsible for late cardiovascular disease. These can be almost completely avoided using modern radiation therapy techniques which avoid irradiating significant amounts of cardiac muscle.

As the use of chemotherapy as an adjuvant increases, it is important to learn how best to combine this with radiation. While optimum timing is unknown, it appears as though concomitant therapy should be avoided since this may limit the dose of chemotherapy and may compromise the cosmetic result. Randomized trials on this matter are not available; however, retrospective analyses indicate that delay in instituting radiation therapy for longer than 16 weeks in order to begin chemotherapy results in a significant increase in local recurrence. These data seem to suggest that radiation should precede chemotherapy, with the possible exception of patients who have a very high likelihood of distant metastases, and even in these patients the radiation therapy should be started sooner rather than later. There appear to be a number of factors which influence the success of radiation in preventing local recurrence. These may be divided into three groups: those that are characteristic of the patient, those that are characteristic of the tumor, and those that are characteristic of the treatment. The most important patient characteristic which influences recurrence is patient age. In a number of studies it appears that younger patients have a higher incidence of local recurrence. They also have a higher incidence of an

Recent Results in Cancer Research, Vol. 127

extensive intraductal component of their tumor—the most important tumor factor which influences recurrence. While these variables are somewhat confounded, when they are separated, they are still independently important. The most important factor with regard to local treatment is the extent of surgery. While it appears that quadrantectomy is unnecessary, those patients who have disease extending to the surgical margins appear to have a higher incidence of local recurrence. It is therefore recommended that the surgical margin should be examined as a part of the treatment of the local disease.

It appears clear from this session that radiation, surgery, and chemotherapy may be combined satisfactorily; however, this requires appropriate attention to the technical aspects of all the specialties and an integrated management team with a consistent management plan.

V. Adjuvant Systemic Therapy: Overview and Improvement of Therapy

Systemic Treatment of Early Breast Cancer by Hormonal, Cytotoxic, or Immune Therapy:133 Randomised Trials involoving 31 000 Recurrences and 24 000 Deaths Among 75 000 Women (Summary)*

Early Breast Cancer Trialists' Collaborative Group (R. Peto)

In a worldwide collaboration, information was sought and centrally checked on mortality and recurrence for each woman in any randomised trial that began before 1985 of any aspect of systemic adjuvant therapy for early breast cancer. Checked data were available for 75 000 women (about 90% of those ever randomised), of whom 32% had died and another 10% had experienced recurrence. The parts now reviewed include 30 000 women in tamoxifen trials, 3000 in ovarian ablation trials, 11 000 in polychemotherapy trials, 15 000 in other chemotherapy comparisons, and 6000 in immunotherapy trials.

Highly significant reductions in the annual rates both of recurrence and of death are produced by tamoxifen (25% SD 2 recurrence and 17% SD 2 mortality: $2p < 0.00001$; Figs. 1, 2), by ablation below age 50 (26% SD 6 recurrence and 25% SD 7 mortality: $2p = 0.0004$; Figs. 3, 4), and by polychemotherapy (28% SD 3 recurrence and 16% SD 3 mortality: $2p < 0.00001$; Figs. 5, 6), but not by ablation at older ages or by immunotherapy. (Tamoxifen also reduced the risk of development of contralateral breast cancer by 39% SD 9: $1p < 0.00001$.) For tamoxifen and for polychemotherapy the avoidance of recurrence is chiefly during years 0–4 (this difference being maintained but not increased afterwards), but the avoidance of mortality is highly significant both during and after years 0–4, so the cumulative differences in survival produced by these relatively brief treatments (median: 2 years tamoxifen, 1 year polychemotherapy) are larger at 10 than at 5 years.

*This contribution represents the summary and Figs. 3, 8, and 12 of an article originally published in *Lancet* (1992) 339: 1–15, 11–85. The authors gratefully acknowledge the permission to reprint it here.

Recent Results in Cancer Research, Vol. 127

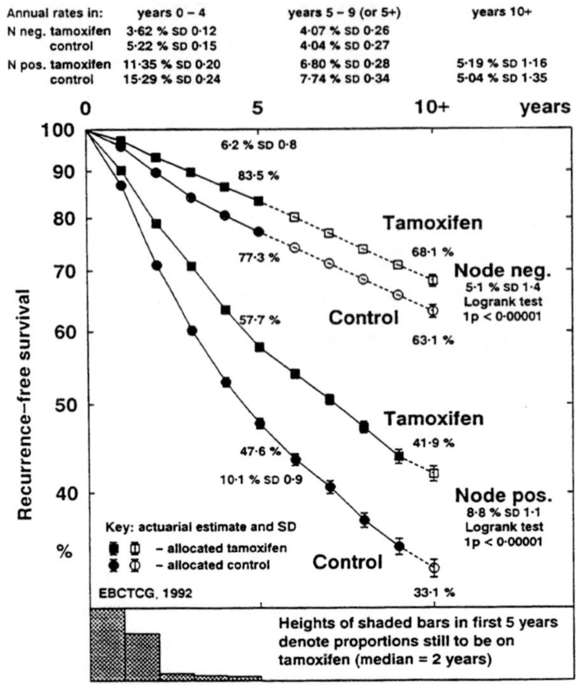

Fig. 1. Recurrence (all ages) in tamoxifen trials

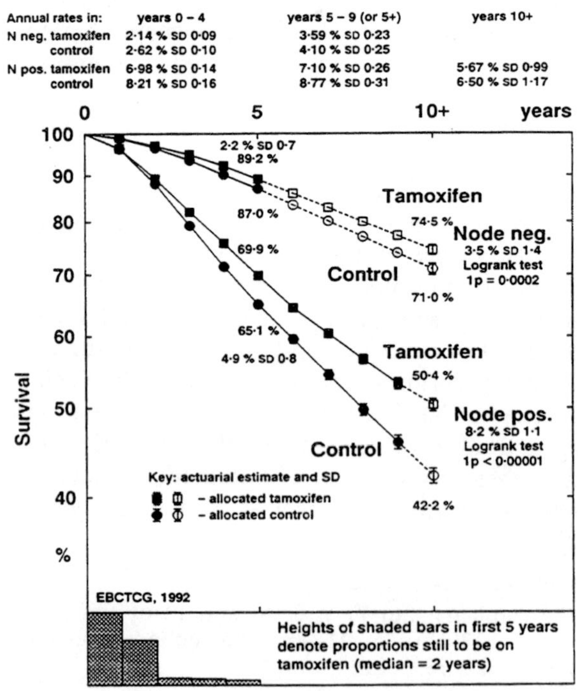

Fig. 2. Mortality (all ages) in tamoxifen trials

Fig. 3. Recurrence (entry age <50) in ovarian ablation trials

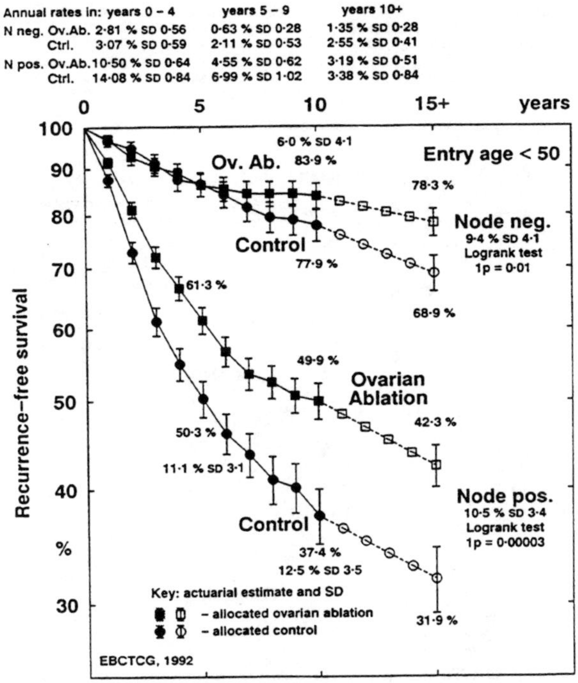

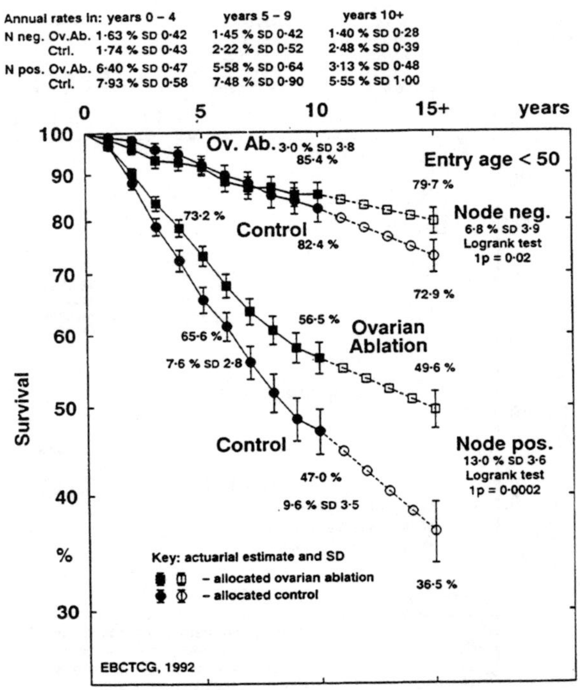

Fig. 4. Mortality (entry age <50) in ovartian ablation trials

Annual rates in:		years 0 – 4	years 5 – 9 (or 5+)	years 10+
N neg.	Cytotoxic	6·06 % SD 0·37	4·08 % SD 0·51	
	Control	8·50 % SD 0·44	3·99 % SD 0·52	
N pos.	Cytotoxic	12·70 % SD 0·32	6·98 % SD 0·44	5·57 % SD 0·94
	Control	17·82 % SD 0·41	8·37 % SD 0·54	4·98 % SD 1·11

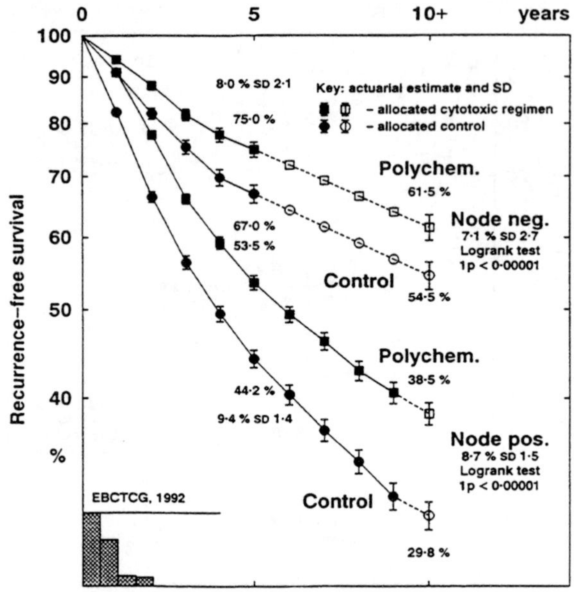

Fig. 5. Recurrence (all ages) in polychemotherapy trials

Annual rates in:		years 0 – 4	years 5 – 9 (or 5+)	years 10+
N neg.	Cytotoxic	3·23 % SD 0·26	4·59 % SD 0·49	
	Control	3·99 % SD 0·29	4·85 % SD 0·52	
N pos.	Cytotoxic	7·47 % SD 0·23	7·47 % SD 0·40	4·94 % SD 0·79
	Control	8·73 % SD 0·26	9·90 % SD 0·49	7·65 % SD 1·14

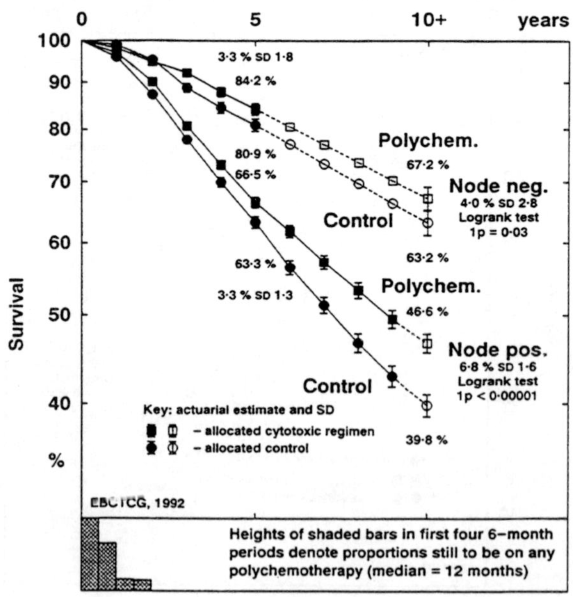

Fig. 6. Mortality (all ages) in polychemotherape trials

There is little information beyond year 10 (except for ovarian ablation, which produces separately significant mortality reductions both during and after years 0–9). Both direct and indirect randomised comparisons show long-term polychemotherapy (e.g., 12 months) to be no better than shorter (e.g., 6 months) regimens, but do show polychemotherapy to be significantly better than single-agent chemotherapy. Indirect randomised comparisons do not reveal significant differences between different forms of polychemotherapy or differences between different tamoxifen doses but do show that long-term tamoxifen (e.g. 2 years, or even 5 years) is significantly more effective than shorter tamoxifen regimens.

In old age (70+) tamoxifen is of demonstrated efficacy, but chemotherapy has not been evaluated. Between ages 50 and 69 direct comparisons show that chemotherapy plus tamoxifen is better ($1p < 0.00001$) than chemotherapy alone both for recurrence and for mortality, and better ($1p < 0.00001$) than tamoxifen alone for recurrence. In women aged under 50 chemotherapy and ovarian ablation appear, by an indirect comparison, to be of comparable efficacy, and the combination may be still better.

The 30%–40% proportional risk reductions that can be produced by combined chemo-endocrine therapy in middle age are similar for node-positive and for node-negative patients, but the absolute improvement in 10-year survival is about twice as great for the former (at least 12 deaths avoided per 100 women treated) as for the latter.

What Did We Learn from the Results of the International Overview about the Effects of Endocrine Therapy?

G. Bonadonna

Istituto Nazionale Tumori, Milan, Italy

The simple answer to the question posed in the title to this chapter is that we have learned, as already expected, that adjuvant endocrine therapy is effective. Indeed, both ovarian ablation and tamoxifen have improved the relapse-free and overall survival rates. The actual clinical problems concern the magnitude of benefit and whether endocrine therapy and chemotherapy should be combined to further improve current adjuvant results. The essential findings of the updated international overview [1] (reprinted in part in this volume) can be summarized in the following points.

1. The long-term (10-year) results essentially confirmed the intermediate (5-year) results.
2. The cumulative difference in total survival was larger at 10 than at 5 years.
3. Tamoxifen produced the highly significant mortality reduction during the first 5 years and an additional mortality reduction during the next 5 years. For polychemotherapy the absolute mortality difference at 5 years was doubled at 10 years.
4. Longer chemotherapy (e.g., 12 months) was not better than shorter chemotherapy (e.g., 6 months).
5. At the 10-year analysis polychemotherapy was documented to reduce tumor mortality also in women $\geqslant$50 years (14 $\pm$ 5%).
6. For those of all ages who were characterized as estrogen receptor poor (i.e., <10 fmol/mg cytosol in total protein) the 10-year mortality reduction following adjuvant tamoxifen was 11% compared to 21% for the estrogen receptor positive subset.
7. Among the 1817 women aged under 50 years, ovarian ablation was associated with a highly significant improvement in recurrence-free survival (26%) and in overall survival (25%).
8. The proportional risk reductions were similar for node-positive and for node-negative patients, but the absolute improvement in 10-year survival was about twice as great for the former than for the latter subset.

Recent Results in Cancer Research, Vol. 127

9. Regarding adjuvant immunotherapy there was no significant difference between treatment and control in recurrence-free survival or in overall survival.

From these mentioned findings we can conclude that both chemotherapy and endocrine therapy are useful adjuvant treatment modalities in high-risk breast cancer.

Does the international overview provide an adequate measure of that which a practicing physician can expect from adjuvant therapy? The crucial point is how properly to read the results of a meta-analysis. In fact, the advantage of assembling a large amount of information may be outweighed by the disadvantages of improper interpretation or the reasonableness of the calculation of average effect. When the studies being pooled are similar with regard to therapy delivered, patient population, and data quality, the averaging of results is quite valuable for detecting moderate treatment effects. This is the case for adjuvant tamoxifen because the majority of study patients were managed with 20 mg/day for a minimum of 2 years. This may also apply to ovarian ablation. As regards the latter modality we should add that most studies were actually conducted between the end of the 1950s and the beginning of the 1960s.

By contrast, when the studies differ with regard to therapeutic interventions (drugs, doses), one must recognize that average results may not be representative of the components making up the average. For example, substantial effectiveness of one chemotherapeutic regimen may be masked by pooling with ineffective treatments. This observation also applies to treatment with cyclophosphamide, methotrexate, and fluorouracil (CMF), the most widely tested drug combination, although this drug regimen was "the only one with separately demonstrated survival advantage in the present overview" [1]. In addition, recent chemotherapy trials delivered through full doses and utilizing anthracycline-containing regimens have improved the intermediate results over those observed in the early trials and failed to detect a different treatment outcome between younger and older women [2–4].

Considering the tumor heterogeneity of breast cancer, we do believe that future studies should rather exert reasonable efforts to make chemotherapy and endocrine therapy effective partners rather than competitors. The indirect estimations of the updated overview clearly suggest that even larger effects can be expected when chemotherapy and endocrine therapy are combined. Research clinicians have attempted to test these modalities in the hope of obtaining an additive if not synergistic effect. However, in vitro studies have illustrated that, when given concurrently, endocrine therapies may decrease the cytotoxic effect of some chemotherapeutic drugs by altering their cell kinetics. An attractive hypothesis to be tested in properly designed clinical trials would thus be the sequential administration of the two modalities. Relatively short, intensive, and optimal chemotherapy should be given first to kill rapidly proliferating tumor cells. Endocrine therapy (e.g., tamoxifen) could then be administered for prolonged periods of time to further improve treatment outcome.

References

1. Early Breast Cancer Trialists' Collaborative Group (1992) Systemic treatment of early breast cancer by hormonal, cytotoxic, or immune therapy: 133 randomised trials involving 31 000 recurrences and 24 000 deaths among 75 000 women. Lancet 339:1–15, 71–85
2. Fisher B, Brown AM, Dimitrov NV et al. (1990) Two months of doxorubicin-cyclophosphamide with and without interval reinduction therapy compared with 6 months of cyclophosphamide, methotrexate and fluorouracil in positive-node breast cancer patients with tamoxifen-noresponsive tumors: results from the National Surgical Adjuvant Breast and Bowel Project 13–15. J Clin Oncol 8: 2483–2496
3. Buzzoni R, Bonadonna G, Valagussa P et al. (1991) Adjuvant chemotherapy with doxorubicin plus cyclophosphamide, methotrexate, and fluorouracil in the treatment of resectable breast cancer with more than three positive axillary nodes. J Clin Oncol 9:2134–2140
4. Bonadonna G, Valagussa P, Zambetti A et al. (1992) Sequential Adriamycin (ADM)-CMF in the adjuvant treatment of breast cancer with more than 3 positive axillary nodes. Proc Am Soc Clin Oncol 11:61

The World Overview at 10 Years: What Did We Learn about the Results of Chemotherapy?

M. Baum

Department of Surgery, The Royal Marsden Hospital, Fulham Road, London SW3 6JJ, UK

Introduction

The publication of the 10-year follow-up world overview of adjuvant systemic therapy for early breast cancer [1] is an historic event representing three remarkable achievements. Firstly, the success of the overview process was dependent on achieving worldwide collaboration among fiercely independent national groups (each of which is organised on feudal rather than democratic principles). Persuading such groups from as far afield as the United States the Soviet Union, Sweden and Australia to pool their data and forget their differences is an example to the puny efforts of the United Nations in working together for the benefit of mankind.

The world overview also represents a bravura statistical achievement by the Oxford Clinical Trials Service Unit. Alone the detective work necessary to identify approximately 150 trials from the four corners of the earth is worthy of acknowledgment. Then to collate and check individual patient data referring to more than 70 000 women followed-up at intervals of 5–15 years, pushed the statistical and computing capacity to its limits. In other words, this study is likely to be a model for the evaluation of any intervention that is likely to produce modest benefits for common diseases. Last but not least, the data themselves vindicate the conceptual and biological revolution concerning the nature of breast cancer that emerged in the 1960s and 1970s following the seminal studies of Fisher in Pittsburgh [2]. These new data suggest that hundreds of thousands of women's lives can be saved worldwide over the next decade.

An accountant wishing to read the bottom line of this audit would conclude that the appropriate use of adjuvant systemic therapy following surgical treatment of early breast cancer will lead to approximately a 25% reduction in the relative risk of death at a constant rate over a period of at least 10 years. This can be translated into absolute gains according to a relatively simple formula. Say that for an average prognosis of women with

Recent Results in Cancer Research, Vol. 127

early breast cancer, the annual risk of death is 8%; in each year this will lead to a gain of 2% amongst those still alive at the beginning of that year. This then translates to approximately 10% net gain after an interval of 10 years. In the United Kingdom alone we expect 150000 deaths over this period; thus we can anticipate the net salvage of 15000 lives before the year 2000. However, this is not the only way of interpreting the bottom line. Even amongst those who are ultimately doomed to die, it is likely that there will be a prolongation of life, with the median survival extended by approximately 2–3 years. Furthermore, as the relative risk reduction following the use of adjuvant systemic therapy appears to be fairly constant across all clinicopathological sub-groups, it is likely that these extra years of life will be shared out amongst all groups.

With the exception of ovarian ablation for the premenopausal group, there does not appear to be any qualitative interactions between treatment and outcome across these clinicopathological sub-groups, although it is likely that some will benefit quantitatively more than others.

The Question of Choice

What then is the "appropriate" use of adjuvant systemic therapy for different patients with early breast cancer? The overview process is not intended to tell us how to treat individual patients but is intended to provide hard objective data based on powerful statistical inferences upon which physicians and patients can make sensible value judgements on the benefits and costs of a particular intervention. Furthermore, any advice or commentary based on the data will inevitably reflect either the prejudice or the intellectual investment of the individual clinician.

For example, collaborative groups in United States, Italy and Japan have a major intellectual investment in the investigation of adjuvant systemic chemotherapy, whereas the rest of the world, in particular, the United Kingdom, Canada and the Scandinavian countries, have been more interested in the endocrine approach to this disease. My own prejudice in favour of an endocrine approach, and muted hostility towards, adjuvant chemotherapy is a matter on record, but I flatter myself that I have sufficient intellectual honesty (or agility) to accept that these new data demand that I re-examine my prejudices.

In retrospect, the variety of prejudgements has been scientifically rewarding and of enormous clinical value, allowing some choice for physicians and their patients, particularly in the developing world who may not have access to or confidence with complex polychemotherapy regimens. However, this variety of approachs also has its inbuilt hazard for the overview process, which is dependent on certain assummptions concerning interaction between treatments. For example, the "main effect" analysis for endocrine therapy summates the trials that are confounded by concomitant chemotherapy with those unconfounded studies that compared the endocrine regimen versus an untreated control group.

Putting this aside for the moment, the individual clinician must now grapple with some rather complex concepts if he is to make intelligent recommendations for his patient. This could be approached at two levels of understanding. Even a most simplistic approach to these data demands an understanding of the difference between relative risk reductions and absolute benefits and also of how these statistics enable sensible cost-benefit analyses to be calculated. Thus the greater the risk of relapse calculated from the clinicopathological details of the patient, the greater is the absolute benefit. Looking upon it another way, the smaller the risk of relapse for the individual patient, the smaller would be the absolute benefit of adjuvant therapy, and the greater would be the significance of the toxic side effects of that therapy. With these principles in mind, some simple guidelines might emerge. For example, a premenopausal woman judged to have a poor prognosis, based either on the nodal status or a variety of biological prognostic markers following analysis of the primary tumour, would benefit from six cycles of polychemotherapy, whereas for a postmenopausal woman who appears to have a preferential benefit from tamoxifen compared with chemotherapy, one might consider adjuvant tamoxifen for 2 years or more even if she has a relatively good prognosis because of the low toxicity of this approach.

Biological "Fall-out" from Trials

Many readers may safely and wisely stop at this point, comfortable with these simple recommendations; however, a more sophisticated understanding of the overview process throws up some interesting paradoxes. Adjuvant chemotherapy does indeed appear to have some long-term benefit in postmenopausal women; (contrary to my prejudice) this might suggest that the addition of chemotherapy to tamoxifen would produce a greater net benefit. At the same time there does appear to be a quantitative interaction between adjuvant tamoxifen and the estrogen receptor (ER) status of the primary tumour, with almost twice the benefit for the ER-positive compared to ER-negative cases. Yet the ER status itself does not identify a sub-group of women who are wholly unresponsive to adjuvant tamoxifen, which might suggest that in countries without access to polychemotherapy, tamoxifen could be an alternative to chemotherapy in ER-negative cases.

Furthermore, the surprising observation that long-term follow-up of the early ovarian ablation trials demonstrates an advantage of the same order as that achieved by polychemotherapy once again raises the question of whether chemotherapy in premenopausal women exerts its influence via an indirect chemical castration [3]. However, we must not jump to conclusions and even hope that different mechanisms are at work so that combined therapy might be addictive. Finally, the fact that the benefits of either approach persist or improve with time is in itself a remarkable observation that cannot be explained adequately in conventional biological models.

Conclusion

From these observations, the next generation or two of clinical trials suggest themselves. For premenopausal women, polychemotherapy needs to be compared directly with ovarian ablation; however, of equal importance, it is necessary to determine whether any additional benefit is obtained by ovarian ablation in patients pre-treated with polychemotherapy. For postmenopausal women, it is necessary to define the optimum duration of tamoxifen comparing 2-year regimens with those in which the drug is given for a longer period or until relapse. Furthermore, the benefits of adding polychemotherapy to 2 years or more of tamoxifen need to be clearly defined.

These trials are currently recruiting well in the portfolio of studies coordinated by the United Kingdom Coordinating Committee for Cancer Research in Great Britain.

References

1. Early Breast Cancer Trialists' Collaborative Group (1992) Systemic treatment of early breast cancer by hormonal, cytotoxic, or immune therapy. Lancet 339:1–15, 71–85
2. Fisher B (1980) Laboratory and clinical research in breast cancer—a personal adventure: the David Kasnofsky Memorial Lecture. Cancer Res 40:3863–3841
3. Bianco AR, del Mastro L, Gallo C, Perrone F, Matano E, Pagliarulo C, de Placido S (1991) Prognostic role of amenorrhea induced by adjuvant chemotherapy in premenopausal patients with early breast cancer. Br J Cancer 63:799–803

From the Overview to the Patient: How To Interpret Meta-analysis Data

R.D. Gelber[1] and A. Goldhirsch[2]

[1] Harvard Medical School, Harvard School of Public Health, and Dana-Farber Cancer Institute, Boston, MA 02115, USA
[2] International Breast Cancer Study Group, Ospedale Civico, Lugano, Switzerland

Accepting the Concept of Meta-analysis

Clinical investigators have not easily accepted the concept of meta-analysis. Those who perform these formal statistical combinations of data from several different trials have been referred to as "those burgeoning band of interlopers, the meta-analysts" [1]. Critics have referred to meta-analysis as "pooling, drowning, and floating" in the past [2], and even today many view the exercise as potentially dangerous, and clearly a threat to the integrity and importance of the individual clinical trial [3, 4].

Meta-analysis is performed to determine whether scientific evidence exists that an experimental agent is active. In the context of the overview by the Early Breast Cancer Trialists' Collaborative Group (EBCTCG) [5], this mission was initially expressed in the following terms: "Does tamoxifen reduce the risk of death?" "Does adjuvant chemotherapy reduce the risk of death?" and "Does ovarian ablation reduce the risk of death?" It is interesting that the order in which these questions were first placed on the agenda back in 1983–1984 is opposite to the chronological order in which the adjuvant therapies were studied within randomized clinical trials. Interest in ovarian ablation declined when treatment differences were not observed early during the follow-up period. Chemotherapy was not aggressively studied in many parts of the world because physicians did not want to expose their patients to the toxic effects of the treatment. Only tamoxifen, due to its relative lack of toxic effects, was studied widely as an adjuvant, but even in this case the number of randomized patients in the individual trials was often too small to demonstrate statistically significant differences.

The overview has been an extraordinary success in terms of its impact on the scientific community. Its ability to stimulate international cooperation alone is enough to make it worthwhile. The information indicating the delayed benefit associated with ovarian ablation, the value of combined chemoendocrine therapies (both for premenopausal and for postmenopausal

Recent Results in Cancer Research, Vol. 127

patients), and the increasing impact of the chemotherapy component over time are important contributions of the overview to our scientific knowledge.

Homogenizing for the Sake of Power

In order to have enough data with which to reach statistically powerful conclusions the meta-analysis includes all randomized trials which represent an unbiased evaluation of the treatment component of interest. All trials having the experimental treatment present as a component of one randomized option and absent from the other are included. All patients randomized to each trial are also included in the analysis. The separate results of the treatment comparison within each study are accumulated in order to provide an overall unbiased estimate for the effectiveness of treatment in terms of reducing the number of events relative to expectation. This procedure is scientifically and experimentally valid to test the null hypothesis that the experimental treatment has zero effect on the endpoint of interest. The primary goal is to include as many patients as possible in the analysis without regard to differences between studies, treatments, or patients. The estimate of treatment effect derived in this way represents a homogenization of these differences for the sake of increasing statistical power. The challenge now is to explore the components of the overview analysis in order to move the results closer to the patient.

Getting Closer to the Patient

After the primary question of the overview is convincingly answered, and the null hypothesis of no treatment effect is soundly refuted by the available data, the consumer of these results will want to use the findings for treatment of his/her patients. In fact, the data must be used for this purpose, as the ultimate goal of clinical research is to improve patient care. It is therefore the responsibility of those who conduct and participate in the meta-analysis to explore ways in which the data can and cannot be reliably used for this purpose.

Some issues deserve to be raised to clarify the reliability of findings for the consumer: these are the role of the arithmetic construct, quantitative interactions between treatment and patient subpopulations, the importance of baseline prognosis, and the use of indirect comparisons.

Sorting Out Treatment Comparisons and Patient Subpopulations

The homogenization of treatment comparisons and patient subpopulations produces estimates of the magnitude of treatment effects which represent results averaged over a wide range of clinical scenarios. Two features that have been previously described are the arithmetic construct which ignores adjuvant treatment interactions and the mixing of patient subgroups which might have different responsiveness to the experimental treatment [6, 7].

The arithmetic construct is used in order to provide a valid test, with as much statistical power as possible, for the null hypothesis that an experimental treatment (treatment A) has no effect. The meta-analysis to determine the effectiveness of treatment A includes those randomized studies which are designed for a comparison of A versus nil (surgical control with no adjuvant therapy in the case of operable breast cancer) and those in which the randomized option is A plus else versus the same else. This means that we consider the trial as if it were an arithmetic equation, cancelling those treatments which are the same in both the experimental and the control groups. For example, trials of chemotherapy plus radiation therapy versus radiation therapy alone are included together with trials of chemotherapy versus no adjuvant treatment to evaluate the effect of chemotherapy alone. Similarly, trials of chemotherapy plus endocrine therapy versus the same endocrine therapy are used for exactly the same objective despite the fact that none of the patients actually received chemotherapy alone in these trials. For the purpose of estimating the magnitude of effect for chemotherapy alone, the arithmetic construct assumes no interaction between the chemotherapy and endocrine therapy or between the chemotherapy and the radiation therapy. It is clear, however, that the combination with chemotherapy cannot be split based on the arbitrary decision related to the names of its components. In fact, chemotherapy and radiation therapy have an interaction related to cosmesis, and chemotherapy and endocrine therapy have an interaction related to efficacy, especially in premenopausal women.

Table 1 shows the influence of the arithmetic construct in the 10-year results from the tamoxifen overview [8] (reprinted in part in this volume) for both younger and older women. The results for older women are similar whether or not chemotherapy was included in both groups. The effect of tamoxifen as adjuvant for the younger women, however, seemed to be reduced by concomitant chemotherapy based on an indirect comparison with the effect of tamoxifen studied against a surgical control.

Homogenization of overview estimates across patient subpopulations must also be sorted out to move the results closer to the patient. The tamoxifen overview provides treatment results for this endocrine therapy according to estrogen receptor (ER) status of the primary tumor (Table 2). A clear increasing effect of tamoxifen was noted for subgroups defined as ER poor, ER unknown and ER positive. The ER-unknown group is obviously a mixture of a population with ER-positive and ER-poor tumors and therefore not surprisingly yields an intermediate result. ER status of the primary tumor is a strong treatment responsiveness factor for tamoxifen adjuvant therapy. This indicates that the magnitude of the tamoxifen effect is indeed greater for patients with ER-positive tumors, but does not

Table 1. Effect of tamoxifen: an arithmetic construct in the EBCTCG overview [8]

		Typical reduction in annual odds	
Patient population	*n*	Recurrence or prior death (% ± SD)	Death from any cause (% ± SD)
Age <50 years			
Tam versus nil	2216	27 ± 7	17 ± 10[a]
CTX + Tam versus CTX	6362	7 ± 4	3 ± 5
Tam overview (<50)	8578	12 ± 4	6 ± 5
Age ⩾50 years			
Tam versus nil	13114	30 ± 2	19 ± 3
CTX + Tam versus CTX	8148	28 ± 3	20 ± 4
Tam overview (⩾50)	21262	29 ± 2	20 ± 2

Tam, Tamoxifen; CTX, chemotherapy.
[a] Data from Tables V, VI of [8].

Table 2. The role of estrogen receptor status on the magnitude of tamoxifen effect: results from the EBCTCG overview [8]

		Typical reduction in annual odds	
Patient population	*n*	Recurrence or prior death (% ± SD)	Death from any cause (% ± SD)
Age <50 years			
ER poor (or <10 fm/mg)	2055	3 ± 8	−5 ± 9[a]
ER unknown	2401	12 ± 7	8 ± 8
ER positive (or ⩾10 fm/mg)	4127	19 ± 6	13 ± 8
Tam overview (<50)	8612	12 ± 4	6 ± 5
Age ⩾50 years			
ER poor (or <10 fm/mg)	3311	16 ± 5	16 ± 6
ER unknown	7153	26 ± 3	17 ± 4
ER positive (or ⩾10 fm/mg)	10845	36 ± 3	23 ± 4
Tam overview (⩾50)	21280	29 ± 2	20 ± 2

ER, estrogen receptor.
[a] Data from Table III of [8].

necessarily mean that tamoxifen provides no benefit for patients with ER-poor tumors.

It is also interesting to note that even among younger patients those with ER-positive tumors show response to tamoxifen which is of similar magnitude to that for older patients with ER-poor tumors (indirect comparison). For purposes of treatment decision making for younger patients it would be interesting to see whether the results for ER-positive tumors are obtained primarily from the studies which did or did not include chemotherapy in both arms.

An analysis which does not rely on the arithmetic construct, and which separates patient subgroups according to ER status might be most useful for patient care purposes. The problem with such an analysis is that too few patients might be available to provide reliable information. Nevertheless, subgroup analysis is the only way to bring the overview results closer to the individual patient.

Baseline Prognosis

It is common for the consumer to look at the large number of patients evaluated and to conclude that the baseline prognosis of the "controls" in the overview represents an accurate and universal estimate of outcome for an untreated group. Little consideration is usually given to the fact that the patients are those who were selected into the trials, and that many of the "controls" actually received some form of adjuvant therapy. In addition, the homogenization of patient and disease characteristics provides an average result based on cohorts likely to have very different prognoses.

The effectiveness of treatment for reducing the risk of an event (relapse or death) can best be estimated by evaluating the relative reduction of risk for treatment compared with control. Not only are the statistical properties of such measures superior to those of the absolute difference in percentage of patients, but the evaluation of treatment effect across patient subgroups is not confounded by subgroup differences in the risk of avoidable events [9]. However, 100% of patients who are prescribed an adjuvant therapy are exposed to the potential adverse effects of the treatment. Therefore, the "usefulness' of an "effective" treatment depends upon the absolute number of patients who can benefit. If a treatment is equally effective for two patient subpopulations having different baseline prognoses, the treatment provides a greater benefit to the subpopulation with the worse prognosis. Thus, the relative effects of treatment as defined in the overview must be brought closer to the patient by considering the impact upon quality of life for the entire population against the absolute benefit achieved for those who would have relapsed if not treated.

Table 3 shows the mortality results from the tamoxifen, ovarian ablation, and polychemotherapy overviews including the 10-year survival percentage estimates as well as the proportional reduction in annual death rates. Much of the treatment effect in the ovarian ablation overview was observed after 10 years; therefore the 10-year values shown had to be approximated from the original report [8]. The table illustrates how the average baseline prognosis differed for the three overviews, suggesting that different patient cohorts and control groups were evaluated. It also indicates how the absolute gain in terms of additional number of patients who remain alive for 10 years

Table 3. Relationship between "control group" prognosis, absolute and proportional reductions in mortality from the EBCTCG overview [8]

Overviews	10-year survival Control (%)	10-year survival Treatment (%)	Absolute reduction in 10-year mortality (% ± SD)	Proportional reduction in annual odds of death (% ± SD)
Overall				
Ovarian ablation (age <50)[a]	56.0	61.9	5.9 ± 2.5	17 ± 7[b]
Tamoxifen (all ages)	52.6	58.8	6.2 ± 0.9	17 ± 2
Polychemotherapy (all ages)	45.0	51.3	6.3 ± 1.4	17 ± 3
Node negative				
Ovarian ablation (age <50)[a]	82.4	85.4	3.0 ± 3.8	20 ± ≥9[b]
Tamoxifen (all ages)	71.0	74.5	3.5 ± 1.4	17 ± 5
Polychemotherapy (all ages)	63.2	67.2	4.0 ± 2.8	18 ± 8
Node positive				
Ovarian ablation (age <50)[a]	47.0	56.5	9.6 ± 3.5	22 ± ≥9[b]
Tamoxifen (all ages)	42.2	50.4	8.2 ± 1.1	18 ± 2
Polychemotherapy (all ages)	39.8	46.6	6.8 ± 1.6	18 ± 3

[a] All values for the ovarian ablation overview are for age <50 years and are approximated at 10 years from annual rates given in Figs. 7M, 8M of [8].
[b] From Figs. 2M, 3M, 7M, 8M, 11M, 12M, and Tables III, IV of [8].

depends on the baseline risk of death for the population. While the overall percentage reduction in annual odds of death is virtually identical for each overview, the treatment difference in percent of patients surviving at 10 years ranges from three to nine depending on baseline prognosis. As patient cohorts are more precisely defined, the absolute gains from treatment might be the deciding factor for therapeutic decision making.

Competing Treatments, Or "The Quest To Find the Winner"

During the past decade an international competition evolved between proponents of endocrine therapies and advocates of cytotoxic drugs. In the overview this competition continues by use of indirect comparisons between the different meta-analyses that were conducted. Table 4 shows the overall summary results in terms of reduction in the odds of recurrence and death for the tamoxifen overview, polychemotherapy overview, and ovarian ablation overview. As a 25% reduction in the odds of death was estimated from both the ovarian ablation and polychemotherapy overviews, some investigators might argue that "ovarian ablation is as good as polychemotherapy for younger patients." Furthermore, some will take this equality of estimated effect in the overviews as evidence that polychemotherapy is merely "a toxic form of ovarian ablation" for younger

Table 4. Results from three separate overviews derived from the EBCTCG data illustrating indirect comparisons between overviews (from [8])

		Typical reduction in annual odds	
Overviews	*n*	Recurrence or prior death (% ± SD)	Death from any cause (% ± SD)
Age <50 years			
Ovarian ablation	1817	26 ± 6	25 ± 7
Polychemotherapy	3363	36 ± 5	25 ± 5
Tamoxifen	8578	12 ± 4	6 ± 5
Age ⩾50 years			
Polychemotherapy	7677	23 ± 3	12 ± 4
Tamoxifen	21262	29 ± 2	20 ± 2

Data from Figs. V and VI of [8].

patients. Equality of estimated effects from two separate overviews, however, does not imply equality of the treatments being studied in terms of the mechanism of action or the patient subpopulations deriving benefit. In fact, polychemotherapy has been shown to be effective in patients with ER-poor tumors. Furthermore, in premenopausal patients polychemotherapy effects were observed early in follow-up, while the effect of ovarian ablation appeared later (indirect comparison). In addition, the overview of studies comparing ovarian ablation plus chemotherapy versus chemotherapy alone suggested an additional effect of the endocrine treatment over and above that achieved for the cytotoxic regimen alone (Table 5). Thus, equality of overview results, at least in the case of competition between chemotherapy and ovarian ablation for younger women, does not indicate equality of the experimental treatments being studied.

Searching for a "winner" among single therapeutic modalities might not be the best way to improve overall patient care. For example, many patients received combination chemotherapy and endocrine therapy as the experimental treatment within a randomized study. In the overview these trials were used to evaluate the effect of the single components (chemotherapy or endocrine therapy) using the arithmetic construct. In contrast, Table 5 shows the results of an overview of combined chemoendocrine therapies relative to the single modalities. This meta-analysis uses information from trials of chemotherapy plus tamoxifen versus chemotherapy alone, chemotherapy plus tamoxifen versus tamoxifen alone, and chemotherapy plus ovarian ablation versus chemotherapy alone. In each case the chemoendocrine therapy was actually better than the individual modality given alone. One could therefore conclude that combined chemoendocrine therapy has a good chance of being the most effective among available options for reducing the risk of recurrence and death.

Table 5. Overview of chemoendocrine therapy (relative to single modality). Derived from the EBCTCG overview [8]

Patient population	n	Typical reduction in annual odds: Recurrence or prior death (% ± SD)	Typical reduction in annual odds: Death from any cause (% ± SD)
Age <50 years			
CTX + Tam versus CTX	6362	7 ± 4	3 ± 5[a]
CTX + Tam versus Tam	386	32 ± 16	−6 ± 23
CTX + ablation versus CTX	939	21 ± 9	19 ± 11
CTX + ablation versus ablation	n/a	n/a	n/a
Age ⩾50 years			
CTX + Tam versus CTX	8148	28 ± 3	20 ± 4
CTX + Tam versus Tam	3932	26 ± 5	10 ± 7

CTX, chemotherapy; Tam, tamoxifen; n/a, not available.
[a] Data from Figs. V, VI of [8].

Patient- and disease-related factors do, however, influence the usefulness of this proven most effective approach. As each of the modalities has a different type and severity of side effects, the therapeutic index is an important consideration when judging whether the combined treatment offers enough additional benefit, especially in comparison with endocrine therapy alone. For example, since the magnitude of benefit from tamoxifen increases for ER-positive tumors, it might be true that the additional benefits from adding chemotherapy for these patients is relatively small and might not justify the additional side effects. Similarly, as tamoxifen is less effective for patients with ER-poor tumors, the chemotherapy effect of the combined regimen predominates. Thus, an analysis of the chemoendocrine overview according to ER status, despite the limited number of events available from the overview of 75 000 randomized women, might be useful in order to bring the results of the overview closer to the patient. Such an analysis should definitely be planned for the next (15-year) update of the EBCTCG.

In Table 5 we note that trials of chemotherapy plus ovarian ablation versus ovarian ablation alone for patients aged under 50 years are not available. Obviously, the lack of early benefit in the ovarian ablation trials and the early, strikingly positive results from chemotherapy trials for younger women convinced most investigators with the resources to conduct these trials to abandon ovarian function suppression in favor of chemotherapy. This issue might be important to study in the future, especially for both node-negative and node-positive premenopausal patients with ER-positive tumors.

Table 6. Summary results from the *New York Times* to illustrate the effects of the *Lancet* paper upon the public perception: "Estimated number of extra survivors 10 years after surgery or radiation for breast cancer, based on an analysis of 133 studies involving 75 000 women. The estimates are for stage 2 cancer, benefits might be about half as great in stage 1 cases."

Follow-up treatment	Additional survivors per 100 women
Women 50 and older	
Tamoxifen alone for 2 years (longer treatment may have more effect)	8
Multiple drug chemotherapy alone	5
Tamoxifen plus chemotherapy	12
Women under 50	
Ovarian ablation alone	11
Multiple-drug chemotherapy alone	10
Ovarian ablation plus chemotherapy	at least 12

A presentation of the overview results in the media stressed the number of "lives saved" and also focused on describing the competing alternatives of chemotherapy and endocrine therapy in an effort to define the "winning treatment." Table 6 illustrates such a summary which appeared in the *New York Times* in January 1992 [10]. The table appeared with an invitation to choose the single modality which yields the best treatment results, without providing enough information on the complexities involved in choosing a most appropriate therapy for patients.

Concluding Remarks

The 10-year update of the EBCTCG overview has provided an important example for international cooperation. Those of us who have had the privilege to participate actively in the process have learned a lot about our own biases and those of others. We find that as long as we keep the best interests of the patient in mind, both in terms of the short-term and the long-term costs and benefits of available adjuvant treatments, we will be able to bring the results of the overview closer to the patient.

The overview suggests that chemoendocrine therapy, in general, provides optimal effect from among the treatments studied to date. The next series of questions to be addressed in future trials and overviews relate to (a) how best to combine cytotoxic treatments and endocrine therapies so as to maximize the benefit, and (b) how to determine the relative improvement due to the combination in patient subgroups defined by ER content of the primary tumor. Translating effects of treatment in terms of relative reduction in the risk of events to patient benefit in terms of absolute gains for the treated population is also needed to bring the results of the overview closer to the patient. This requires better assessment of quality-of-life oriented endpoints and further refinement of methods to evaluate costs and benefits of adjuvant therapies.

References

1. Horton R (1991) Conference report: double dealing with your data. Lancet 337:784–785
2. Goldman L, Feinstein AR (1979) Anticoagulants and myocardial infarction: the problems of pooling, drowning, and floating. Ann Intern Med 90:92–94
3. Wachter K (1988) Disturbed by meta-analysis? Science 241:1407–1408
4. Mann C (1990) Meta-analysis in the breech. Science 249:476–480
5. Early Breast Cancer Trialists' Collaborative Group (1988) Effects of adjuvant tamoxifen and of cytotoxic therapy on mortality in early breast cancer: an overview of 61 randomized trials among 28896 women. N Engl J Med 319:1681–1692
6. Gelber RD, Goldhirsch A (1986) The concept of an overview of cancer clinical trials with special emphasis on early breast cancer. J Clin Oncol 4:1696–1703
7. Gelber RD, Goldhirsch A (1987) The evaluation of subsets in meta-analysis. Stat Med 6:371–388
8. Early Breast Cancer Trialists' Collaborative Group (1992) Systemic treatment of early breast cancer by hormonal, cytotoxic or immune therapy: 133 randomised trials involving 31000 recurrences and 24000 deaths among 75000 women. Lancet 339:1–15, 71–85
9. Gelber RD, Goldhirsch A, for the International Breast Cancer Study Group (formerly Ludwig Group) (1992) Reporting and interpreting adjuvant therapy clinical trials. J Natl Cancer Inst Monogr 11:175–180
10. Altman LK (1992) Study on breast cancer finds therapy is effective for years. New York Times, Jan 4

High-Dose Adjuvant Chemotherapy for High-Risk Breast Cancer

M.D. Abeloff

The Johns Hopkins Oncology Center, Baltimore, MD 21287, USA

As has been noted in the previous papers on individual clinical trials and the latest overview update [1] (reprinted in part in this volume), systemic adjuvant therapy has resulted in a significant and long-lasting reduction in mortality due to early breast cancer. However, it is also apparent from these analyses that many patients develop metastatic disease and die of breast cancer despite having received standard adjuvant therapeutic regimens. In order to achieve further improvement in survival with systemic adjuvant therapy, several hurdles must be surmounted, including (a) enhanced ability to identify patients who are unlikely to respond to current treatments and (b) development of more effective therapies. This paper focuses on the latter issue and specifically the use of high-dose cytotoxic chemotherapy as an approach to improving systemic adjuvant therapy.

In view of the considerable toxicity that results from cytotoxic therapy, and high-dose therapy in particular, it is important to be able to select patients for these vigorous new therapies who do not benefit from more conventional approaches. There are well-established prognostic factors (such as extent of pathologic axillary lymph node involvement, tumor size, quantitative estrogen and progesterone receptor status, tumor histology) which help to predict the natural history of breast cancer. With the advent of recombinant DNA technology, a plethora of new potential prognostic factors have been identified, including determination of proliferative capacity and ploidy, expression of cathepsin D, c-*erbB2*/*HER2-neu*, epidermal growth factor receptor, and nm23. However, at the present time the magnitude of the predictive contribution of these new markers to the information obtained by review of classic prognostic factors is uncertain [2, 3], particularly in the node-positive setting. Moreover, the ability of these new biologic factors to predict responsiveness to specific therapies is virtually untested.

Despite the limitations of current predictive markers, it is generally accepted that patients with more than three positive nodes, and ten or more

Recent Results in Cancer Research, Vol. 127

nodes in particular, constitute a high-risk category. Patients with ten or more positive axillary lymph nodes account for 15%–20% of patients with node-positive breast cancer, and their 5-year relapse-free survival after local therapy alone is estimated at 10%–20% [4]. In a recently published adjuvant study in women with more than three positive axillary nodes, Buzzoni et al. [5] reported that the sequential administration of four courses of doxorubicin (Adriamycin, ADM) followed by eight courses of cyclophosphamide, methotrexate, and 5-fluorouracil (CMF) yielded superior results compared to two courses of CMF alternated with one course of ADM for a total of 12 courses. In the patients with more than ten positive nodes, the 5-year relapse-free survival with sequential ADM→CMF was 50% compared to 24% with alternating CMF/ADM. Thus, although there is considerable biologic, pathologic, and clinical heterogeneity even within the group with ten or more positive nodes, 50% or more of these patients develop recurrence within 5 years of follow-up. With the recognition of considerable heterogeneity within this high-risk group and the understanding that lymph node status does not appear to be a good *predictor of response* to adjuvant systemic therapy, this manuscript focuses on new high-dose therapies in patients with ten or more histologically positive axillary nodes.

Concepts currently undergoing investigation in the adjuvant therapy of breast cancer include (a) dose intensity, (b) chemoendocrine approaches, (c) neoadjuvant therapy, (d) kinetics-based sequencing, and (e) mathematical modeling, including the Goldie-Coldman hypothesis and the Norton-Simon hypothesis. The strategy of increasing dose intensity of chemotherapy, i.e., the amount of cytotoxic drugs given per unit of time, has been one of the most attractive for theoretical as well as practical reasons. There is ample evidence for a steep dose-response relationship for chemotherapy, particularly alkylating agents, in experimental breast cancer systems [6]. The provocative retrospective analyses of Hryniuk and Bush [7] greatly stimulated interest in this area with the demonstration that there is a positive correlation between dose delivered per unit of time and survival in the adjuvant setting. The findings from these laboratory models and retrospective studies plus significant improvements in supportive care set the stage for a number of pilot investigations of new high-dose regimens as well as randomized evaluations of the efficacy of established dose-intense regimens.

In the development of new adjuvant therapy regimens, an operating principle has been that the regimens must first be shown to be effective in metastatic disease. Two randomized trials of higher dose intensity versus lower dose intensity chemotherapy regimens in metastatic breast cancer have received considerable attention. Tannock et al. [8] have shown that conventional-dose CMF resulted in a superior objective response, disease-free and overall survival, and improved quality of life compared to low-dose CMF. However, Hortobagyi et al. [9] demonstrated no improved outcome with high-dose 5-fluorouracil, doxorubicin, and cyclophosphamide (FAC; requiring protected environment and prophylactic antibiotics) compared to conventional FAC. Reanalysis of this trial revealed that as a result of treatment toxicity the actual dose received by patients was not significantly different between the two arms [10]. Review of these two studies and other prospective trials does not clearly resolve the issue of the importance of high-dose cytotoxic therapy in metastatic breast cancer.

Although the benefit of increased dose intensity in metastatic disease is not fully established, the rationale for high-dose chemotherapy and the inherent difficulties in adequately assessing tumor kill in metastatic disease appeared more than adequate to justify studies in the adjuvant setting. At the Johns Hopkins Oncology Center, we have developed and piloted a novel, multidrug, dose-intense regimen which is administered over a 16-week period. A total of 64 patients with operable breast cancer and ten or more histologically positive axillary nodes were treated with this five-drug regimen that incorporated the concepts of weekly chemotherapy, sequential administration of antimetabolites, and continuous infusion of fluorouracil. The chemotherapy regimen consisted of eight cycles (each of 2-week duration) of $100\,mg/m^2$ cyclophosphamide orally on days 1–7, $40\,mg/m^2$ doxorubicin intravenously on day 1, $100\,mg/m^2$ methotrexate intravenously on day 1 with $10\,mg/m^2$ leucovorin rescue every 6h for six oral doses on day 2, 1 mg vincristine intravenously on day 1, and $600\,mg/m^2$ fluorouracil intravenously at hour 20 over 2h. A continuous infusion of $300\,mg/m^2$ fluorouracil per day was given intravenously on days 8 and 9 of each 2-week cycle. The doses and schedule of drug administration were designed to minimize dosage reduction and treatment delay.

The initial results and detailed toxicity analysis have been published elsewhere [11]. An updated analysis indicates that at a median follow-up of 40 months the disease-free survival for these 64 patients is 53% (95% C.I. 38%–65%) and overall survival 81% (95% C.I. 70%–90%). Subset analysis yields the provocative finding that the relapse-free survival is 44% (95% C.I. 28%–59%) for patients with estrogen receptor positive tumors compared with 73% (95% C.I. 44%–89%) for those with estrogen receptor negative tumors. This type of single-institution pilot study cannot establish efficacy, but the initial results were judged sufficiently encouraging to merit further investigation in a phase III randomized study. To that end, the Eastern Cooperative Oncology Group with the collaboration of the Southwestern Oncology Group and Acute Leukemia Group B are comparing in Intergroup Trial 0108 the relative efficacy and toxicity of cyclophosphamide, doxorubicin, and 5-fluorouracil (CAF) and the 16-week regimen in pre- and postmenopausal, node-positive, steroid receptor negative patients.

Intergroup Trial 0108 is a comparison of two dose-intense regimens but is not a test of the concept of dose intensity. Two well-designed cooperative group trials in women with node-positive breast cancer have been completed and will significantly enhance our understanding of the relative contributions of dose intensity and total dose in determining outcome with adjuvant therapy. National Surgical Breast and Bowel Program B-22 compares three regimens: (a) "standard" doxorubicin plus cyclophosphamide (AC) therapy, (b) AC therapy in which the cyclophosphamide is intensified while the cumulative dose remains the same, and (c) AC therapy in which both intensity and cumulative dose of cyclophosphamide are increased. Similarly, a trial of Acute Leukemia Group B compares CAF at high dose for 4 months, moderate dose for 6 months, and low dose for 4 months.

Another important potential application of dose-intense chemotherapy in the management of breast cancer is late intensification (or consolidation therapy) with high-dose chemotherapy followed by autologous bone marrow rescue (HDC-ABMT). In vitro studies with breast cancer cell lines have demonstrated greatly increased log tumor cell kill with alkylating agents such as cyclophosphamide, thiotepa, and cisplatin [6]. Interest in HDC-ABMT in breast was also stimulated by studies in chemotherapy-responsive diseases such as Hodgkin's and non-Hodgkin's lymphoma, which demonstrated that such aggressive therapy can result in long-term remission for approximately 25% of patients who have relapsed after first-line therapy [12].

The first report on autologous bone marrow transplantation in breast cancer was published in 1977, but it is only in the past 5 years that HDC-ABMT has become a serious treatment option for patients with metastatic breast cancer or high-risk operable primary disease. As noted by Henderson [13], there now are five published trials which have adequately reported results in metastatic breast cancer with the use of HDC-ABMT following a response to conventional-dose chemotherapy. Overall response rates in excess of 80% and complete response rates two to three times those achieved with standard regimens are described in these studies.

In one such trial at the Johns Hopkins Oncology Center [14] thirty women with hormone-unresponsive metastatic breast cancer, previously

Table 1. Results of therapy: comparison of CAMFV versus high-dose chemotherapy (n = 30)

	n	%
Response after CAMFV		
Complete response	8	27
Partial response	16	53
No response	3	10
Disease progression	3	10
Response after high-dose chemotherapy		
Complete response	11	37
Partial response	13[a]	43

CAMFV, Cyclophosphamide, doxorubicin, methotrexate, vincristine, leucovorin, fluorouracil.
[a] Two patients had complete response at all sites except bone.

untreated with adjuvant doxorubicin or any chemotherapy for metastatic disease, received induction therapy with the 16 week multidrug regimen. Those patients who achieved a complete or partial response proceeded to marrow harvest and treatment with 6000 mg/m^2 cyclophosphamide and 800 mg/m^2 thiotepa given by continuous infusion over 4 days. Harvested marrow was purged with 100 µg/ml 4-hydroperoxycyclophosphamide, and all patients engrafted satisfactorily. The initial results have been published elsewhere; the therapeutic results are summarized in Table 1. Updated analysis shows that the median time to disease progression for all patients in this study is 11 months, and median survival is 21 months. Four of the original 30 patients remain without disease progression at a median of 47 months from entry into this study. Although there were no toxic deaths in this particular study, the morbidity of this generation of HDC-ABMT studies was considerable (predominantly myelosuppressive and gastrointestinal), and the overall mortality was in the range of 5%–10%.

The impressive overall and complete response rates and the estimate of 10%–20% long-term survivors achieved with HDC-ABMT in metastatic breast cancer have led to the application of this approach to patients in the high-risk adjuvant setting. In a pilot study [15] Peters et al. have investigated the role of high-dose cyclophosphamide, cisplatin, and carmustine in conjunction with autologous bone marrow rescue as consolidation therapy following four cycles of CAF adjuvant therapy in 53 patients with stage II or stage III breast cancer involving ten or more axillary nodes. Hormone receptor positive patients also received tamoxifen for 5 years following transplant, and all but the first eight patients received local-regional radiation therapy. Four of the first 35 patients died of treatment-related toxicity, and there have been six relapses, with a median follow-up of 14 months and lead follow-up of 40 months. The actuarial relapse-free survival at 3 years is reported to be 80%. In addition, in a separate pilot trial, Tajima et al. [16] reported a 79% probability of 5-year disease-free survival in 20 patients with at least ten axillary nodes who received HDC-ABMT. Again, the preliminary nature of the results from both of these studies must be emphasized.

These initial results, combined with the enhancement in hematologic reconstitution which can be achieved with the use of colony-stimulating factors and peripheral blood stem cells, have led to the initiation of two multi-institutional trials which will assess the role of high-dose chemotherapy in high risk patients with ≥10 positive axillary nodes. Acute Leukemia Group B Study 9082 compares adjuvant chemotherapy with four cycles of CAF followed by high-dose cyclophosphamide, cisplatin, and carmustine to CAF for four cycles followed by outpatient doses of the same three alkylating agents in patients with operable breast cancer involving ten or more axillary nodes. In Intergroup Trial 0121 women with early breast cancer with at least ten positive lymph nodes will be randomized to receive adjuvant CAF for six cycles or CAF for six cycles followed by high-dose cyclophosphamide and thiotepa. Although there is considerable uncertainty about the optimal duration of antiestrogen therapy and the impact of tamoxifen on survival in these high-risk patients, tamoxifen therapy for 5 years has been incorporated into both of these studies in steroid receptor positive patients following the completion of the chemotherapy phase of the treatment. Likewise, postoperative irradiation of the chest wall and draining lymphatics in mastectomy patients after completion of chemotherapy is being utilized. Its use in this setting is based on the data of Fowble et al. [17], who have suggested that improved survival may be observed in a subset of patients with multiple positive nodes and/or large primary tumors who undergo postmastectomy irradiation in addition to chemotherapy.

These cooperative group randomized studies will surely answer major questions regarding the relative efficacy of HDC-ABMT in high-risk early breast cancer, and it is my firm opinion that such therapy should not be currently employed outside of the investigational setting. Furthermore, the results in metastatic disease with HDC-ABMT clearly indicate that there is considerable room for improvement in our current high-dose regimens. Our investigational efforts at the Johns Hopkins Oncology Center are focusing on means of inducing a greater proportion of patients with metastatic breast cancer into remission prior to consolidation therapy as well as augmenting the potency of the consolidative high-dose chemotherapy. For example, we are testing the utility of incorporating the semisynthetic vinca alkaloid navelbine into the 16-week multidrug dose-intensive induction regimen. From the standpoint of consolidation therapy, we are assessing whether a controlled graft-versus-host immunologic phenomenon induced by cyclosporine A and interferon-γ can augment the antitumor effect of high-dose chemotherapy with autologous bone marrow rescue [18]. In addition, we are studying pharmacologic means of increasing the potency of high-dose chemotherapy by utilizing the coumeromycin antibiotic novobiocin to reverse alkylating agent resistance during high-dose chemotherapy [19]. Other groups are assessing the feasibility and efficacy of the use of two or more cycles of the high-dose chemotherapy.

References

1. Early Breast Cancer Trialists' Collaborative Group (1992) Systemic treatment of early breast cancer by hormonal, cytotoxic or immune therapy. Lancet 339: 1–15, 71–84
2. Levine MN, Browman GP, Gent M et al. (1991) When is a prognostic factor useful? A guide for the perplexed. J Clin Oncol 9:348–356
3. Callahan R, Campbell G (1989) Mutations in human breast cancer: an overview. J Natl Cancer Inst 81:1780–1786
4. Bonadonna G, Valagussa P, Zambetti N et al. (1987) Milan adjuvant trials for stage I–II breast cancer. In: Salmon S (ed) Adjuvant therapy of cancer V. Grune and Stratton, New York, pp 211–221
5. Buzzoni R, Bonnadonna G, Valagussa P, Zambetti M (1991) Adjuvant chemotherapy with doxorubicin plus cyclophosphamide, methotrexate and

fluorouracil in the treatment of resectable breast cancer with more than three positive axillary nodes, J Clin Oncol 9:2134–2140

6. Teicher BA, Cucchi CA, Lee JB et al. (1986) Alkylating agents: in vitro studies of cross-resistance patterns in human cell lines. Cancer Res 46:4379–4383
7. Hryniuk W, Levine MN (1986) Analysis of dose intensity for adjuvant chemotherapy trials in stage II breast cancer. J Clin Oncol 4:1162–1170
8. Tannock IF, Boyd NF, DeBoer G et al. (1988) A randomized trial of two dose levels of cyclophosphamide, methotrexate, and fluorouracil chemotherapy for patients with metastatic breast cancer. J Clin Oncol 6:1377–1387
9. Hortobagyi GN, Buzdar AU, Bodey GP et al. (1987) High-dose induction chemotherapy of metastatic breast cancer in protected environment: a prospective randomized study. J Clin Oncol 5:178–184
10. Hortobagyi GN, Hryniuk WH, Frye D et al. (1989) Dose-intensity (DI) analysis of high-dose (HD) chemotherapy for metastatic breast cancer (MBC). Proc Am Assoc Cancer Res 30:252
11. Abeloff MD, Beveridge RE, Donehower RC et al. (1990) Sixteen-week dose-intense chemotherapy in the adjuvant treatment of breast cancer. J Natl Cancer Inst 82:1220–1221
12. Armitage JO (1990) Bone marrow transplantation in the treatment of lymphoma. Curr Opin Oncol 2:843–848
13. Henderson IC (1991) Window of opportunity. J Natl Cancer Inst 83:894–896
14. Kennedy MK, Beveridge RA, Rowley SD et al. (1991) High dose chemotherapy with reinfusion of purged autologous bone marrow following dose-intense induction as initial therapy for metastatic breast cancer. J Natl Cancer Inst 83:920–925
15. Peters WP (1991) High-dose chemotherapy and autologous bone marrow support for breast cancer. In: Devita VT Jr, Hellman S, Rosenberg SA (eds) Important advances in oncology 1991. Lippincott, Philadelphia, pp 135–150
16. Tajima T, Tokuda Y, Kubota M et al. (1990) Adjuvant chemotherapy with reinfusion of purged autologous bone marrow following dose-intense induction as initial therapy for metastatic breast cancer. Proc Am Soc Clin Oncol 9:31
17. Fowble B, Gray R, Gilchrist K et al. (1988) Identification of a subgroup of patients with breast cancer and histologically positive axillary nodes receiving adjuvant chemotherapy who may benefit from postoperative radiotherapy. J Clin Oncol 6:1107–1117
18. Geller RB, Esa AH, Beschorner WE et al. (1989) Successful in vitro graft versus tumor effect against an Ia bearing tumor using cyclosporin-induced syngeneic graft versus host disease in the rat. Blood 74:1165–1171
19. Eder JP (1989) Effect of novobiocin on the antitumor activity and tumor cell and bone marrow survivors of three alkylating agents. Cancer Res 49:595–598

Maintenance Tamoxifen After Induction Postoperative Chemotherapy in Node-Positive Breast Cancer Patients: The Eastern Cooperative Oncology Group Trials

D.C. Tormey[1], R. Gray[2], H.C. Falkson[3], K. Gilchrist[1], M.D. Abeloff[4], G. Falkson[3], and Participating Investigators

[1] University of Wisconsin Comprehensive Cancer Center, Madison, WI, USA
[2] Dana-Farber Cancer Institute, Boston, MA 02115, USA
[3] University of Pretoria, Pretoria, South Africa
[4] Johns Hopkins Oncology Center, Baltimore, MD 21205, USA

Introduction

The use of systemic chemotherapy for 1 or more years to treat women with postoperative ipsilateral node-positive (N+) breast carcinoma was begun in 1972 and 1973. The initial results from these early trials suggested an advantage for treatment with both L-phenylalanine mustard (L-Pam) and for a cyclophosphamide, methotrexate, 5-fluorouracil (CMF) combination [1, 2]. During this period the Eastern Cooperative Oncology Group (ECOG) metastatic disease trials demonstrated the superiority of CMF over L-Pam [3] and that of CMF plus prednisone (CMFP) over CMF [4]. Simultaneously, tamoxifen (Tam) became accepted as an active hormonal treatment for disseminated disease [5, 6]. The addition of Tam to an advanced-disease chemotherapy regimen was also beneficial [7]. These data led the ECOG to perform adjuvant therapy trials in N+ women that compared the therapeutic effectiveness of 1 year of CMFP plus Tam (CMFPT) to CMFP and CMF in premenopausal women, and to CMFP and observation (Obs) in postmenopausal women. The results showed no significant difference with the addition of Tam to this 1-year chemotherapy regimen [8, 9]. However, early analyses suggested an advantage for the CMFPT regimen in both pre- and postmenopausal patients. This program was thereby chosen as the control regimen for the trials reported here.

The premenopausal trial tested CMFPT against a regimen consisting of CMFPT plus fluoxymesterone in the odd-numbered cycles and a doxorubicin-containing regimen with the addition of Tam in the even-numbered cycles. The latter regimen contained vinblastine, doxorubicin, thiotepa, and fluoxymesterone (VATH). It was chosen because of its effectiveness in advanced disease [10, 11] and its different profile of drugs.

The postmenopausal trial compared 12 months of the CMFPT regimen to a 4-month regimen. Early results from other trials had suggested that 12

Recent Results in Cancer Research, Vol. 127

months was equivalent to 24 months of treatment [12], and that 6 months was equivalent to 12 months [13].

Finally, both trials also evaluated the concept of maintenance Tam therapy beyond 2 years. This concept had its inception in preclinical experiments which strongly suggested Tam to be primarily a cytostatic agent [14, 15]. These data also led to a postoperative clinical study which showed the pharmacologic feasibility and possible benefit of up to 10 years or more of postchemotherapy Tam maintenance [16, 17].

Materials and Methods

Patient Eligibility. Women were considered for entry who had infiltrating breast carcinoma pathologically of 5 cm or less and a radical or modified radical mastectomy, histopathologically N+ and a biochemical estrogen receptor (ER) assay result. Menopausal status and general eligibility criteria were as previously defined [8, 9]. In brief, the patients had surgically resectable disease, no evidence of metastases by clinical examination, laboratory test, and bone scan. They provided appropriate informed consent. Central pathologic and clinical review of eligibility was performed prospectively by the study chairman and cochairmen.

Randomization. Randomized treatment assignments in both trials for North American patients were by telephone to a central office and for others via sealed envelope [8, 9]. North American patients were stratified for induction by one to three, four to ten, or more than ten positive nodes and by ER− (<10 fm/mg protein) versus ER+ (≥10 fm/mg protein) status. The premenoapausal patients were also stratified by induction regimen for the second and third randomizations at years 1 and 5.

Treatment Regimens. Each of the induction treatment regimens consisted of cycles of therapy beginning 1–6 weeks after mastectomy. Drug dosages were as follows:

CMFPT regimen
- Cyclophosphamide 100 mg/m^2 orally, days 1–14
- Methotrexate 40 mg/m^2 intravenously, days 1 and 8
- Fluorouracil 600 mg/m^2 intravenously, days 1 and 8
- Prednisone 40 mg/m^2 orally, days 1–14
- Tamoxifen 10 mg orally, twice daily

VATH regimen
- Vinblastine 4.5 mg/m^2 intravenously, day 1
- Doxorubicin (Adiamycin) 45 mg/m^2 intravenously, day 1
- Thiotepa 12 mg/m^2 intravenously, day 1
- Fluoxymesterone (Halotestin) 10 mg orally, twice daily.

Doses were based on the patient's body surface area, which was calculated from the lesser of the patient's ideal and actual body weights. Premenopausal patients received 12 cycles of induction therapy. The CMFPT regimen was repeated each 28 days. The odd-numbered cycles of the alternating (ALTER) regimen consisted of the 28-day CMFPT regimen with the addition of fluoxymesterone; the prednisone was omitted after cycle 3. The even-numbered cycles consisted of 22-day courses of VATH and Tam. After 12 cycles of induction therapy, patients were randomized to continue Tam or to Obs for 4 additional years. In postmenopausal patients treatment consisted of the CMFPT regimen delivered for 4 or 12 cycles or 12 cycles followed by Tam for 4 additional years. In patients older than 60 years, the methotrexate dose was modified if creatinine clearance was abnormal. For creatinine clearances of more than 70 ml/min, 40 mg/m^2 was administered; for 50–69, 30 mg/m^2, for 30–49, 20 mg/m^2; and for less than 30,10 mg/m^2. In both studies patients disease-free on Tam 5 years after initial randomization were again randomized to continue Tam or to Obs. Analysis of the data from this latter randomization is still too imcomplete to report.

Drug Dosage Modifications. The CMF and VAT doses in subsequent cycles were reduced by 25% if the nadir WBC was under 2000/mm^3 or nadir platelet count under 75 000/mm^3, and increased by 25% if the nadir WBC was over 3500/mm^3 and nadir platelet count over 125 000/mm^3. Treatment delays of up to 2 weeks were allowed prior to each cycle to allow for recovery from hematologic toxicity. On days 1 and 8 of each cycle CMF and VAT doses were reduced to 50% if the WBC was no higher than 4000/mm^3 or platelet count no higher than 100 000/mm^3, and omitted if the WBC was under 2500/mm^3 or platelet count under 75 000/mm^3. Dosage modification guidelines for gastrointestinal, bladder, renal, hepatic, and neurologic toxicity were also specified but seldom required. If steroid-related toxicity occurred, the prednisone dose was reduced.

Patient Evaluation. During the 1st year follow-up included a history and physical examination, blood counts, BUN or creatinine, and glucose prior to day 1 of each cycle; blood counts prior to day 8 of each cycle; bilirubin, alkaline phosphatase, SGOT, serum calcium, and chest X-ray every 3 months; a bone scan every 6 months; and a mammogram after 12 months. Thereafter, the patients were scheduled for a clinic visit with blood studies every 3 months, a chest X-ray every 6 months, and a bone scan and mammography every 12 months.

Patient Evaluability. There were 658 patients randomized to the premenopausal trial and 962 to the postmenopausal trial. Patients were excluded from the primary analyses due to inadequate data, refusal of all treatment, and ineligibility characteristics. In the majority of these prestudy tests were abnormal or not done, or tumors larger than 5 cm or with muscle or dermal

Table 1. Patient characteristics

Characteristic	Premenopausal Trial				Postmenopausal Trial		
	Induction		Maintenance				
	ALTER	CMFPT	Tam	Obs	×12 → T	×12	×4
Axillary N+ >3	47%	46%	46%	46%	52%	50%	51%
ER positive	63%	63%	67%	64%	70%	68%	71%
PgR positive	57%	52%	55%	59%	43%	43%	39%
Tp <3.0 cm	52%	52%	57%	50%	58%	59%	62%
Age (median, years)	44	42	44	42	60	60	61

lymphatic invasion. The 532 analyzed premenopausal cases were distributed with 262 randomized to CMFPT, 270 to ALTER, and subsequently 201 to continue Tam and 195 to Obs. The median follow-up was 6.1 years for the induction regimens and 5.0 years for the maintenance Tam and Obs randomization. There were CMFPT × 12 → Tam; median follow-up was 5.9 years.

Statistical Methods. Analyses measured both time to relapse (TTR) and survival from the time of randomization to relapse or death. The date of relapse was taken as that of the first evidence of subsequently documented relapse. Amenorrhea was defined as at least 6 months without menstrual activity. Separate TTR and survival treatment comparisons were also performed analyzing all randomized entries and again by counting non-disease-related deaths as failures. The results of these analyses were similar to those obtained from the major analyses. The statistical methods and definitions used were similar to those previously described [8, 9]. All p values are from two-tailed tests, and the level of significance was set at $p \leq 0.05$.

Patient Characteristics. The major patient characteristics were well balanced among the treatment ragimens (Table 1). These and other characteristics were controlled for in the treatment comparison analyses, where appropriate.

Results

TTR Treatment Comparisons

The estimated 5-year relapse-free survival of premenopausal patients was 71% among those receiving ALTER therapy and 64% in the CMFPT group ($p = 0.03$; Table 2). The strongest trend among the stratified subgroups

Table 2. Five-year relapse-free survival in the premenopausal trial

Group	Induction				Maintenance			
	n	ALTER	CMFPT	Log rank *p* value	*n*	Tam	Obs	Log rank *p* value
Overall	532	71%	64%	0.03	396	74%	64%	0.03
ER status								
Positive	334	78%	69%	0.06	258	80%	69%	0.02
Negative	198	59%	55%	0.24	138	61%	56%	0.48
No. positive nodes								
1–3	284	77%	74%	0.22	214	81%	70%	0.04
>3	248	63%	51%	0.07	182	65%	57%	0.28

Table 3. Five-year relapse-free survival in the postmenopausal trial

Group	*n*	×12 → T	×12	×4	Log rank *p* value
Overall	804	65%	57%	56%	0.02
ER status					
Positive	561	68%	60%	57%	0.02
Negative	243	58%	52%	53%	0.56
No. positive nodes					
1–3	393	84%	70%	65%	0.003
>3	411	48%	45%	47%	0.60

favored ALTER therapy among the ER+ patients (78% versus 69%; $p = 0.06$).

During maintenance those premenopausal patients randomized to continue Tam had an estimated 5-year relapse-free survival of 74% compared to 64% for those randomized to Obs ($p = 0.03$; Table 3). This difference was significant in the ER+ strata (80% versus 69%; $p = 0.02$) but not in the ER− strata (61% versus 56%; $p = 0.48$).

The estimated TTR in the postmenopausal patients was longer for patients on CMFPT × 12 plus continuous Tam than for those on CMFPT × 4 ($p = 0.005$) or CMFPT × 12 ($p = 0.08$). As in the premenopausal trial, the results were significantly different in the ER+ strata ($p = 0.02$) but not in the ER− strata ($p = 0.56$). The difference between 4 or 12 cycles of CMFPT was not significant. The 5-year estimated relapse-free rates were 65% for CMFPT × 12 plus continuous Tam, 57% for CMFPT × 12, and 56% for CMFPT × 4 (Table 3).

Survival Treatment Comparisons

The overall estimated 5-year survival rate in the premenopausal trial was 80% for the ALTER group and 76% for the CMFPT group ($p = 0.31$).

The 5-year overall survival rate was 83% for the Tam-maintained group compared with 76% for the Obs group ($p = 0.38$). The differences among the various induction and maintenance strata were also not significant at this time. The survival results in the postmenopausal trial were similar in that there were currently no significant differences in survival between the three regimens or among the stratified subgroups. The overall 5-year survival rates were 71% for CMFPT × 12 → Tam, 73% for CMFPT × 12, and 72% for CMFPT × 4.

Effect of Prognostic Factors

The effect of pretreatment characteristics upon TTR were analyzed, unadjusted by the log rank procedure and then by a proportional hazards multivariate model. A shorter TTR in the premenopausal trial was associated with increasing number of positive nodes ($p < 0.001$), ER− status ($p < 0.001$), decreasing age ($p = 0.001$), induction CMFPT ($p = 0.04$), and progesterone receptor negative (PgR−) status ($p = 0.09$). Patients developing amenorrhea for 6 months or longer during therapy had a longer TTR (log rank, $p = 0.04$), with the effect being qualitatively similar in ER+ and ER− patients. The disease-free proportion at 5 years with amenorrhea versus without was: overall 74% versus 63%; ER+ 79% versus 69%; and ER− 64% versus 52%. Shorter survivals in a proportional hazards multivariate model were associated with increasing number of positive nodes (<0.001), ER− assay ($p = 0.006$), PgR− assay ($p = 0.007$), and increasing primary tumor size ($p = 0.02$). Patients developing amenorrhea during therapy had a better survival (log rank, $p = 0.04$) with qualitatively similar effects in ER+ and ER− patients. The proportion alive at 5 years with amenorrhea versus without was: overall 86% versus 78%; ER+ 94% versus 87%; and ER− 71% versus 63%.

The association of hormone receptor status and number of positive nodes with TTR and survival was also highly significant in the postmenopausal trial. A shorter TTR and survival are associated with increasing number of positive nodes ($p < 0.0001$, $p < 0.0001$), ER− status ($p = 0.0004$, $p = 0.0003$) and PgR− status ($p = 0.02$, $p = 0.0001$). Because the administration of at least 5 years of Tam was part of the initial randomization, this variable was also analyzed and was found to be associated with an improved TTR ($p = 0.03$).

Sites of First Relapse and Causes of Death

The sites of first relapse with each regimen were categorized as local-regional or distant. There were no statistical differences in the relapse patterns between the premenopausal induction regimens, although the ALTER regimen tended to have fewer local-regional (6% versus 9%) and distant (18% versus 23%) only recurrences. The Tam maintenance regimen in premenopausal patients was associated with fewer local-regional relapses (4.0%) than the Obs group (10.2%; $p = 0.02$). In the postmenopausal patients there was also a trend toward fewer local-regional relapses with maintenance Tam (7%) than with Obs (14% and 11%).

The major cause of death in all groups in both trials was breast cancer (336 patients). Only 49 patients died from other causes.

Side Effects During Treatment

In the premenopausal patients a significantly higher incidence of the following side effects were observed with the ALTER regimen: acne/skin, allergic, nausea/emesis, alopecia, hirsutism, peripheral nervous system, and joint pains. The CMFPT regimen was associated with a significantly higher incidence of anemia, thrombocytopenia, infection, cushingoid changes, insomnia, weight gain, and eye complaints. Various mild or moderate side effects were observed in 40% of the CMFPT group and 40% of the ALTER group, whereas severe or life-threatening events occurred in, respectively, 60% and 58%. There was one death on CMFPT associated with a WBC of 900/mm^3 and a mesenteric venous occlusion occurring in cycle 3. The ALTER regimen was associated with four deaths due to intracranial vascular events (cycles 1, 1, 3, and 7). The percentage of patients not completing induction therapy for reasons other than relapse was 21% for CMFPT and 18% for ALTER therapy.

The use of maintenance Tam in the premenopausal trial was associated with significantly more hot flashes (67% versus 53%; $p = 0.008$) but less bone pain (6% versus 12%; $p = 0.05$). Three patients developed amenorrhea during maintenance Tam and five on Obs; however, of the patients developing amenorrhea during induction or maintenance, 15% of the Obs and 18% of the Tam patients resumed menstruating.

Nine second non-breast cancers were reported in the premenopausal trial. These were endometrial carcinomas [2], sarcoma, colorectal carcinoma, left conjunctival squamous cell carcinoma in situ, ovarian, melanoma, basal cell carcinoma, and leukemia.

The most common side effects in the postmenopausal trial were hematologic, nausea and vomiting and alopecia. In general, there were fewer side effects among those patients receiving four courses of CMFPT than in those receiving 12. In addition, 31% of patients receiving 12 cycles and 22% of those receiving 4 cycles had hot flashes. There were 77 cases reported with life-threatening toxicity and 7 with lethal toxicities. In three patients death was attributed to a thromboembolic event, three other patients died with severe hemopoietic depression and septicemia, and one died of acute pancreatitis. Thrombotic or embolic events occurred in 10.6%

of patients receiving 12 cycles and 6.9% of those receiving 4 cycles. Side effects reported for patients on continuous Tam after 12 months were qualitatively similiar to those reported in the Obs groups.

There were 27 cases of second primaries other than breast cancer reported in the postmenopausal trial with 11 on CMFPT × 4, 7 on CMFPT × 12, and 9 on CMFPT × 12 → T. On the CMFPT × 4 and ×12 programs these were colorectal (5), head and neck (1), leukemia (1), melanoma (1), skin (4), cervical (2), uterine (1), endometrium (1), and kidney (1). The second cancers on the CMFPT × 12 → T regimen were pancreas (1), colorectal (1), lung (1), skin (3), uterine (1), endometrium (1), and kidney (1).

Drug Dosing During Treatment

In the premenopausal trial at least six cycles of induction therapy was delivered to 88% of patients on ALTER and 89% of those on CMFPT. Twelve cycles were delivered to 78% on ALTER and 74% on CMFPT. Drug dosing in individual patients was evaluated in random order for 392 of the 533 eligible premenopausal patients. The average dose of CMF delivered during the odd-numbered cycles in each of the induction regimens was similar (Wilcoxon ranked sums test). The average dose of prednisone in cycles 1 and 3 was 95.1% and 80.9% with CMFPT and 97.1% and 83.0% with ALTER therapy. These analyses indexed all analyzable patients regardless of whether they received therapy as long as they had not relapsed. Treatment interruption due to relapse led to censoring of the subsequent data. The percentage ideal dose was 100 times the actual dose divided by the protocol ideal dose, where the protocol ideal did not take into account dose modifications. For CMF these were calculated separately for each drug and averaged. The proportion of premenopausal patients discontinuing Tam for reasons other than relapse during induction was 14%, most due to stopping all therapy. The proportion discontinuing Tam during the first 5 years of maintenance was 9%, and during years 1–5 after the maintenance randomization was, respectively, 1.6%, 3.2%, 0.6%, 0.7%, and 2.1%.

For postmenopausal patients randomized to receive four cycles, 10.7% were given one to three cycles, 87% were given four cycles, and 2.3% were given more than four cycles. For patients randomized to receive 12 cycles, 10.3% were given 1 to 4 cycles, 16.8% were given 5 to 11 cycles, and 72% were given all 12 cycles. Disease-free survival and overall survival analyses were based on patients as randomized, not as drugs received. The proportion of postmenopausal patients discontinuing Tam for reasons other than relapse during induction was 14%, most due to stopping all therapy. The proportion discontinuing Tam during years 1–5 of maintenance was, respectively, 3.3%, 0.7%, 1.5%, 2.9%, and 5.9%.

Discussion

An overall TTR benefit was a demonstrated in our trials with a doxorubicin-containing regimen in premenopausal women and with the continuation of Tam maintenance for at least 5 years in both permenopausal and postmenopausal patients. There is also no evidence that treatment of postmenopausal women with 12 courses of CMFPT is superior to that of 4 courses. The results with the doxorubicin-containing regimen provides additional evidence that such regimens are superior to non-doxorubicin-containing regimens in postoperative patients [18, 19]. The Tam maintenance results verifies preclinical experiments [14] as well as the early clinical suggestions of its effectiveness [16]. The relative reduction of local-regional relapses in the Tam-maintained patients also suggests a role for the drug in the preventing of second breast cancers or of breast cancer in high-risk cohorts of women. Despite this observation it appears that the incidence of distant recurrences continues to be the major therapeutic problem following the diagnosis of breast carcinoma.

Several trials [12, 13, 20, 21] addressing the issue of duration of adjuvant therapy have shown no advantage for more than 6 months of chemotherapy. However, one study showed a significant survival advantage for patients randomized to 36 weeks of CMFVP compared with those given 12 weeks of CMFVP followed by single-agent doxorubicin [22]. The results reported here show that neither TTR nor survival are significantly different for 4 or 12 months of CMFPT in postmenopausal patients.

The results from the present trials further support reports of the prognostic importance of the number of nodes involved, ER status, and size of the primary tumor [23–26]. In keeping with our previous data [8], we observed a greater therapeutic effect among premenopausal patients developing amenorrhea. This implies that the induction of an ovarian ablation contributes to the therapeutic effect of adjuvant therapy in premenopausal patients and should be explored prospectively.

Side effects with the various regimens were as expected from previous ECOG trials, including the non significant reduction of side effects with 4 as compared to 12 courses of therapy.

Based on the results of these and other studies, ECOG is currently participating in trials to further evaluate the role of maintenance hormone therapy in both N− and N+ pre- and postmenopausal patients. The N− trial also includes an evaluation of CMF versus CAF. In ER− N+ patients an "aggressive" CAMF plus leucovorin factor chemotherapy regimen is compared to a standard CAF regimen.

In summary, the present premenopausal trial provides evidence that the incorporation of a doxorubicin-containing regimen in the induction chemotherapy program provides an improvement in the therapeutic effect. Both the pre- and postmenopausal trials provide strong evidence for incorporating a maintenance program using at least 5 years of Tam. The benefit from this approach appears to be most pronounced in ER+ patients.

Acknowledgements. The authors gratefully acknowledge the participation of all the involved ECOG investigators and their patients. These studies were conducted by the Eastern Cooperative Oncology Group (Douglass C. Tormey, M.D, Ph.D., Chairman) and was supported by Public Health Service grants from the National Cancer Institute, the National Institutes of Health, and the Department of Health and Human Services.

References

1. Fisher B, Carbone P, Economou SG, Frelick R, Glass A, Lerner H, Redmond C, Zelen M, Band P, Katrych DL, Wolmark N, Fisher ER (1975) L-Phenylalanine mustard (L-PAM) in the management of primary breast cancer. N Engl J Med 292:117–122
2. Bonadonna G, Brusamolino E, Valagussa P, Rossi A, Brugnatelli L, Brambilla C, DeLena M, Tancini G, Bajetta E, Musumeci R, Veronesi V (1976) Combination chemotherapy as an adjuvant treatment in operable breast cancer. N Engl J Med 294:405–410
3. Canellos GP, Pocock SJ, Taylor SG III, Sears ME, Klaasen DJ, Band PR (1976) Combination chemotherapy for metastatic breast carcinoma. Prospective comparison of multiple drug therapy with L-phenylalanine mustard. Cancer 38:1882–1886
4. Tormey DC, Gelman R, Band PR, Sears M, Rosenthal SN, DeWys W, Perlia C, Rice MA (1982) Comparison of induction chemotherapies for metastatic breast cancer: An Eastern Cooperative Oncology Group trial. Cancer 50:1235–1244
5. Ward HWC (1973) Anti-oestrogen therapy for breast cancer: a trial of tamoxifen at two dose levels. Br Med J 1:13–14
6. Tormey DC, Simon RM, Lippman ME, Bull JM, Myers CE (1976) Evaluation of tamoxifen dose in advanced breast cancer: a progress report. Cancer Treat Rep 60:1451–1459
7. Tormey DC, Falkson G, Crowley J, Falkson HC, Voelkel J, Davis TE (1982) Dibromodulcitol and Adriamycin ± tamoxifen in advanced breast cancer. Cancer Clin Trials 5:33–39
8. Tormey DC, Gray R, Gichrist K, Grage T, Carbone PP, Wolter J, Woll JE, Cummings FJ (1990) Adjuvant chemohormonal therapy with cyclophosphamide, methotrexate, fluorouracil, prednisone (CMFP) or CMFP plus temoxifen compared to CMF for premenopausal breast cancer patients – An Eastern Cooperative Oncology Group trial. Cancer 65:200–206
9. Taylor SG IV, Knuiman M, Olson JE, Tormey DC, Gilchrist KW, Falkson G, Rosenthal SN, Sleeper LA, Carbone PP, Cummings FJ (1989) Six year results of the Eastern Cooperative Oncology Group trial of observation versus CMFP versus CMFPT in postmenopausal patients with node positive breast cancer. J Clin Oncol 7:879–889
10. Hart RD, Perloff M, Holland JF (1981) One-day VATH (vinblastine, Adriamycin, thioTEPA, and halotestin) therapy for advanced breast cancer refractory to chemotherapy. Cancer 48:1522–1527
11. Skeel RT, Andersen JW, Tormey DC, Benson AB III, Asbury RF, Falkson G (1989) Combination chemotherapy of advanced breast cancer: comparison of

dibromodulcitol, Adriamycin, vincristine, and halotestin to thiotepa, Adriamycin, vinblastine, and halotestin. An Eastern Cooperative Oncology Group study. Cancer 64:1393–1399

12. Jungi WF, Alberto P, Brunner KW, Mermillod B, Barrelet L, Cavalli F (1984) Short- or long-term chemotherapy for node positive breast cancer: LMF 6 versus 18 cycles. SAKK study 27/76. Recent Results Cancer Res 96:175–177
13. Bonadonna G, Valagussa P, Rossi A, Tancini G, Brambilla C, Zambetti M, Veronesi U (1985) Ten-year experience with CMF-based adjuvant chemotherapy in resectable breast cancer. Breast Cancer Res Treat 5:95–115
14. Jordan VC, Dix CJ, Allen KE (1979) The effectiveness of long-term tamoxifen treatment in a laboratory model for adjuvant hormone therapy of breast cancer. In: Jones SE, Salmon SE (eds) Adjuvant therapy of cancer II. Grune and Stratton, New York, pp 19–26
15. Green MD, Whybourne AM, Taylor IW, Sutherland RL (1981) Effects of antioestrogens on the growth and cell cycle kinetics of cultured human mammary carcinoma cells. In: Sutherland RL, Jordan VC (eds) Nonsteroidal antioestrogens: molecular pharmacology and antitumour activity. Academic, Sydney, pp 397–412
16. Tormey DC, Jordan VC (1984) A long-term tamoxifen adjuvant therapy in node positive breast cancer – a metabolic and pilot clinical study. Breast Cancer Res Treat 4:297–302
17. Langan-Fahey SM, Tormey DC, Jordan VC (1990) Tamoxifen metabolites in patients on long-term adjuvant therapy for breast cancer. Eur J Cancer 26:883–888
18. Misset JL, de Vassal F, Jasmis C et al. (1984) Five-year results of the French adjuvant trial for breast cancer comparing CMF to a combination of Adriamycin (ADM), vincristine (VCR), cyclophosphamide (CPM), and 5-fluorouracile (5FU). In: Jones SE, Salmon SE (eds) Adjuvant therapy of cancer IV. Grune and Stratton, Orlando, pp 243–251
19. Fisher B, Redmond C, Wicherham DL, Bowman D, Schipper H, Wolmark N, Sass R, Fisher ER, Jochimsen P, Legault-Poisson S, Dimitrov N, Wolter J, Bornstein R, Elias EG, Licalzi N, Sutherland CM, Paterson AHG (1989) Doxorubicin-containing regimens for the treatment of stage II breast cancer: the National Surgical Adjuvant Breast and Bowel Project experience. J Clin Oncol 7:572–582
20. Henderson IC, Gelman RS, Harris JR, Canellos GP (1986) Duration of therapy in adjuvant chemotherapy trials. Natl Cancer Inst Monogr 95–98
21. Velez-Garcia E, Moore M, Vogel CL, Marcial V, Ketcham A, Raney M, Smalley R (1984) Post-surgical adjuvant chemotherapy in women with breast cancer and positive axillary nodes. The Southeastern Cancer Study Group (SECSG) experience. In: Jones SE, Salmon SE (eds) Adjuvant therapy of cancer IV. Grune and Stratton, Philadelphia, pp 273–282
22. Levine M, Bush H, Gent W, Hryniuk W, Levin L (1988) A randomized controlled trial comparing 12 weeks with 36 weeks of adjuvant chemotherapy in stage II breast cancer (Abstr) Proc Am Soc Clin Oncol 7:8
23. Tormey DC, Weinberg VE, Holland JF, Weiss RB, Glidewell OJ, Perloff M, Falkson G, Falkson HC, Henry PH, Leone LA, Rafla S, Ginsberg SJ, Silver RT, Blom J, Carey RW, Schein PS, Lesnick GJ (1983) A randomized trial of five and three drug chemotherapy and chemoimmunotherapy in women with operable node positive breast cancer. J Clin Oncol 1:138–145
24. Tancini G, Bonadonna G, Valagussa P, Marchini S, Veronesi U (1983) Adjuvant CMF in breast cancer: comparative 5-year results of 12 versus 6 cycles. J Clin Oncol 1:2–10

25. Glucksberg H, Rivkin SE, Rasmussen S, Tranum B, Gad-El-Mawla N, Costanzi J, Hoogstraten B, Athens J, Maloney T, McCracken J, Vaughn C (1982) Combination chemotherapy (CMFVP) versus L-phenylalanine mustard (L-PAM) for operable breast cancer with positive axillary nodes. Cancer 50:423–434
26. Fisher B, Slack NH, Bross DJ (1969) Cancer of the breast: size of neoplasm and prognosis. Cancer 24:1071–1080

Adjuvant Systemic Therapy: Overview

I.C. Henderson

University of California San Francisco, San Francisco, CA 94143, USA

Seeing the results of a meta-analysis or overview for the first time is somewhat like a first peep through a microscope. One's initial reaction is likely to be awe, disorientation, or a combination of these. Because of the large number of patients studied in many trials addressing an identical or nearly identical question, an overview that includes all of these patients allows us to detect small or modest effects of therapy that are not always apparent when the data from a single study are evaluated. The increased statistical power resulting from so many events means that differences between the treated and control groups that might not have been apparent at all in a single study of ordinary size, or which would not have been statistically significant in a very large study are not only easily seen but are associated with a *p* value preceded by many zeros. This level of statistical significance provides assurance that these differences are unlikely to have occurred by chance alone. However, this level of statistical significance may also lead us erroneously to conclude that the differences are much larger than they really are. Confusion arises not only because the process is new to most of us, but because such a large data set allows multiple analyses of the effects of therapy in subsets of patients. To the physician accustomed to absorbing a few major conclusions from a single clinical trial, this enormous buffet of data is often difficult to digest and, at the very least, requires a substantial expenditure of time.

The first overviews of adjuvant system therapy were performed 8 years ago. Prior to that time it was apparent from individual studies that the use of either adjuvant chemotherapy or adjuvant tamoxifen significantly prolongs the time to recurrence in both younger and older women. However, it was not so certain that the survival of these patients was prolonged, as well. The overviews have confirmed the survival advantage resulting from the use of chemotherapy in younger women, and the size of the effect is nearly as large as that suggested by the first Milan trial. The survival advantage from the use of adjuvant tamoxifen in older women is now equally well established,

Recent Results in Cancer Research, Vol. 127

and the size of the benefit is similar to that of the NATO study in the United Kingdom, the first group to report a survival advantage from using adjuvant tamoxifen. It seems likely that the greatest impact of the overviews on the practice of medical oncology has been the nearly universal acceptance of tamoxifen as adjuvant treatment for older women, at least for the approximately 80% of older women whose tumors are estrogen receptor positive. The overview effectively eliminated doubts about the power of relatively nontoxic endocrine therapy to kill a large enough number of tumor cells and to prolong patient survival. It is not clear that the worldwide use of adjuvant chemotherapy has increased proportionately, probably because it is associated with greater acute toxicity and is more difficult to administer than tamoxifen.

Other results suggested by individual trials and confirmed by the overviews include:

- Chemotherapy is one half to one third as effective in older as it is in younger women.
- The effects of tamoxifen are less striking in younger than older women, and thus far the use of tamoxifen among women aged under age 50 years has not been shown to result in a statistically significant overall survival advantage, especially when it is used in conjunction with chemotherapy.
- The benefits derived from shorter courses of chemotherapy are at least as great as those from longer courses.
- Combinations of cytotoxic agents are more effective than the use a single drug.
- The benefits of adjuvant tamoxifen are considerably larger in women whose tumors have an estrogen receptor, but no group of *older* women for whom there is no benefit from the use of adjuvant tamoxifen can be identified.
- The *proportional* effects of this therapy are nearly the same in all groups defined by the presence or absence of histologically involved lymph nodes, but the greatest *absolute* benefits are in those patient groups with the greatest likelihood of having disease recurrence.

Some of the results of the overview were largely unanticipated by all but a few prescient investigators. These include:

- The survival benefits from both adjuvant chemotherapy and adjuvant tamoxifen have persisted for up to 10 years at levels as large or larger than those observed at the end of the first 5 years of follow-up.
- The survival benefits from adjuvant ovarian ablation are statistically significant and persist well beyond the first decade of follow-up.
- Adjuvant tamoxifen reduces the probability of developing a new breast cancer in the contralateral breast.
- Adjuvant tamoxifen significantly reduces nonbreast cancer mortality, especially mortality from vascular disease, as well as reducing thc probability of recurrence and death from breast cancer.

Almost as long as there have been physicians, comparisons have been made between the results obtained by one physician, by one group of investigators, or in one trial with those of another. These are called *indirect* comparisons, and in general they are less reliable than direct comparisons obtained by randomizing patients to one or another treatment. Differences in outcome between groups compared indirectly are as likely to result from confounding factors, such as the patient mix, as they are from differences in the therapy used. Although some investigators would argue that indirect comparisons made between two randomized trials or within the context of an overview are more valid than indirect comparisons made between nonrandomized trials or between other types of studies, few, if any, would argue that indirect comparisons have as much validity as direct comparisons. In the recently published overview (reprinted in part in this volume) there are multiple opportunities for such indirect comparisons, and this is a valuable source of new hypotheses that can be formally evaluated in future randomized trials. However, there is also considerable danger that these indirect comparisons will remove uncertainty in the minds of most physicians, lead to premature or inappropriate changes in clinical practice, and actually discourage the conducting of formal trials to evaluate the hypothesis. Among the most important of these indirect comparisons are;

- Adjuvant ovarian ablation appears to be as effective as adjuvant chemotherapy among younger women.
- Longer durations of adjuvant tamoxifen appear to be more effective than shorter durations. When these comparisons are made separately among younger and older women, however, the optimal duration of tamoxifen treatment appears to be somewhat different. Among older women, there is a substantially greater effect of tamoxifen in those trials utilizing 2 years of tamoxifen compared to those using 1 year, but no additional benefit was apparent in those trials utilizing more than 2 years of tamoxifen compared to those using only 2 years. The number of younger women enrolled in tamoxifen studies is smaller and the results less certain, but no significant benefits from adjuvant tamoxifen therapy were seen among younger women in trials utilizing either 1 or 2 years of adjuvant tamoxifen. However, there was an apparent effect in those trials in which tamoxifen therapy was continued beyond 2 years.
- The results of trials using a combination of adjuvant chemotherapy plus tamoxifen were superior to those using either tamoxifen alone or chemotherapy alone in older women; trials of adjuvant ovarian ablation plus chemotherapy produced a greater survival benefit than those using either alone in younger women. On the other hand, these indirect comparisons suggest that tamoxifen plus chemotherapy is no better than chemotherapy alone in younger women. Multiple trials addressing these issues are ongoing in various parts of the world, and the data from these studies should serve as the basis of a direct comparison in the next overview. Thus far, the overviews have not assessed the relative effects of a com-

bination of hormone therapy plus chemotherapy compared to hormone therapy alone (either tamoxifen or ovarian ablation) among younger women because no randomized trials have been performed addressing this question.

As a result of the overview, some questions hotly debated only a few years ago can be considered to have been answered definitely. The survival benefits of adjuvant tamoxifen in older women and adjuvant chemotherapy in younger women are both real and large enough that few physicians would withhold these therapies, especially from women with a substantial risk of recurrence. Remaining questions, such as those suggested by the indirect comparisons, should and are being subjected to randomized trials. Under the best or circumstances, the additional months or years of life that a woman gains from undergoing adjuvant therapy is modest, and there is considerable room for the introduction of much more effective treatments. However, there are important issues that cannot be addressed by an overview, and that require the traditional judgment of the clinician at the bedside weighing the observed benefits against the toxicities, known and as yet unknown, that the patient is likely to experience. Is a 10% reduction in the odds of death, which might equal an average prolongation of life in the range of 6–12 months, worth the side effects of chemotherapy? Is it reasonable to use these treatments in a woman who has a 90% likelihood of 10 year survival without additional treatment? Overviews are not meant to address these questions but rather to provide additional information of value to the individual physician answering these questions with his/her patient.

VI. Quality-of-Life Considerations in the Adjuvant Setting

Assessment of Quality of Life and Benefits from Adjuvant Therapies in Breast Cancer

N.K. Aaronson

The Netherlands Cancer Institute, Division of Psychosocial Research and Epidemiology, Plesmanlaan 121, 1066 CX Amsterdam, The Netherlands

Introduction

The traditional outcome parameters employed in clinical research in oncology include tumor response, local recurrence rate, development of metastatic disease, disease-free and overall survival, and, in the case of palliative therapies, the control of major physical symptoms. Increasingly, however, there is interest in incorporating a broader set of evaluation criteria that reflect the impact of the disease and of its treatment on the functional, psychological, and social health of the individual patient.

Nowhere is this interest in cancer patients' quality of life more evident than in the field of breast cancer research. Over the past 15 years an extensive body of both descriptive and evaluative research has been generated that details the range of physical and psychosocial effects, both acute and chronic, of breast cancer and its treatment. The large majority of these studies has concerned the impact of surgery alone or, more recently, of limited surgery plus radiotherapy on patients' quality of life (see [26, 29] for recent reviews).

Increasing attention has been directed toward the quality of life of patients undergoing adjuvant therapy following primary surgical treatment [16, 30, 32]. This seems particularly appropriate given the significant patient burden associated with such therapies, both in the short-term (i.e., acute drug toxicity) and long-term (e.g., chronic fatigue, premature onset of menopause with concomitant emotional, psychosexual, and interpersonal problems). As the potential population of patients deemed eligible for adjuvant therapy expands (e.g., node-negative patients), the relevance of quality-of-life considerations becomes all the greater. Targeted information on the quality-of-life impact of such therapies can aid clinicians and patients alike in the complex task of weighing the costs of treatment against the potential benefits in terms of disease-free and overall survival.

Recent Results in Cancer Research, Vol. 127

To be of optimal value, however, quality-of-life data need to be generated in as standardized a manner as possible. This is particularly important in the realm of clinical trial-based quality-of-life investigations. Only by employing common methodologies can we ever hope to build a coherent database for comparison of results across studies. Yet, a review of the limited number of clinical trials of adjuvant therapy in breast cancer in which quality of life has been evaluated reveals a striking lack of standardization of methodology. This is particularly the case in those studies that employ a classical psychometric approach (i.e., the use of questionnaires) to quality-of-life assessment. Across nine such studies, 14 different measures were used to assess various aspects of the patients' quality of life. Four of these studies relied primarily on ad hoc, study-specific, quality-of-life measures. While the remaining investigations employed instruments with known validity and reliability, there is virtually no overlap across these studies in terms of the measures used [3, 7, 22, 24, 31, 33, 34, 36, 43].

In the hope of fostering greater standardization of methods in assessing the quality of life of breast cancer patients undergoing adjuvant therapy, this paper provides a brief review of some of the more salient methodological considerations involved in such assessments. Areas are identified in which a fair degree of consensus has been achieved, as well as those in which controversy still exists. Where appropriate, recommendations are made for improving the feasibility and practically of clinical trial-based quality-of-life investigations.

Sources of Quality-of-Life Data

The quality of life of breast cancer patients can be assessed by the health care provider, by the patient herself, or by someone close to the patient such as a partner or other family member. Historically, it has most often been the physician who has provided such assessments, albeit in a limited way. Thus, for example, in oncological trials clinicians are asked routinely to rate the performance status of their patients and the acute side effects of treatment. Other physician-based rating systems have been developed that address a broader set of quality-of-life issues, including emotional and social functioning [41].

While it may require significantly less time and effort to complete a rating form oneself than to arrange for patients to be interviewed or to fill out a questionnaire, the available evidence suggests that such efficiency is achieved at a high cost in terms of methodological rigor. Numerous studies have documented low levels of interobserver reliability and, perhaps more importantly, low levels of agreement between ratings provided by physicians and those by patients themselves [25, 37].

For this reason, it is widely acknowledged today that the patient herself should be the principle source of information on her quality of life. This is clearly appropriate when one is interested in assessing such subjective experiences as pain, fatigue, or emotional distress. Yet, even in the case of more readily observable symptoms (e.g., chemotherapy-induced alopecia), direct patient feedback may provide important insights into their meaning and impact on the patient's daily life.

Patients may sometimes underreport the problems that they are experiencing due to feelings of embarrassment (e.g., sexual dysfunction) or out of a desire to be seen as a "good" patient (e.g., by stoically accepting physical side effects of treatment). In such cases, feedback provided by a partner or other family member can yield useful supplementary information regarding the patient's level of functioning. Typically, however, the use of such informants is reserved for studies involving very young or very ill patients who are not able or willing to provide such information themselves, or for descriptive studies focused specifically on the impact of cancer on the family system. In clinical trials, where resources are limited and logistics complicated, such forms of "triangulated" data collection are seldom feasible.

Defining Quality of Life

Just as cancer is a collective term for some 100 forms of disease [6], so is quality of life a nonspecific term referring to a set of related, interacting issues. Indeed, quality of life is an elusive concept that defies precise definition. As Feinstein [14] has stated: "the idea has become a kind of umbrella under which are placed many different indexes dealing with whatever the user wants to focus on."

One way of circumventing the definitional problem is to leave the task up to the individual patient. For example, Gough et al. [20] suggested that one need ask only a single question in evaluating cancer patients' quality of life: "How would you rate your quality of life today?" While perhaps seductive in its simplicity, such an approach begs the issue of utility. While it may be useful to generate a summary quality-of-life score for certain tasks (e.g., for calculating quality-adjusted life years; see below), more specific information is required in order to understand such global ratings. How are we to make sense of a patient reporting a low overall quality of life? Does it imply limitations in functional capacity, intolerable symptoms levels, depression, social isolation, or a combination of such factors?

The World Health Organization [49] definition of health as "a state of complete physical, mental and social well-being, and not merely the absence of disease and infirmity" has withstood the test of time, providing a useful conceptual anchor for those working in the field of quality-of-life assessment. In fact, the only real definitional refinement that has been introduced in the past 40 years is the recommendation that, in clinical studies, we restrict ourselves to issues that are both health-relevant and potentially sensitive to health care interventions [40, 46, 47].

Within such a health-related framework, a review of the literature suggests that quality of life is most often approached as a *multidimensional* construct, reflecting minimally the following four domains: (a) disease-related and treatment-related physical symptoms, (b) physical functioning, (c) psychological functioning, and (d) social and role functioning. Beyond this basic set of domains, additional psychosocial topics are often included in assessment batteries that are of relevance to particular patient populations (e.g., sexuality and body image impairment, fear of disease recurrence, etc.) [8, 11].

The use of such a multidimensional approach to quality-of-life assessment carries with it two principal advantages over a more global measurement strategy. First, it allows one to disentangle the positive and negative effects of (competing) treatments. It is seldom the case that one treatment offers clear, consistent advantages over its alternatives. Rather, we are most typically confronted with a number of trade-offs (e.g., heightened acute toxicity versus milder but more chronic treatment side effects). Second, it facilitates the detection of changing patterns of effect over the disease and treatment trajectory. For example, during the initial treatment phase, patients undergoing chemotherapy may be most distressed by acute toxicities (e.g., nausea and vomiting) while other concerns (e.g., chronic fatigue, fear of recurrence, sexual dysfunction) may emerge only much later. Knowledge of the specific, time-dependent psychosocial costs and benefits of treatment, and not only of their average effects, can facilitate effective patient education and treatment planning.

Utility Versus Psychometric Approaches to Quality-of-Life Assessment

The utility approach to quality-of-life assessment, derived from economic theory, involves generating empirical weights (sometimes, but not always based on patients' preferences) for different health states, ranging from 1.0 for "perfect health" to 0.0 for death. In clinical trials these weights, expressed as a single number, can be used to adjust survival data for the quality of life during the period of survival (i.e., quality-adjusted life years, or QUALYs). Utility analyses are particularly well-suited for health policy analyses, where the cost utility of various medical care technologies is of primary interest [28, 44].

The International Breast Cancer Study Group has developed a variant on utility analysis for use specifically in adjuvant breast cancer trials [18, 19]. Basically, their method involves calculating the time that patients spend with(out) symptoms of disease and with(out) subjective toxic effects of therapy (TWiST). By attaching weights or utilities to these time periods (Q-TWiST), survival data can be discounted for quality-of-life impairment (see Gelber et al., this volume, for a full description of this approach).

The TWiST methodology, as well as the other types of utility analysis hold a great deal of promise for resolving the problems associated with synthesizing quality of life and survival data generated within clinical trials. At the same time, however, they present a new set of challenges, both conceptually and methodologically. In particular, additional attention needs to be devoted to the procedures employed to generate utilities (sometimes arbitrary, often quite complex), to demonstrating the stability of utilities across populations and over time, and to demonstrating their responsiveness to small but important changes in patients' health status [5, 15, 21].

The psychometric approach to quality-of-life assessment involves the use of patient interviews, questionnaires, or daily diaries. In contrast to the utility methods outlined above, this more classical assessment approach cannot be easily integrated with other evaluative endpoints (e.g., survival data) but rather provides a parallel stream of data. In this sense, psychometric studies do not simplify the evaluative process. On the contrary, their value lies in their ability to capture, hopefully with a high degree of accuracy, the complexity of issues involved in evaluating health and health care interventions.

Interviews represent the most flexible means of collecting patient-based quality-of-life data. They can be applied across the broadest range of patients, including those who might otherwise be unable to participate in our studies (e.g., the elderly, the poorly educated). Interviews also facilitate sophisticated question branching and can minimize the problem of missing data by incorporating probes for clarification or amplification of patients' responses. Offsetting these advantage is the fact that interviews require more staff involvement than may be available in clinical settings. Particularly in multicenter trials it cannot be expected that sufficient resurces will be available to permit interviewing as the standard means of data collection.

Although self-administered questionnaires sacrifice some of the flexibility of interviews, they represent the most practical, efficient, and inexpensive method of obtaining quality-of-life data from patients. A particularly important advantage of questionnaires is that, if designed with simplicity in mind, they can be administered serially over the course of a study without creating unacceptable levels of patient burden. While some patients may need assistance in completing a questionnaire, this is often the case only with the first administration.

Diaries are particularly useful if one is interested in frequent (e.g., daily) assessment of changes in symptom experience. For example, the British Medical Research Council has developed a diary card for use among patients receiving chemotherapy or radiotherapy which includes ratings of nausea and vomiting, activity level, mood state, anxiety, and overall health [13]. The major limitation of diaries is that, due to the frequency of administration, the number of questions asked must remain quite limited. Further, patient compliance can be a significant problem which may remain undetected if patients complete the diary retrospectively (e.g., for an entire week).

A Taxonomy of Quality-of-Life Instruments

In assessing health-related quality of life one can employ a battery of unidimensional questionnaires, each measuring a distinct quality-of-life component (e.g., physical functioning, psychological distress) or, alternatively, a single instrument incorporating a range of quality-of-life issues. The primary advantage of the battery approach is that it allows one to select the best available measure for each distinct quality-of-life domain of interest. However, because the best (i.e., most valid and reliable) unidimensional instruments are often fairly lengthy, use of the battery appproach can quickly result in an unacceptable level of patient burden.

For this reason, much of the recent work on instrument development has focused on single, comprehensive measures that include questions pertaining to each of the major quality-of-life domains, and that, preferably, yield subscale scores for each separate domain (often termed "health profiles"). Such instruments can be organized along a continuum reflecting their intended spectrum of application: (a) generic measures designed for use across a broad range of chronic disease populations, (b) disease-specific instruments for use across a related class of diagnoses (e.g., cancer-specific), and (c) diagnosis-specific measures (e.g., designed for primary breast cancer patients).

Generic instruments are particularly well-suited for large scale, population-based studies where a range of chronic disease populations are under investigation. Their broad coverage of basic psychosocial issues facilitates a stepwise process of instrument development, validation, and revalidation in a variety of research settings. Generic measures such as the Sickness Impact Profile [4], the Nottingham Health Profile [23], and the McMaster Health Index Questionnaire [10] have well-documented validity and reliability. However, generic instruments carry with them several important limitations. First, they tend to be quite lengthy. Second, they may contain a relatively large number of items that are not particularly relevant for a given population of patients and, conversely, may fail to address issues that are highly relevant for that population. Finally, their responsiveness to small but clinically significant changes in patients' health status is often less than optimal. Several recently published generic measures–Medical Outcome Study (MOS) Short-form General Health Survey [42] and the SF-36 Health Status Questionnaire [48]–hold promise for resolving these various methodological problems.

A great deal of recent effort has been devoted to developing cancer-specific instruments that can be employed across a broad range of diagnostic groups. These include the Functional Living Index–Cancer [38], the Cancer

Rehabilitation Evaluation System (CARES) [17] the EORTC QLQ C-36 [2], the Functional Assessment of Cancer Therapy (FACT) [9], the Rotterdam Symptom Checklist [12], and the Quality of Life Index [35] (see [8, 45], for reviews of these and other cancer-specific instruments). Some of these instruments have already been employed extensively in clinical studies while others are still in a developmental stage. While none of these measures has undergone sufficient field testing to recommend its use above the others, the measurement strategy common to these instruments offers the possibility of cross-study comparisons while providing a relatively targeted assessment of quality-of-life issues specifically relevant to cancer patient populations.

Finally, several measures have been developed specifically for use with breast cancer patients. These include the Linear Analog Self-Assessment [39] and the Breast Cancer Chemotherapy Questionnaire (BCG) [31]. While these measures have acceptable levels of psychometric robustness, one can question whether it is necessary or desirable to move in the direction of such diagnosis-specific instruments.

To balance the trade-offs inherent in choosing between generic and more specific measures, it may be possible to synthesize these approaches in a single *modular* assessment strategy [1]. By this is meant the use of a *core* instrument (perhaps one of the cancer-specific or shorter, generic measures), supplemented by brief, standardized, disease-specific (e.g., breast cancer) or treatment-specific (e.g., chemotherapy, radiotherapy) assessment modules. While the development of such a modular system would require a well-coordinated and sustained research effort, the rewards could be substantial. One would have the flexibility to tailor quality-of-life assessments to the needs of specific clinical trials while maintaining a high degree of standardization across investigations.

Conclusion

In a 1985 report, the United States Food and Drug Administration formally recognized the relevance of quality-of-life data for the evaluation of anticancer drugs [27, p. 1155]: "Survival and quality of life are the key efficacy parameters. In the past, new anticancer drugs were approved solely on the basis of objective tumor response, but this is no longer the case. Biological activity (tumor shrinkage) and efficacy (patient benefit) are not necessarily synonymous."

To our knowledge, no drug has yet to be approved on the basis of its quality-of-life impact. Nevertheless, both university- and industry-based scientists appear to be increasingly willing to invest the additional resources necessary to generate such data within their clinical investigations.

As quality-of-life studies become ever more common place, it is critical that methodological standards be established that are acceptable to the international research community. Of particular importance is the need to develop a common approach to quality-of-life assessment. In this paper a number of basic guidelines have been suggested in this regard:

- Rely primarily on patients themselves to provide feedback regarding their quality of life.
- Assess quality of life in terms of patients' physical, psychological, and social functioning.
- While in descriptive studies the use of patient interviews may be appropriate, rely on self-administered questionnaires as the primary mode of data collection in clinical trials.
- Employ instruments that are generic or cancer-specific, that have been designed with an eye toward brevity and simplicity, that have clearly demonstrated reliability and validity and, perhaps most importantly, that are responsiveness to clinically meaningful changes in health status.

Finally, it is important to emphasize that one need not "reinvent the wheel" in conducting quality-of-life studies. A number of well-designed instruments are currently available from which one can choose. At the same time, however, we should not necessarily be searching for a "gold standard" in quality-of-life assessment. Due to the many extrascientific considerations that are involved in selecting such standards, we may run the risk of adopting a quality-of-life measure that, while useful in the short term, may prove resistant to legitimate criticism and attempts at refinement. With sustained intellectual and financial commitment, continued advances can be expected in this young and dynamic field.

References

1. Aaronson NK, Bullinger M, Ahmedzai S (1988) A modular approach to quality of life assessment in cancer clinical trials. Recent Results Cancer Res 111: 231–249
2. Aaronson NK, Bullinger M, Ahmedzai S et al. (1991) The EORTC core quality-of-life questionnaire: interim results of an international field study. In: Osoba D (ed) Effect of cancer on quality of life. CRC, London, pp 185–203
3. Berglund G, Bolund C, Fornander T, Rutqvist LE, Sjödén P (1991) Late effects of adjuvant chemotherapy and postoperative radiotherapy on quality of life among breast cancer patients. Eur J Cancer 27:1075–1081
4. Bergner M, Bobbitt RA, Carter WB, Gilson BS (1981) The sickness impact profile: development and final revision of a health status measure. Med Care 19:787–805
5. Brunner KW (1989) Adjuvant therapies in breast cancer and quality of life: a critical review of the TWIST concept. Recent Results Cancer Res 115:239–243
6. Cairns J (1985) The treatment of disease and the war against cancer. Sci Am 253:31–39
7. Cassileth BR, Knuiman MW, Abeloff MD, Falkson G, Ezdinli EZ, Mehta CR (1986) Anxiety levels in patients randomized to adjuvant therapy versus observation for early breast cancer. J Clin Oncol 4:972–974

8. Cella DF, Tulsky DS (1990) Measuring quality of life today: methodological aspects. Oncology 4:29–38
9. Cella DF, Lee-Riordan D, Silberman M et al. (1989) Quality of life in advanced cancer: three new disease-specific measures (Abstr). Proc Am Soc Clin Oncol 8:315
10. Chambers LW, MacDonald LA, Tugwell P, Buchanan W, Kraag G (1982) The McMaster health index questionnaire as a measure of quality of life for patients with rheumatoid disease. J Rheumatol 9:780–784
11. De Haes JCJM, van Knippenberg FCE (1985) The quality of life of cancer patients: a review of the literature. Soc Sci Med 20:809–817
12. De Haes JCJM, van Knippenberg FCE, Neijt JP (1990) Measuring psychological and physical distress in cancer patients: structure and application of the Rotterdam symptom checklist. Br J Cancer 62:1034–1038
13. Fayers PM, Jones SDR (1983) Measuring and analyzing the quality of life in cancer clinical trials: a review. Stat Med 2:429–446
14. Feinstein AR (1987) Clinimetric perspectives. J Chronic Dis 40:635–640
15. Feldstein ML (1991) Quality-of-life-adjusted survival comparing cancer treatments. Cancer 67:851–854
16. Ganz PA, Polinsky MI, Schag CAC, Heinrich RL (1989) Rehabilitation of patients with primary breast cancer: assessing the impact of adjuvant therapy. Recent Results Cancer Res 115:244–254
17. Ganz PA, Coscarelli Schag CA, Cheng HL (1990) Assessing the quality of life – a study in newly diagnosed breast cancer patients. J Clin Epidemiol 43:75–86
18. Gelber RD, Goldhirsch A (1986) A new endpoint for the assessment of adjuvant therapy in postmenopausal women with operable breast cancer. J Clin Oncol 4:1772–1779
19. Goldhirsch A, Gelber RD, Simes RJ, Glasziou P, Coates AS (1989) Costs and benefits of adjuvant therapy in breast cancer: a quality-adjust survival analysis. J Clin Oncol 7:36–44
20. Gough IR, Furnival CM, Schilder L, Grove W (1983) Assessment of the quality of life of patients with advanced cancer. Eur J Cancer Clin Oncol 19:1161–1165
21. Guyatt G, Feeny D, Patrick D (1991) Issues in quality-of-life measurement in clinical trials. Controlled Clin Trials 12:81S–90S
22. Hughson AVM, Cooper AF, McArdle CS, Smith DC (1986) Psychological impact of adjuvant chemotherapy in the first two years after mastectomy. Br Med J 293:1268–1271
23. Hunt SM, McEwen J (1980) The development of a subjective health indicator. Sociol Health Jll 2:231–246
24. Hürny C, Bernhard J, Gelber RD et al. (1992) Quality of life measures for patients receiving adjuvant therapy for breast cancer: an international trial. Eur J Cancer (in press)
25. Hutchinson TA, Boyd NF, Feinstein AR (1979) Scientific problems in clinical scales as demonstrated by the Karnofsky index of performance status. J Chronic Dis 32:661–666
26. Irvine D, Brown B, Crooks D, Roberts J, Browne G (1991) Psychosocial adjustment in women with breast cancer. Cancer 67:1097–1117
27. Johnson JR, Temple R (1985) Food and Drug Administration requirements for approval of new anticancer drugs. Cancer Treat Rep 69:1155–1157
28. Kaplan RM, Buksh JW (1982) Health-related quality of life measurement for evaluation research and policy analysis. J Healt Econ 5:1–30
29. Kiebert GM, de Haes JCJM, van de Velde CJH (1991) The impact of breast-conserving treatment and mastectomy on the quality of life of ealry-stage breast cancer patients: a review. J Clin Oncol 9:1059–1070

30. Knopf T (1990) Symptoms and rehabilitation needs of patients with early stage breast cancer during primary therapy. Cancer 66:1392–1401
31. Levine MN, Guyatt GH, Gent M et al. (1988) Quality of life in stage II breast cancer: an instrument for clinical trials. J Clin Oncol 6:1798–1810
32. Love RR, Leventhal H, Easterling DV, Nerenz DR (1989) Side effects and emotional distress during cancer chemotherapy. Cancer 63:604–612
33. Maguire GP, Tait A, Brooke M, Thomas C (1980) Psychiatric morbidity and physical toxicity associated with adjuvant chemotherapy after mastectomy. Br Med J 281:1179–1180
34. Mcardle CS, Calman KC, Cooper AF, Hughson AVM, Russell AR, Smith DC (1981) The social, emotional and financial implications of adjuvant chemotherapy in breast cancer. Br J Surg 68:261–264
35. Padilla GV, Presant C, Grant MM, Metter G, Lipsett J, Heide F (1983) Quality of life index for patients with Cancer. Res Nurs Health 6:117–126
36. Palmer BV, Walsh GA, McKinna JA, Greening WP (1980) Adjuvant chemotherapy for breast cancer: side effects and quality of life. Br Med J 281:1594–1597
37. Schag CC, Heinrich RL, Ganz PA (1984) Karnofsky performance status revisited: reliability, validity and guidelines. J Clin Oncol 2:187–193
38. Schipper H, Clinch J, McMurray A, Levitt M (1984) Measuring the quality of life of cancer patients: the functional living index–cancer. J Clin Oncol 2:472–483
39. Selby PJ, Chapman JA, Etazadi-Amoli J, Dalley D, Boyd NF (1984) The development of a method of assessing the quality of life for cancer patients. Br J Cancer 50:13–22
40. Spitzer WO (1987) State of science 1986: quality of life and functional status as target variables for research. J Chronic Dis 40:473–480
41. Spitzer WO, Dobson AJ, Hall J, Chesterman E, Levi J, Shepherd R, Battista RN, Catchlove BR (1981) Measuring the quality of life cancer patients: a concise QL-index for use by physicians. J Chronic Dis 34:585–597
42. Stewart AL, Hays RD, Ware JE (1988) The MOS short-form general health survey: reliability and validity in a patient population. Med Care 26:724–735
43. Tamburini M, Brambilla C, Ferrari L, Bombino T, Gangeri L, Rosso S (1991) Two simple indexes used to evaluate the impact of therapy on the quality of life of patients receiving primary chemotherapy for operable breast cancer. Ann Oncol 2:417–422
44. Torrance GW (1986) Measurement of health state utilities for economic appraisal. J Health Econ 5:1–30
45. van Knippenberg FCE, de Haes JCJM (1988) Measuring the quality of life of cancer patients: psychometric properties of instruments. J Clin Epidemiol 41:1043–1053
46. Ware JE Jr (1984) Conceptualizing disease impact and treatment outcomes. Cancer 53:2216–2326
47. Ware JE Jr (1987) Standards for validating health measures: definitions and content. J Chronic Dis 40:473–480
48. Ware JE Jr, Sherbourne CD (1992) The MOS 36-item short form health survey (SF-36). I. Conceptual framework and item selection. Med Care (in press)
49. World Health Organization (1947) The constitution of the World Health Organization. WHO Chronicle 1:2

Coping and Survival in Early Breast Cancer: An Update

C. Hürny

Medical Division Lory, Inselspital, 3010 Bern, Switzerland

Introduction

From a theoretical point of view biomedical, psychological, and social factors may define outcome in breast cancer [14]. On the biomedical level some tumor-related prognostic factors are well established: nodal status, size of the primary, and, less powerfully estrogen and progesterone receptor status and histological grading. Besides the prognostic impact of menopausal status host-related factors such as immune and differential endocrine status are discussed but are not evident.

The known biological factors explain only part of the large outcome variance. On the psychological and social levels prognostic factors are so far mainly hypothetical. One clearcut fact is that survival is substantially better in (breast) cancer patients with high as compared to low socioeconomic status. The two main hypotheses emerging from the available studies are, that (a) patients with "adaptive coping" survive longer than patients with "maladaptive coping." and (b) that patients with perceived or actual good social support survive longer than patients lacking social support. No consensus exists about the definition of adaptive versus maladaptive coping. According to personality style and individual biography one way of coping may be adaptive for one patient but maladaptive for another one. Furthermore, the coping pattern may change over time. For this reason no standard method for coping assessment has yet been established. Similar conceptual problems exist in the assessment of social support.

Without a standardized assessment methodology findings are not easily replicated, and a clearcut impact of coping and social support on survival is difficult to demonstrate. Further reasons that the findings must be regarded as hypothetical for the moment are important methodological shortcomings regarding study design, small sample sizes with large numbers of variables, lack of control for confounding variables such as sociodemographic characteristics, and, most importantly, biomedical characteristics carrying prognostic

Recent Results in Cancer Research, Vol. 127

power. To exemplify the methodological pitfalls I have analyzed in 1989 [14], the two most frequently cited studies in the field with contradictory findings [4, 10]. In this chapter I discuss several new studies with impact on research methodology.

Follow-up on the Two Indicator Studies with Contradictory Findings

The group of Greer at Kings College Hospital in London, prospectively investigating a sample of 57 stage I and II breast cancer patients, found that those patients reacting to the diagnosis at 3 months from surgery with "active denial" or "fighting spirit" had significantly longer disease-free (DFS) and overall survival (OS) than those reacting with "stoic acceptance" and "hoplessness/helplessness" at 5, 10, and 15 years of follow-up [10, 11, 24]. The main methodological shortcoming of this study is that at the time of patient accrual no surgical clearing of the axilla with histological staging was performed. Since nodal status is the most powerful prognostic factor in early breast cancer, an unequal distribution of stage I and stage II patients among the psychologically defined groups could explain the survival difference. Reporting the 10- and 15-year follow-up of the study the authors claim by citing Fentiman et al. [8], that nodal status is less important for predicting survival beyond 5 years. However, in other series nodal status and size of the primary tumor retain their prognostic relevance up to 30 years after diagnosis.

To determine whether Greer's findings are real or artifactual, replications of the study controlling for confounding variables are needed. Dean and Surtees [6] from the Royal Edinburgh Hospital assessed 121 stage I and II breast cancer patients preoperatively and at 3 months with an extensive psychiatric interview defining cases of depressive and anxiety disorders according to Spitzer's Research Diagnostic Criteria (RDC), the four coping categories of Greer, the General Health Questionnaire (GHQ), and the Eysenck Personality Inventory (EPI). At a mean follow-up of 6.7 years patients defined as RDC cases preoperatively, i.e., showing high levels of depression and/or anxiety, had longer DFS ($p < 0.01$) and OS ($p < 0.1$), and those reacting preoperatively with stoic acceptance and/or hoplessness/helplessness had longer DFS ($p < 0.05$), but there was no effect on OS, and those showing high levels of distress in the GHQ had longer DFS and OS ($p < 0.01$). Unemployment preoperatively predicted shorter DFS ($p < 0.01$) and as a trend OS ($p < 0.1$). Low social class predicted poor OS ($p < 0.05$). The only psychosocial factor predicting longer survival at 3 months was denial (DFS, $p < 0.05$; OS, $p < 0.1$) as compared to fighting spirit, stoic acceptance, and helplessness/hopelessness [6].

At the first glance these results seem to be puzzling. One finding of the Greer et al. study, denial at month 3 predicting survival has been confirmed. The other three responses to the diagnosis at month 3 had no predictive value in terms of DFS and OS. Since in the Dean and Surtees study biomedical and sociodemographic variables were well controlled, one explanation for the different findings could be the removal of a selection bias (nodal status), leaving denial as the only predictive variable at month 3. Another explanation could be a difference in assessment of the four response categories. In their initial study Greer et al. [10] defined the four categories with short statements; since then they have further operationalized their constructs [9]. Unfortunately this work was not available when Dean assessed her patients. She rated all patients herself into the four coping categories as described by Greer et al. initially. A systematic rating difference could explain the result difference. Preoperative expression of distress (anxiety, depression, helplessness/hopelessness) was associated with better prognosis across instruments except for the EPI. This is in accordance with earlier findings [7, 18, 20] but seems to conflict with the results of Greer et al. [10]. However coping is a process over time, and initial distress followed by denial to restore psychological equilibrium corresponds to the normal grief reaction. Along this line of thinking the association of a normal psychological response to cancer diagnosis over time with a good prognosis seems plausible.

As I have stated previously, the main positive findings of psychosocial factors predicting survival in breast cancer patients are based on interview data [14]. In the study of Dean and Surtees [6] this is confirmed. A further confirmation is the negative study of Buddeberg et al. [2], assessing 107 stage I and II breast cancer patients at 6 months from surgery with the Zurich Coping Questionnaire and the Freiburg Coping Questionnaire. Coping did not predict survival at 3.5 years follow-up.

As in previous population-based studies low social class predicted shorter survival in the Dean and Surtees [6] study. According to their findings this could be due to low compliance with treatment.

The group of Cassileth et al. [4, 5] at the University of Pennsylvania Cancer Center in Philadelphia, investigating prospectively 155 consecutive patients (93 with stage II breast cancer, 62 with stage I melanoma) found no predictive value for survival of 7 psychosocial factors assessed by questionnaire (social ties, job satisfaction, psychotropic drug use, life satisfaction, subjective view of adult health, hopelessness, and perceived adjustment to chronic illness). The main shortcoming of this study was the assessment instrument, a 32-item questionnaire attempting to assess seven complex psychosocial constructs, not validated except for one subscale. It is unlikely that this questionnaire adequately assesses relevant aspects of the coping process. No further follow-up of this study has been published.

In the International Breast Cancer Study Group (IBCSG) trials VI and VII, the Cassileth 1985 study was replicated in part, in that one subscale, the perceived adjustment to chronic illness scale (PACIS) was used to assess one aspect of quality of life among others. The PACIS has been shown to be a reasonable indicator of coping [3] and to be sensitive to time from diagnosis, language, and medical treatment [15]. In the ongoing IBCSG trials VI and VII evaluating different strategies of adjuvant treatment in stage II breast cancer patients, the PACIS among other measures is administered to the patients within 6 weeks of surgery and every 3 months thereafter. At a median follow-up of 21 months on 1391 patients with complete data initial coping did not predict DFS. However, when changes in coping scores between baseline and month 3 were considered in the patient subgroup initially receiving tamoxifen only, patients with smaller change had shorter DFS than those with greater change ($p < 0.02$) [16]. This is the largest available study; biomedical and sociodemographic variables are well controlled.

From this point of view the essentially negative finding must be acknowledged. However, assessment of coping by the PACIS, a one-item, self-rated scale is relatively superficial, and although being a reasonable indicator of coping for quality-of-life assessment, it may not reflect the complexity of the coping process. In a Swiss subgroup of the IBCSG study 150 patients were assessed in more depth regarding the coping process, but the data are not yet ready for analysis. Furthermore, a follow-up of 21 months is very short in stage II breast cancer, and the analysis is therefore very preliminary. As in adjuvant treatment early impact may have late effects. The preliminary finding of major change in coping scores between baseline and month 3 in one subgroup predicting longer survival is in accordance with the findings of Dean and Surtees [6]. Flexible copers may have a better prognosis than rigid copers. However, these findings must also be considered as very preliminary.

New, Possibly Confounding Variables

Besides the above-mentioned and previously described, possibly confounding biomedical and sociodemographic variables in the assessment of coping as a prognostic factor, some new factors are appearing in the literature. Breast cancer patients undergoing adjuvant treatment show substantial weight gain. Weight gain may have a prognostic impact and is differentially associated with coping style [19]. This factor must be assessed in future studies.

In an elegant case control study Ramirez et al. [25] found an association between severely threatening-life events and difficulties with prognosis in operable breast cancer patients. The relative risk of relapse associated with severe life events was more than five times higher. In future studies life events must be recorded throughout the follow-up period.

Intervention Studies

If coping has an impact on survival, a psychotherapeutic intervention aiming at improving coping and adaptation to the disease may also improve survival.

Although there is only conflicting evidence of the prognostic influence of coping on survival, several intervention studies are currently ongoing. The main goal of psychotherapeutic intervention studies in breast cancer patients is to show improvement of subjective well-being and quality of life. Only in a second line is impact on survival of interest.

The first intervention study in breast cancer showing an impact on survival was published by Spiegel et al. [29] at Stanford University in California. In this study 86 patients with metastatic breast cancer were randomly assigned to an intervention group (n = 50) or to a control group (n = 36). The intervention group had weekly group therapy (90 min) aimed at symptom control and improvement of adjustment and was lead by a psychiatrist or social worker with a therapist who herself had breast cancer in remission. The intervention was effective in terms of symptom relief and improvement of psychological well-being [28]. The mean survival time for the intervention group was 36.6 months as compared to 18.9 months for the control group. Although medical factors possibly confounding these results, such as initial disease stage, disease-free interval, and medical treatments, were well controlled, reservation towards these findings is still appropriate. The psychotherapeutic intervention doubles survival time. No medical treatment has ever had such a huge effect in metastatic breast cancer. In contrary, the survival time in breast cancer, once there are distant metastases, is usualiy not affected by treatments. This makes it unlikely that another treatment modality should have such an enormous effect. Since there are large individual differences in survival in breast cancer (from a few months to over 30 years), which are explained only in part by known biomedical prognostic factors, the results of Spiegel et al. [29] are likely to be the effect of a selection bias. At a median time of survival of about 20 months there is no difference. The difference started to appear at about 32 months, 8 months after the end of the intervention and when more than half of the patients had died, leaving about 20 patients per group. Although the two groups were similar in terms of numbers of metastases per site, one factor possibly contributing to the selection bias was the type of metastatic spread, not controlled for. The prognosis of women with soft tissue metastases only is substantially better compared to visceral, especially liver or CNS, involvement or worse, involvement of more than one metastatic site [13]. Further well-controlled studies are needed to elucidate the impact of a psychotherapeutic intervention on survival in breast cancer.

Psychobiological Studies

If coping has an effect on survival, mediating factors between environment, psychological processes, CNS, and malignant cell growth must be postulated. In breast cancer the main hypothetical mediators are the immune and endocrine systems. Many psychosocial stressors and psychological reactions have been shown to influence immune function in healthy and in acutely and chronically ill individuals [27]. However, it is not known whether the observed changes in immune function are normal fluctuations, or whether they contribute to the development or the progression of disease. Although the concept of immune surveillance in malignant disease is quite popular, the role of the immune system in malignant diseases is not clear yet.

In spite of these uncertainties Levy, in a series of studies, has developed a different approach to the problem of psychosocial influence on survival in breast cancer, concurrently assessing hypothetical psychosocial and immunological factors [20–22]. In the most recent study in a sample of 61 stage I and II breast cancer patients examined within about 6 weeks of diagnosis higher natural killer cell (NK) activity was predicted by – in order of relevance – perception of positive social support from the spouse and physician, estrogen receptor (ER) negative tumor status, receiving an excisional biopsy only, and utilizing social support as a coping strategy. Perception of high-quality social support from the spouse or significant other alone accounted for almost one third of the variance explained in NK activity [23]. In this study perceived social support seemed to enhance NK activity, possibly a protective factor against tumor growth. At the same time an interaction between ER status and NK activity emerges. These are only a few pieces in a complex puzzle that is difficult to understand at the moment. The outcome of the study will probably clarify whether the findings reflect physiological changes or do have an impact on disease course.

Another interesting observation in this area by Razavi et al. [26] is the correlation of ER and progesterone receptor status with psychosocial adjustment in 93 patients with primary breast cancer. Patients with receptor-positive tumors were better adjusted than those with receptor-negative tumors. These findings have been confirmed in part in a larger patient sample [17]. The expression of hormone receptors is primarily defined by the genetics of a particular tumor but also by the levels of circulating hormones. Hormone levels are well known to influence psychological functioning, such as in premenstrual syndrome. On the other hand, psychological stress may induce temporary amenorrhea, showing a possible interaction in the other direction. The correlation of receptor status with psychosocial adjustment opens new possibilities of fairly direct interactions between coping and tumor growth. It may also explain some of the contradictory findings in regard to coping and survival, since receptor status as a prognostic factor could be a confounding variable, one rarely controlled for in psychosocial studies.

Conclusions

As noted above [14], there is still no clearcut evidence of coping and – related to this – social support predicting survival in early breast cancer.

However, some interesting new aspects are emerging. Changes in coping over time appear to be more important than actual reactions at one moment. An initial crisis with high emotional distress at diagnosis followed by adaptive denial 3 months later may have a positive impact on survival. Psychosocial interventions targeted at improving adjustment and psychological well-being have shown survival benefits for metastatic breast cancer patients in one study. This finding must be taken with caution and will be tested by currently ongoing studies. However, this is a novel way of indirect testing of the hypothesis. Patients with individually different coping styles may profit from psychotherapy. The intervention may enhance adaptation irrespective of coping. A survival benefit would then depend on the result of coping: adaptation.

Concerning mediators between coping and disease process some major but ill-defined pathways are becoming somewhat clearer, for example the endocrine pathway, through a correlation of receptor status of the tumor to psychosocial adjustment, and the immune pathway, through a differential association of social support and immune function, especially NK activity. There is also some evidence of an interaction between NK activity and receptor status, pointing to hypothetical highly complex interactions.

The major reasons for the lack of clearcut positive or negative evidence of the coping process predicting survival are still methodological shortcomings of the available studies, mainly problems in the assessment of coping and lack of control for confounding psychosocial and biomedical variables. Recently described, possibly confounding variables are weight gain on the biomedical side and life events on the psychosocial side.

In regard to coping assessment it is striking that most positive findings are based on interview data. Psychometric assessments rarely predict survival. This phenomenon may be explained in two ways. First, for an appropriate assessment of coping a physician-patient relationship is necessary because patients reveal more intimate information and use less avoidance than in psychometric tests. Second, interviewers intuitively and subconsciously pick up prognostic factors not necessarily related to coping. This bias could be removed by recording the interviews for rating by others.

The assessment of coping and social support must be further refined and possibly standardized. This may not be easy since the coping process and the perception of social support probably are highly individual, even if a rough pattern over time is observable. The individuality of the coping process may be another reason for the conflicting results of the studies comparing groups of patients. Effects may be shown in one sample and not in another. One possibility to resolve the dilemma would be not to assess the ways of coping only, but to include an expert judgment as to whether the individual coping is adaptive considering the patient's personality and biography. Adaptation, an equivalent to homeostasis, may be assessed more easily.

Individuality of the coping process may go beyond the psychological level. Adler and von Uexküll [1] have postulated and individual physiology defined by genetic factors, early childhood experience, biography, and life events, resulting in highly specific interactions between the biological, psychological, and social levels. For example, in one patient social support could be associated with high estrogen levels and low NK activity but in another with high estrogen levels and high NK activity. In this model the individually specific interactions are determinants of health and disease. Biopsychosocial interactions can no longer be denied, but they are difficult to assess. A definite methodology is not yet available. We are accustomed to investigating within a particlar level of organization defined by a specific scientific discipline (e.g., sociology, psychology, immunology, molecular biology) but not between such levels.

Considering the complexity of the problem, I propose two main research strategies for the future. On the one hand, longitudinal indepth studies of individual patients at the social, psychological, and biological levels assessing all available parameters are needed, with the goal of detecting individual patterns of biopsychosocial interactions. If patterns of such interactions are detected, they may be operationalized and tested in large-scale studies. The other approach is the longitudinal assessment of patients with simple indicators on the biological, psychological, and social levels in very large-scale studies in which individual differences are possibly washed out and common patterns may emerge. This strategy could possibly be adopted in clinical trials, where optimal biomedical assessment is already performed. The current research strategy of one assessment on the psychosocial level around the time of diagnosis in a small sample of patients will not give the answer to the question of whether coping has an impact on survival in breast cancer or not.

References

1. Adler RH, von Uexküll T (1987) Individuelle Physiologie als Zukunftsaufgabe der Medizin. Schweiz Rundsch Med PRAX 76:1275–1280
2. Buddeberg C, Wolf C, Sieber M et al. (1991) Coping strategies and course of disease of breast cancer patients. Psychother Psychosom 55:151–157
3. Butow P, Coates A, Dunn S et al. (1991) On the receiving end. IV. Validation of quality of life indicators. Ann Oncol 2:597–603
4. Cassileth BR, Lusk EJ, Miller DS et al. (1985) Psychological correlates of survival in advanced malignant disease? N Engl J Med 312:1551–1555
5. Cassileth BR, Walsh WP, Lusk EJ (1988) Psychosocial correlates of cancer survival: a subsequent report 3 to 8 years after cancer diagnosis. J Clin Oncol 6:1753–1759
6. Dean C, Surtees GS (1989) Do psychological factors predict survival in breast cancer? J Psychosom Res 33:561–569
7. Derogatis LR, Abeloff MD, Melisaratos N (1979) Psychological coping mechanisms and survival time in metastatic breast cancer. JAMA 242:1504–1508
8. Fentiman IS, Cuzick J, Millis RR, Hayward JL (1984) Which patients are cured of breast cancer? Br Med J 289:1108–1111

9. Greer S, Watson M (1987) Mental adjustment to cancer: its measurement and prognostic importance. Cancer Surv 6:439–453
10. Greer S, Morris T, Pettingale KW (1979) Psychological response to breast cancer. Effect on outcome. Lancet 2(8146):785–787
11. Greer S, Morris T, Pettingale KW, Haybittle JL (1990) Psychological response to breast cancer and 15 year outcome. Lancet 1(335):49–50
12. Henderson CI, Harris JR, Kinne DW et al. (1989) Cancer of the breast. In: de Vita VT, Hellmann S, Rosenberg SA (eds) Cancer, principles and practice of oncology, vol 1, 3rd edn. Lippincott, Philadelphia, pp 1208–1210
13. Henderson CI, Harris JR, Kinne DW et al. (1989) Cancer of the breast. In: de Vita VT, Hellmann S, Rosenberg SA (eds) Cancer, principles and practice of oncology, vol 1, 3rd edn. Lippincott, Philadelphia, pp 1245–1246
14. Hürny C, Bernhard J (1989) Coping and survival in patients with primary breast cancer: a critical analysis of current research strategies and proposal for a new approach integrating biomedical, psychological and social variables. In: Senn HJ, Goldhirsch A, Gelber RD, Osterwalder B (eds) Adjuvant therapy of primary breast cancer. Springer, Berlin Heidelberg New York, pp 255–271 (Recent Results in Cancer Research, vol 115)
15. Hürny C, Bernhard J, Gelber RD et al. (1992) Quality of life measures for patients receiving adjuvant therapy for breast cancer: an international trial. Eur J Cancer 28:118–124
16. Hürny C, Bernhard J, Peterson H et al. (1992) Psychosocial predictors of survival in stage II breast cancer patients: a preliminary analysis (Abstr). 4th International Conference on Adjuvant Therapy of Primary Breast Cancer, St. Gallen
17. Hürny C, for the International Breast Cancer Study Group IBCSG (1992) Psychosocial correlates of estrogen receptor status in breast cancer (Abstr). Proc Am Soc Clin Oncol 11:57
18. Jensen MR (1987) Psychobiological factors predicting the course of breast cancer. J Pers 55:317–342
19. Levine EG, Raczynski JM, Carpenter JT (1991) Weight gain with breast cancer adjuvant treatment. Cancer 67(7):1954–1959
20. Levy SM, Herberman RB, Malvish AM et al. (1985) Prognostic risk assessment in primary breast cancer by behavioral and immunological parameters. Health Psychol 4:99–113
21. Levy SM, Herberman R, Lippman M, d'Angelo T (1987) Correlation of stress factors with sustained depression of natural killer cell activity and predicted prognosis in patients with breast cancer. J Clin Oncol 5:348–353
22. Levy SM, Lee J, Bagley C et al. (1988) Survival hazards analysis in first recurrent breast cancer patients: seven years follow-up. Psychosom Med 50: 520–528
23. Levy SM, Herberman RB, Whiteside T et al. (1990) Perceived social support and tumor estrogen/progesterone receptor status as predictors of natural killer cell activity in breast cancer patients. Psychosom Med 52:73–85
24. Pettingale KW, Morris T, Greer S, Haybittle JL (1985) Mental attitudes to cancer: an additional prognostic factor. Lancet 1(8431):750
25. Ramirez AJ, Craig TKJ, Watson JP et al. (1989) Stress and relapse of breast cancer. Br Med J 298:291–293
26. Razavi D, Farvacques C, Delvaux N (1990) Psychosocial correlates of estrogen and progesterone receptors in breast cancer. Lancet 2(335):931–933
27. Sabbioni M (1991) Cancer and stress: a possible role for psychoneuroimmunology in cancer research? In: Cooper CL, Watson M (eds) Cancer and stress. Wiley, Chichester, pp 3–26

28. Spiegel D, Bloom JR, Yalom ID (1981) Group support for patients with metastatic breast cancer. Arch Gen Psychiatry 38:527–531
29. Spiegel D, Bloom JR, Kraemer HC et al. (1989) Effect of psychosocial treatment on survival of patients with metastatic breast cancer. Lancet 2(8668): 888–891

How To Compare Quality of Life of Breast Cancer Patients in Clinical Trials

R.D. Gelber[1,2], B.F. Cole[2] and A. Goldhirsch[3] for the International Breast Cancer Study Group, Bern, Switzerland

[1] Harvard Medical School and Harvard School of Public Health, Boston, MA 02115, USA
[2] Dana-Farber Cancer Institute, Boston, MA 02115, USA
[3] International Breast Cancer Study Group, Ospedale Civico, Lugano, Switzerland

Introduction

Quality of life of breast cancer patients receiving systemic therapy has been studied in advanced disease when treatments are given with palliative intent [1–3]. In the adjuvant setting, however, therapies associated with acute toxic effects are administered during a time when patients are free of disease-related symptoms [4]. The expectation is that the investment of this period of toxicity will be balanced by a delay in relapse and improvement in survival for the future. The toxic effects are felt by the entire population of patients, while it is possible that the benefits of treatment might be enjoyed by only some.

Quality of life is a multidimensional and subjective entity which is impossible to measure in absolute quantitative terms. It is influenced by all aspects of life, including general health, psychosocial well-being, and the subjective sense of satisfaction. Measurement of specific treatment effects on quality of life might be more feasible. First attempts at assessing the impact of treatments on quality of life were made by identifying and grading the side effects. Subsequent efforts have been made to measure patients' perceptions of the influence of side effects of adjuvant treatment, and patients' perceptions of symptoms of disease and treatment for relapse.

Other chapters in this volume discuss issues related to the choice of instruments used to measure quality of life for breast cancer patients. We discuss issues relating to the comparison of treatments within clinical trials. Specifically, our approach to quality-of-life analysis begins with the usual measures for treatment comparison (disease-free survival and overall survival) and provides a framework within which quality-of-life measurement can introduce the patients' perceptions into decisions concerning treatment choice.

Quality-of-life measures, indices, and scales take a snapshot of the patient's status at one point in time. Subsequent alterations in the scores

Recent Results in Cancer Research, Vol. 127

obtained can be used to assess changes in the quality-of-life measures over time. Groups of patients who receive different treatments can be compared by evaluating the average changes using standard statistical methods for comparing group means, and multivariate repeated measures for analysis of variance [5]. Issues of missing data and censored observations complicate the treatment comparisons using these methods. Models for longitudinal data analysis can be applied to the quality-of-life measures over time to obtain some treatment comparisons adjusting for missing data [6].

A Decision Analytic Approach

The primary goal of a randomized clinical trial is to compare treatments. Similarly, the decision analyst is interested in comparing various scenarios or strategies to determine under which conditions and assumptions the individual options would be preferred. Treatment comparisons based on disease-free survival and overall survival are most familiar to oncologists who must decide on the best way to treat patients with operable breast cancer. The usual approach to the analysis of these endpoints is to focus on the reduction in relapse or mortality rates in order to describe the benefit that might be achieved from an effective therapy. The patient, however, is likely to be interested primarily in time. A common question from the patient is, "How much longer will I live if I receive the treatment?" An additional question of interest is "How will the treatment influence the quality of my life?"

The Q-TWiST Method

Determining the time without symptoms of the disease and toxicity of treatment (TWiST) and assigning of quality-adjustment weights to the periods involved (Q-TWiST) provide a method to evaluate time periods for comparison of treatment effects [7–12]. This method is designed to incorporate aspects of quality of life into adjuvant chemotherapy and endocrine therapy comparisons. The application of the method proceeds in three steps.

1. The first step is to define quality-of-life oriented endpoints that highlight specific differences between the treatments being compared. For example, time with toxicity (TOX) is the period in which the patient is exposed to subjective side effects of therapy. Time spent living with overt metastatic disease (REL) is all time after the diagnosis of systemic spread of the disease. The definitions of TOX and REL reflect the fact that these periods of time have a negative impact on the overall quality of life of the patient. Furthermore, their definition is designed to highlight the contrasting properties of the different treatments under study. Time without either symptoms of the disease and toxicity of treatment is denoted as TWiST.

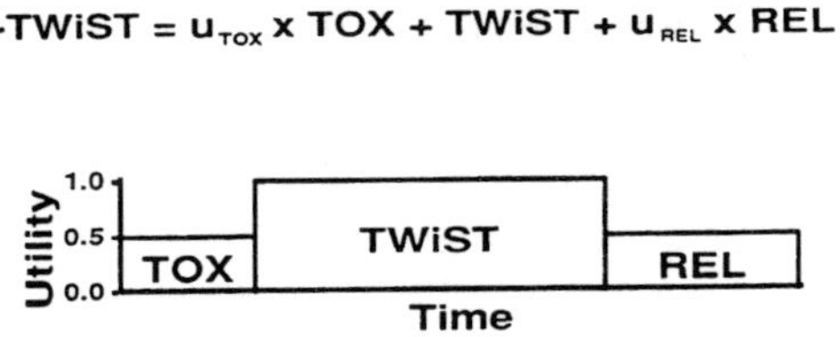

Fig. 1. Components of *Q*uality-adjusted *T*ime *W*ithout *S*ymptoms and *T*oxicity (*Q-TWiST*), illustrating the division of overall survival into TOX (subjective toxic effects), TWiST, and REL (relapse), and the weighting of these time periods using utility coefficients u_{tox} and u_{rel}

2. The second step is to consider each treatment separately and to partition the overall survival time into the defined periods. Areas under the survival curve represent average amounts of time spent in TOX, TWiST, and REL. These are calculated up to a specific point in time determined according to the follow-up time of the study cohort.

3. The third step is to compare the treatment regimens using the weighted averages of the times calculated in step 2. The quality-adjusted comparison offers the opportunity to include utility coefficients to reflect the assumed relative worth of different periods characterized by different circumstances (TOX and REL) relative to TWiST. Figure 1 displays the different time periods according to assumed weights of 1.0 for TWiST, 0.5 for TOX, and 0.5 for REL. This example represents a scenario in which 1 month spent in TOX or REL is equivalent to one-half of a month spent with the better quality of life which characterizes TWiST.

International Breast Cancer Study Group Trial V: Evaluation of Short-Course Chemotherapy Versus Long-Duration Treatment Using Standard Endpoints and Q-TWiST

Trial V of the International Breast Cancer Study Group (IBCSG) investigated in patients with node-positive breast cancer the use of 1 month of perioperative systemic treatment compared with a long-duration adjuvant therapy (6 or 7 months) [11, 13]. The short-duration therapy consisted of a combination chemotherapy with cyclophosphamide, methotrexate, and fluorouracil (CMF) given entirely intravenously on days 1 and 8 after surgery. The majority of patients with perioperative treatment also received leucovorin. The long-duration treatment regimen consisted of CMF plus prednisone (CMFp) for 6 months (cyclophosphamide administered orally, prednisone administered at a low dose given daily for the entire duration of the chemotherapy) either following the single perioperative course or initiated 3–5 weeks after surgery. Postmenopausal women also received tamoxifen for the entire duration of the six cycles of long-duration chemo-

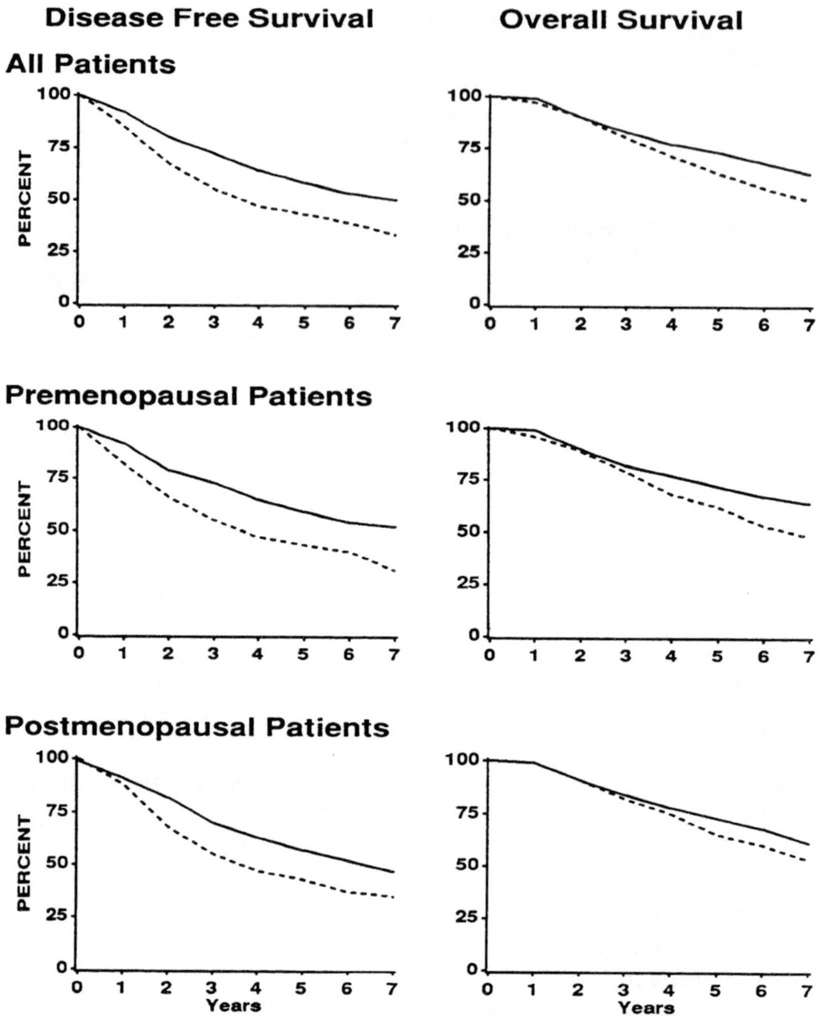

Fig. 2. Disease-free survival and overall survival for 1229 patients with node-positive breast cancer in International Breast Cancer Study Group Trial V at 7 years of median follow-up. Figures are shown for all patients, for 715 premenopausal patients, and for 514 postmenopausal patients. — Long duration; --- short duration

therapy. Thus, the long-duration treatment comprised six cycles of chemotherapy for premenopausal women and six cycles of chemoendocrine therapy for postmenopausal women, either with or without an initial 4-week course of perioperative chemotherapy.

Figure 2 shows the disease-free survival and overall survival comparisions of the long-duration treatment group versus the short-duration group. Results are presented for all 1229 patients and separately for 715 pre-

Table 1. Seven-year disease-free survival (DFS) and overall survival (OS): percentages according to treatment group, menopausal status, number of nodes involved, and estrogen receptor (ER) status in 1229 patients with node-positive breast cancer in IBCSG Trial V

Patient population	*n*		7-year DFS (%)			7-year OS (%)		
	Long[a]	Short	Long[a]	Short	p[b]	Long[a]	Short	p[b]
All patients	816	413	45	27	<0.0001	63	50	0.0002
Premenopausal								
All	475	240	47	25	<0.0001	64	48	0.0001
No. of nodes								
1–3	273	133	60	36	<0.0001	79	59	0.0001
≥4	202	107	29	10	0.0001	44	34	0.10
ER status								
Positive	249	114	47	25	0.0001	70	53	0.02
Negative	168	85	45	22	0.0002	54	37	0.01
Unknown	58	41	52	33	0.07	68	55	0.06
Postmenopausal								
All	341	173	43	30	0.0001	62	53	0.26
No. of nodes								
1–3	193	100	53	40	0.03	74	69	0.97
≥4	148	73	29	15	<0.0001	47	31	0.06
ER status								
Positive	200	101	43	25	<0.0001	67	58	0.43
Negative	102	52	41	30	0.16	50	35	0.19
Unknown	39	20	47	50	0.56	69	69	0.77

[a] For premenopausal patients, long-duration treatment comprised 6 months of CMFp chemotherapy (half also received a perioperative course of intravenous CMF + leucovorin). For postmenopausal patients, long-duration treatment comprised 6 months of CMFp + tamoxifen chemoendocrine therapy (half also received a perioperative course of intravenous CMF + leucovorin).
[b] All p values were calculated using a two-tailed logrank test.

menopausal patients and 514 postmenopausal women. Table 1 describes the 7-year percentages for the two endpoints according to menopausal status, number of lymph nodes involved, and estrogen receptor status of the primary tumor. Median follow-up for this analysis is 7 years. For the premenopausal patients, the long-duration chemotherapy significantly increased both disease-free survival and overall survival compared with the short-duration treatment. For the postmenopausal patients, while differences in terms of disease-free survival are highly significant, those in terms of overall survival appear late during follow-up and are not statistically significant.

The advantage for the long-duration treatment group in terms of the standard endpoints must be balanced against the increased duration of exposure to toxic effects of treatment. For premenopausal patients in whom an overall survival advantage has been demonstrated, the issue of cost-benefit is less pertinent due to the relevant life-years gained by treat-

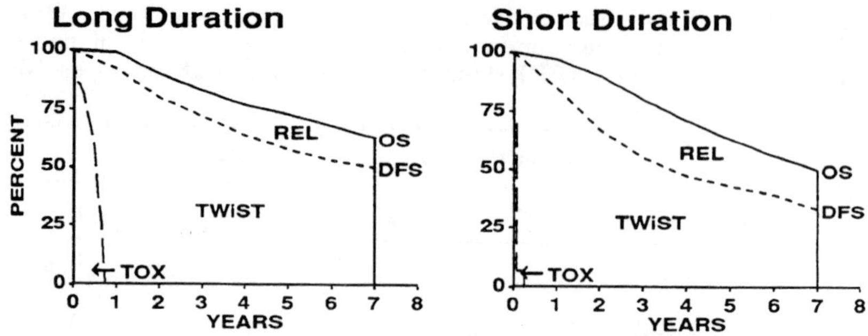

Fig. 3. Partitioned survival for long-duration and for short-duration treatments in 1229 patients with node-positive breast cancer in International Breast Cancer Study Group Trial V at 7 years median follow-up. The areas under the overall survival (*OS*) curves are partitioned by the curves for disease-free survival (*DFS*) and time under adjuvant treatment to obtain average months of time spent in TOX, TWiST, and REL up to 7 years after randomization

ment. For the postmenopausal women, although survival differences are not statistically significant, the improved quality of life associated with a delay in the appearance of overt metastatic disease might nevertheless justify the additional time with toxic effects.

Partitioning the Overall Survival Time

The Q-TWiST analysis of Trial V at 7 years of follow-up is shown in Figs. 3–6 and in Table 2. Figure 3 graphically displays the partitioning of overall survival for each treatment group separately. The larger area of TOX and the smaller area of REL are characteristics of the long-duration treatment in terms of time with reduced quality of life. Seven years (84 months) is obviously the maximum amount of time that patients could remain alive and well if none of them relapsed or died. The three curves for overall survival, disease-free survival, and treatment duration partition this 84-month maximum into average amounts of time spent under treatment, in TWiST, and alive after first relapse.

Table 2 shows the average amounts of time in TOX, TWiST, and REL up to 7 years from randomization; the treatments are compared in terms of differences in the average amount of time that patients spend in the various states under long-duration chemotherapy minus that of the short-duration treatment. The Q-TWiST calculation here attributes the utility coefficient of 0.5 to the average value of both TOX and REL. A patient who assigns these utility coefficients would be willing to trade away 2 months of TOX in return for 1 month of TWiST or 2 months of REL for 1 month of TWiST. These values are selected arbitrarily to illustrate the method and do not represent specific values actually derived from an individual patient preference. Within 7 years the amount of Q-TWiST gained by the long-duration treatment is 5

Table 2. Average time (months) according to quality-of-life endpoints (up to 7 years)

Endpoint	Chemotherapy group		Difference (Long[a] − Short)	95% C.I.
	Long[a]	Short		
All patients				
TOX	6	1	5	5− to 5+
TWiST	53	47	6	3 to 10
REL	9	16	−7	−9 to −5
Q-TWiST[b]	61	56	5	3 to 8
OS	69	64	5	2 to 8
DFS	59	48	11	8 to 15
TFS	62	63	−1	−4 to 2
Premenopausal patients				
TOX	6	1	5	5− to 5+
TWiST	54	47	7	2 to 12
REL	8	15	−7	−10 to −4
Q-TWiST[b]	61	55	6	4 to 8
OS	68	63	5	1 to 9
DFS	60	48	12	2 to 12
TFS	62	62	0	−4 to 4
Postmenopausal patients				
TOX	6	1	5	5− to 5+
TWiST	53	47	6	0 to 12
REL	10	18	−8	−12 to −4
Q-TWiST[b]	61	57	4	−1 to 9
OS	69	66	3	−1 to 7
DFS	59	48	11	5 to 17
TFS	63	65	−2	−6 to 2

OS, Overall survival; DFS, disease-free survival; TFS, adjuvant-treatment-free survival.

[a] For premenopausal patients, long-duration treatment comprised 6 months of CMFp chemotherapy (half also received a perioperative course of intravenous CMF + leucovorin). For postmenopausal patients, long-duration treatment comprised 6 months of CMFp + tamoxifen chemoendocrine therapy (half also received a perioperative course of intravenous CMF + leucovorin).

[b] $u_{tox} = u_{rel} = 0.5$.

months for the entire population: 6 months and 4 months for the two cohorts of pre- and postmenopausal patients, respectively.

Quality-Adjusted Time Gained During Follow-up

Table 2 describes the treatment comparisons at a fixed point in time (7 years). Figure 4 shows the amount of Q-TWiST gained for the long-duration

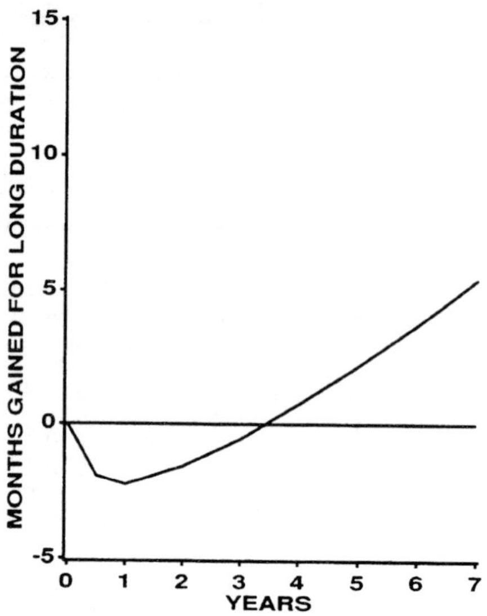

Fig. 4. Quality-adjusted time gained during follow-up. Average months of Q-TWiST (0.5, 0.5) gained for long-duration compared with short-duration treatment in International Breast Cancer Study Group Trial V as a function of years from randomization. The 95% confidence interval at 7 years is given in Table 2

treatment compared with short-duration therapy for times leading up to the 7-year analysis. We call this curve the *Q-TWiST gain function*. Early in the course of follow-up the toxic effects of long-duration treatment reduce the Q-TWiST for this regimen. By 3 years for premenopausal patients and by 4 years for postmenopausal patients, the time lost due to toxic effects is balanced by the time gained due to delay in relapse. The months gained with long-duration therapy will increase still further with additional follow-up provided that the disease-free and overall survival curves for the two treatments remain separated.

The analysis shown in Fig. 4 reflects the arbitrary choice of utility coefficients (0.5) for time spent with toxicity (TOX) and postrelapse survival (REL) to reflect the relative value of these time periods. Figure 5 displays the Q-TWiST gained for long- versus short-duration therapy for a variety of other choices for these coefficients. Specifically, by choosing the coefficients of 1.0 for TOX and 0.0 for REL, treatment comparisons of the average amount of disease-free survival time can be plotted. Similarly, coefficients of 1.0 for TOX and 1.0 for REL define the analysis of average overall survival time. TWiST is displayed when both coefficients are equal to zero. The average time of adjuvant-treatment-free survival is defined by a zero value allocated to TOX but full value allocated to REL. The curves for Q-TWiST gained for long- versus short-duration therapy delineate a region displaying the gains for the entire range of utility coefficients (Fig. 5).

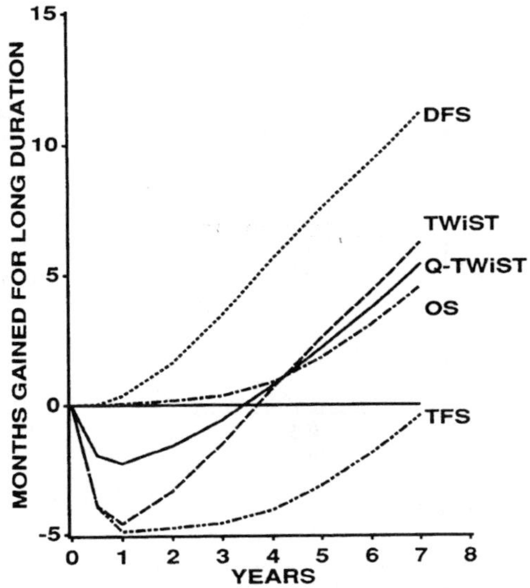

Fig. 5. Quality-adjusted time gained during follow-up. Average months for long-duration compared with short-duration treatment in International Breast Cancer Study Group Trial V using a variety of quality-adjusted endpoints. Each endpoint represents Q-TWiST for specific values of the utility coefficients: disease-free survival (*DFS*; $u_{tox} = 1$, $u_{rel} = 0$); TWiST ($u_{tox} = u_{rel} = 0$); Q-TWiST ($u_{tox} = u_{rel} = 0.5$); survival time (*OS*; $u_{tox} = u_{rel} = 1$); treatment-free survival (*TFS*; $u_{tox} = 0$, $u_{rel} = 1$). The 95% confidence intervals at 7 years are given in Table 2

Threshold Utility Analysis

It is clear that the amount of Q-TWiST gained for the long-duration treatment depends upon the utility values assigned to the time periods having different quality-of-life impact. The threshold utility analysis illustrates this dependence (Fig. 6). The range of utility coefficient values (0 to 1) for TOX and REL are displayed on the vertical and horizontal axes and are denoted by u_{tox} and u_{rel}, respectively. The treatment providing the greatest amount of Q-TWiST for each pair of utility coefficient values can be determined. The dark line in the figure defines a threshold which separates utility values for which the long-duration treatment provides more Q-TWiST from those values for which the short-duration treatment yields more quality-adjusted time. The dashed line delineates those coefficient values for which a statistically significant difference was achieved. Figure 6 shows four threshold utility analyses. The upper two present the results for pre- and postmenopausal patients at 5 years of follow-up, while the lower two represent the same populations at 7 years of follow-up. The differences show that even for postmenopausal patients, a significant Q-TWiST gain is achieved for a large range of choices for the utility coefficients. Furthermore, the range of

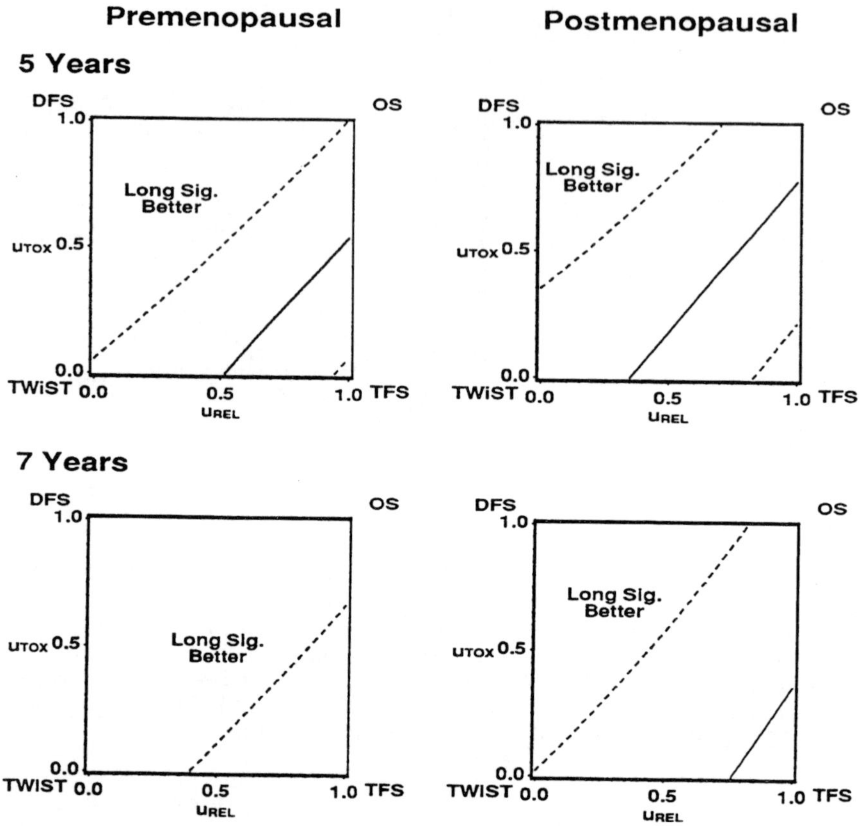

Fig. 6. Threshold utility analyses. *Vertical axis*, u_{tox}; *horizontal axis*, u_{rel}. Both u_{tox} and u_{rel} range between 0 and 1, where the value 1 indicates that the time is worth the same as TWiST, while the value 0 indicates that the time is worth nothing. *Solid line*, the threshold (based on values of u_{tox} and u_{rel}) for which the two treatments have equal Q-TWiST. *Dashed line*, the 95% confidence band for the threshold. *Long Sig. Better*, the values of utility coefficients for which average Q-TWiST 7 years after randomization was statistically significantly greater for long-duration therapy compared with short-duration treatment. Analyses are shown separately for premenopausal and for postmenopausal patients, each at maximum follow-up times of 5 years and 7 years

weights for which a benefit favoring the long-duration treatment is observed increases with additional follow-up time.

The graph in Fig. 6 allows one to determine the treatment preference given a pair of utility coefficient values. For example, for a patient with utility coefficient values of $u_{tox} = u_{rel} = 0.5$, the Long duration treatment is significantly better and, thus, is the preferred treatment in terms of Q-TWiST. On the other hand, for a patient with utility coefficient values of $u_{tox} = 0.1$ and $u_{rel} = 0.9$, for whom the disutility of toxic effects is great

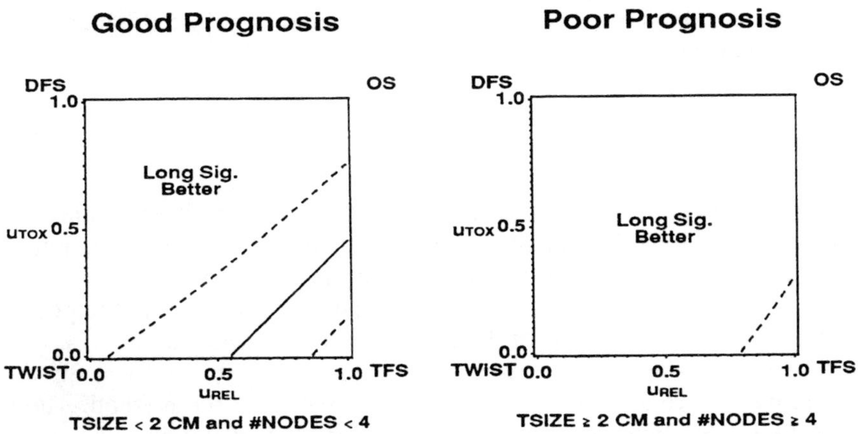

Fig. 7. Threshold utility analyses for subgroups. Threshold diagrams are shown for 59-year-old patients with good prognosis (tumor size <2 cm, number of metastatic nodes <4) and those with poor prognosis (tumor size ⩾2 cm, number of metastatic nodes ⩾4). *Long Sig. Better*, the values of utility coefficients for which average Q-TWiST 7 years after randomization was statistically significantly greater for long-duration therapy compared with short-duration treatment

while the disutility of relapse is minimal, the gain in Q-TWiST at 7 years is not significant. In this case, the treatment preference in terms of Q-TWiST is not conclusive. It is important to note that the threshold utility analysis does not indicate the distribution of the utility coefficients for the population. In other words, the threshold line does not tell us how many patients prefer one treatment over the other. This question must be addressed with additional research.

Threshold Utility Analyses for Subgroups

The amount of average quality time that can be gained by using an effective adjuvant treatment depends upon the baseline prognosis of the cohort. The worse the prognosis, the greater is the potential gain within a fixed follow-up time period. This can be illustrated by displaying separate threshold utility analyses for different patient subgroups. Figure 7 shows such an analysis for two prognostic subgroups in Trial V defined by a Cox proportional hazard regression model including factors for tumor size, number of nodes involved, patient age, and treatment. The range of utility coefficients favoring the more toxicity-intensive long-duration therapy is larger for the poor-prognosis group. This is the case even though the relative effectiveness of treatment is similar for the two patient subgroups (i.e., the same percentage reduction in the risk of an event). This clearly illustrates how, from the patient's point of view, the Q-TWiST method summarizes the quality-adjusted benefits of an effective therapy.

Conclusions

In order to express benefits of adjuvant therapies for breast cancer that incorporate aspects of quality of life for treatment decision making we have developed a quality-adjusted survival analysis. The usefulness of the method, as illustrated by the example of Trial V, is to translate the potential treatment benefit into terms of the amount of useful time gained by applying one treatment program compared with a less intensive (and less effective) alternative. There are two key descriptive elements of the method. The first is the Q-TWiST gain function which describes the evaluation of gains and loses of one treatment compared with the other over time. This gives the physician the possibility to determine when treatment costs of a more toxic program begin to "yield benefits." The second is the threshold utility analysis which, for a given point in time, illustrates the range of utility coefficients for which one treatment is preferred to the other in terms of a greater amount of Q-TWiST. This display is particularly useful for showing the different results within the subgroups of patients that might influence treatment choice based upon a quality-of-life adjusted survival analysis. By showing the range of utility values over which the more intensive or less intensive therapy would by preferred, the physician is given a tool that can be used to determine appropriate treatment for individual patients depending upon their willingness to accept treatment side effects. Additional research is needed to define appropriate utility coefficient values that might be estimated for the impact of toxic effects and relapse on the patient's quality of life.

Acknowledgements. We thank the patients, physicians, nurses, and data managers of the International Breast Cancer Study Group who contributed to the clinical trial described in this paper. Financial support for the clinical trial was provided by the Swiss Cancer League, the Cancer League of Ticino, the Ludwig Institute for Cancer Research, the Swedish Cancer Society, the Australia-New Zealand Breast Cancer Group, the Frontier Science and Technology Research Foundation, and the Swiss Group for Clinical and Epidemiological Cancer Research. Support for the methodological development was provided by grant PBR-53 from the American Cancer Society and grant CA-06516 from the National Cancer Institute.

References

1. Brunner KW, Sonntag RW, Martz G et al. (1975) Controlled study in the use of combined drug therapy for metastatic breast cancer. Cancer 36:1208–1219
2. Priestman TJ, Baum M (1976) Evaluation of quality of life in patients receiving treatment for advanced breast cancer. Lancet i:899–901
3. Coates AS, Gebski V, Bishop JF et al., for the Australian New Zealand Breast Cancer Trials Group (1987) Improving quality of life during chemotherapy for advanced breast cancer: a comparison of intermittent and continuous treatment strategies. N Engl J Med 317:1490–1495
4. Coates AS, Glasziou P, McNeil D (1990) On the receiving end. III. Measurement of quality of life during cancer chemotherapy. Ann Oncol 1:213–217
5. Marrow GR, Black PM, Dudgeon DJ (1991) Advances in data assessment: application to the etiology of nausea reported during chemotherapy, concerns about significance testing, and opportunities in clinical trials. Cancer 67:780–787
6. Schumacher M, Olschewski M, Schulgen G (1991) Assessment of quality of life in clinical trials. Stat Med 10:1915–1930
7. Gelber RD, Goldhirsch A (1986) A new endpoint for the assessment of adjuvant therapy in postmenopausal women with operable breast cancer. J Clin Oncol 4:1772–1779
8. Gelber RD, Gelman RS, Goldhirsch A (1989) A quality-of-life-oriented endpoint for comparing therapies. Biometrics 45:781–795
9. Goldhirsch A, Gelber RD, Simes RJ et al., for the Ludwig Breast Cancer Study Group (1989) Costs and benefits of adjuvant therapy in breast cancer: a quality-adjusted survival analysis. J Clin Oncol 7:36–44
10. Glasziou PP, Simes RJ, Gelber RD (1990) Quality adjusted survival analysis. Stat Med 9:1259–1276
11. Gelber RD, Goldhirsch A, Cavalli F, for the International Breast Cancer Study Group (1991) Quality-of-life-adjusted evaluation of a randomized trial comparing adjuvant therapies for operable breast cancer. Ann Intern Med 114:621–628
12. Gelber RD, Goldhirsch A, Hürny C, Bernhard J, Simes RJ, for the International Breast Cancer Study Group (1992) Quality of life in clinical trials of adjuvant therapies. Natl Cancer Inst Monogr 11:127–135
13. Ludwig Breast Cancer Study Group (1988) Combination adjuvant chemotherapy for node-positive breast cancer: inadequacy of a single perioperative cycle. N Engl J Med 319:677–683

Psychosocial Issues in Breast Cancer Clinical Trials

W.S. Schain

Memorial Cancer Institute, Long Beach, CA, USA

Introduction

We are at a critical juncture in breast cancer care, where treatment decisions are complex, conflicted, and often challenged by the consumer. Never before in the history of medicine has there been such vocal demands for a working partnership between provider and patient or such intense outcries for more information about risks and benefits regarding cancer therapies or prevention programs.

The historical precedent for physician-patient interaction has been characterized by an authoritarian physician recommending a specific treatment based on personal experience, and the grateful patient generally complying with few questions asked. This image of the accepting and grateful patient has been supplanted by a much more sophisticated and inquisitive woman. Today's physician-patient communication is generally more egalitarian and interactive than even 5 years ago. Today's scenario often contains a demanding patient who wants to know not only what treatment is recommended for her disease, but also what the benefits and risks are. She may even request this information be explained in quantitative terms with special references both to her survivorship and the impact which a given treatment may have on her quality of life. In the last decade of the twentieth century, approximately 1 300 000 women will develop breast cancer. Many of these patients, thousands of family members who love them, and hundreds of physicians will be seeking answers to such questions as: Which treatment is the optimal therapy for a given woman? What are its benefits and risks, and what are possible trade-offs between survival outcome and quality of life?

The effectiveness of cancer treatments is determined primarily by clinical trials. To be accepted as the standard of care by the medical community, treatment efficacy must be demonstrated in a well-conducted randomized trial [1]. Recommendations for primary surgery, adjuvant treatments, and

Recent Results in Cancer Research, Vol. 127

now cancer chemoprevention are based on the results gathered in this manner. Benson et al. [2] have asked:

> [If] evidence from therapeutic results achieved from clinical trial research provide the basis for treatment decisions for all, why are not clinical trials the treatment of choice for all eligible patients? Why is it that . . . nationwide, only about 3% of cancer patients receive treatment in a clinical trial [1, p. 2067]. The answer to this question is quite complicated and is influenced by such factors as physician beliefs about trials [3], their reluctance to enroll patients [4] as well as attitudes of patients who may think a clinical trial is a good idea for a hypothetical person but would resist enrollment personally [5].

This issue requires a separate treatise and is not the subject of this chapter but does need to be kept in mind in the present context.

This chapter discusses the role of psychosocial issues in clinical trials and how that which has been learned from this type of work as well as research in psychosocial oncology can be applied to help increase the usefulness of clinical trials in breast cancer. The following critical questions are discussed:

- What is the distinction between psychosocial issues and quality of life?
- Why are psychosocial issues and quality-of-life data important in breast cancer clinical trial research?
- What is meant by a dynamic versus a static approach to clinical trial research?
- How can we use knowledge about psychosocial issues to improve the clinical effectiveness of breast cancer trials?

Differences Between Psychosocial Issues and Quality of Life

The distinction between psychosocial issues and quality of life is quite vague as each of these two areas overlap with the other. For the most part, the two constructs are interdependent, and one may be seen as having an impact on the other. In a number of instances, however, the two terms can be used interchangeably. For purposes of clarity, I make a small distinction between the two. The concept of psychosocial issues is a broad construct which both encompasses quality of life and also impacts on it. Specifically, psychosocial factors are those conditions and circumstances in life that are universal in everyone's day-to-day functioning, and that influence his/her psychological, social, physical, functional, and spiritual state. Quality of life, especially as it relates to health, is a more narrowly defined construct [6]. While it appears vague and somewhat ambiguous, there are specific domains which have some general agreement among experts in the field of oncology throughout North America and Europe [7–10]. While the specific number and areas which constitute quality-of-life domains differ among trials and research investigators, the following factors enter the equation in some proportion [11, 12]: functional status, psychological distress, fatigue/malaise, fears and concerns [13], nausea and vomiting, pain, social functioning, existential or spiritual concerns, cognitive functioning [14], and sexuality [15, 16].

Another area of consensual agreement among psychosocial oncology researchers is that most clinical studies must contain a combination of assessment tools which measure both global aspects of quality of life and those conditions which are unique and specific to a given trial, type of medication, or organ site malignancy [17]. A general quality-of-life measure does not elicit the special reactions of a breast cancer patient's reaction to her loss of ovarian function, hair, or stamina as a result of chemotherapy. Only a specially designed modular questionnaire can identify these psychosocial responses and therefore must be included in the assessment battery [12].

Why are Psychosocial Issues or Quality-of-Life Data Important in Breast Cancer Clinical Trials?

Recommendations for therapy today are determined not merely by theory but in part also by an understanding of the biology of the disease and the expectations of the woman's psychosocial and functional outcome. This situation is reflected most poignantly today in the frequently encountered interaction between a physician and a breast cancer patient in whom the biological parameters of her disease make her a candidate for either mastectomy or breast conservation surgery. The individual physician may respond to her by saying the following: "Medically you cannot make a wrong decision; the choice is really a psychological one." Physicians and patients are increasingly faced with choices between different treatments which are associated with similar survival rates but different toxicities or impact on quality of life. Sometimes patients are willing to trade off a few months of survival for an increase in quality of life [18]. Schipper [19] has emphasized that something is lost if one focuses solely on survival information to the exclusion of quality of life data. We also know that longevity could be compromised if we are to make judgments on dose or duration of certain systemic therapies based only on quality of life or psychosocial reactions. Neither outcome today can be the final measure by which we judge treatment efficacy. "The success of therapy for a patient is measured in the eyes of the patients who (may) live longer or live better. What our psychosocial methodologies lack in precision, they may to a certain extent, compensate for in relevance" [19].

Specifically, psychosocial issues and quality-of-life data are essential in clinical trials for breast cancer because they:

- Define and describe treatment morbidity.
- Provide information for decision making.
- Guide decisions about modifications in treatment protocols.

- Provide the necessary information to develop support services.
- Assist in giving us information for patient education and professional development.
- Stimulate hypotheses for the next generation of clinical trials.

In summary, treatment strategies must consider conclusions from clinical trial research which combine biological and behavioral sciences to look for more effective and humane ways to reduce mortality and morbidity from breast cancer. In order to accomplish this end we must move the design and implementation of this type of research from a static to a dynamic perspective.

Static Versus Dynamic Perspective of Clinical Trial Research

Most clinical trial research is driven by a "static" view of clinical investigation. Such a perspective pays close attention to the formal rules of a trial, such as inclusion and exclusion criteria, quality control, and rules for stopping. The "dynamic" view of a clinical trial emphasizes certain behavioral aspects of the patient's participation and the ways in which such variables may affect the actual outcome of the trial [20]. In the static interpretation of research one assumes that the biological differences noted in the endpoints are a result of the two different treatments, and that all other factors in the experiment are likely to be randomly distributed across the two conditions. The dynamic view, however, assumes that other variables are very likely to be interactive and may indeed confound the perceived outcome.

Since the Breast Cancer Chemoprevention Trial is a the next frontier of clinical trial research and one which clearly reflects the ways in which participants' behaviors may confound the identified biological endpoints, it is essential that this be discussed. As Leventhal et al. [20] observe, "If behavioral factors interact differently with treatment and control conditions, they can introduce serious confounding . . . by adding to, subtracting from or multiplying the (main) effects . . ." (p. 133). In a double-blind prevention trial of this type, psychosocial factors which must be identified in order to account for confounding of the outcome include (a) the participant's reasons for entering the trial (e.g., altruism, financial, self-protection), (b) her beliefs about the treatment arm to which she is randomized, (c) her perception of the treatment impact and its side effects, and (d) her performance of specific behaviors which might affect the study outcome variables (e.g., breast self-examination, diet, adherence to medication).

Some women believe that in taking the active agent tamoxifen they may feel safe and "protected" from a possible breast cancer. They may then feel that they are free to eat fatty foods, drink excessive alcohol, and not exercise. On the other hand, there may be a subset of women on the active agent who, unlike the former group, intensify their efforts to remain healthy and well, reducing dietary fat, exercising, performing breast self-examination scrupulously every month, and paying great attention to signs and symptoms of gynecological problems. Such behavioral manifestations related to beliefs about certain conditions of the trial may have profound implications for conclusions to be drawn from these and other clinical investigations. Careful attention must be paid to these types of psychosocial issues, from the conception of the clinical trial design through its final analysis.

How Can Psychosocial Issues Help in Expanding the Usefulness of Breast Cancer Clinical Trials?

Feinstein [27] has noted that, "From a static view, the ability to study treatment efficacy is confounded by noncompliance. From a behavioral perspective any non-adherence is something that must be understood in determining the drug's effectiveness for cancer prevention (or cancer treatment)." Bell et al. [22] observe that "There may be greater benefit in disease reduction with a less efficacious treatment that is fully utilized than a more efficacious treatment that is under utilized." One of the ways to ensure that adherence is optimal, and that there is internal validity to a trial's objectives is to incorporate knowledge of psychosocial and behavioral issues into the design, implementation, and analysis of research on breast cancer, irrespective of whether it is of cancer treatment or prevention.

The primary focus of the treatment's impact on biological endpoints must be of paramount importance in any clinical trial. While this is absolutely essential to advance medical care, it is no longer enough. Biological outcome measures are necessary but not sufficient to obtain the answers that are needed in the real world and to transfer the knowledge to patients who will be treated in the community. We need to develop research protocols which are patient centered in terms of primary objectives, intervening variables, and ultimate endpoints. One example is the possibility, in the very near future, of a clinical trial to evaluate the efficacy of hormone replacement therapy in previously treated breast cancer patients (United States Food and Drug Administration FDA Hearing, Rockville, Maryland, Feb. 14, 1992). In a study of this type, quality of life is not just an endpoint or even an integral component of the trial; it is the source and substance of the research. Commitment to this type of clinical research is likely to expand the usefulness of breast cancer clinical trials by asking questions in such a way that addresses psychosocial issues are prominent. In constructing studies of this type it may be possible to attract more patients to research and to retain them more successfully because of their recognition of the study's attention to psychosocial and behavioral concerns. In this manner we are likely to increase enrollment, be able to deal more successfully with compliance difficulties, and increase the retention of study subjects on the trial. All these conditions will lead to higher statistical power, more reliable cnclusions, and greater confidence that the types of psychosocial variables likely to confound the medical endpoints have been appropriately addressed and managed.

In conclusion, the marriage of behavioral and biological sciences is crucial for the next generation of clinical trial research in order to ensure its efficacy and effectiveness. Ways to facilitate this outcome include: (a) providing professional education about the need and value of psychosocial issues in clinical trial research, (b) requiring that all clinical trials have dual leadership which combines the expertise of biological and behavioral scientists, and (c) including psychosocial theory in the design, execution, and analysis of clinical trials.

References

1. Benson AB, Pregler JP, Bean JA et al. (1991) Oncologists' reluctance to accrue patients onto clinical trials. J Clin Oncol 9(11):2067–2075
2. Gelber R, Goldhirsh A (1988) Can a clinical trial be the treatment of choice for patients with cancer? J Nate Cancer Inst 80(12):886–887
3. Lind SE, Good MJ, Delvecchio, Minkovitz CS, Good BJ (1991) Oncologists' vary in their willingness to undertake anti-cancer therapies. Br J Cancer 64: 391–395
4. Taylor K, Margolese RG, Soskolne CL (1984) Physicians reasons for not entering eligible patients in a randomized clinical trial of surgery for breast cancer. N Engl J Med 310(21):1363–1367
5. Cassileth BR, Lusk EJ, Miller DS et al. (1982) Attitudes toward clinical trials among patients and the public. JAMA 248(8):968–970
6. Ware JE Jr (1987) Standards for validating health measures. Definition and content. J Chronic Dis 40:473–480
7. Moinpour CM, Feigl P, Metch B et al. (1989) Quality of life endpoints in cancer clinical trials: review and recomendations. J Nate Cancer Inst 81:485–495
8. Ganz PA, Schag CA, Cheng HL (1990) Assessing the quality of life: a study in newly diagnosed breast cancer patients. J Clin Epidememiol 43(1):75–86
9. De Haes JCJM, van Knippenberg FCE (1985) Quality of life of cancer patients. Soc Sci Med 20:809–817
10. Cella DF, Cherin EA (1987) Measuring quality of life in patients with cancer. In: Proceedings of the Fifth National Conference on Human Values and Cancer. NY Amer Can Soc, pp 23–31
11. Coscarelli CS, Heinrich RL (1988) CARES: cancer rehabilitation evaluation system. Cares Consultants, Los Angeles
12. Aaronson NK (1990) Quality of life research in cancer clinical trials: a need for common rules and language. Oncology 4(5):59–66
13. Meyerowitz BE (1986) Assessing the quality of breast cancer patients: a review of recent literature. In: Ventafridda V, van Dam FSAM, Yanick R et al. (eds) Proceedings of the International Workshop on Quality of Life Assessment and Cancer Treatment. Excepta Medica, Amsterdam, pp 127–138
14. Levine MN, Guyatt GH, Gent M et al. (1988) Quality of life in stage II breast cancer. An instrument for clinical trials. J Clin Oncol 6:1798–1810
15. Sugarbaker PH, Barofsky I, Rosenberg SA et al. (1982) Quality of life assessment of patients in extremity sarcoma clinical trials. Surgery 91:17–23
16. Schain WS (1988) A sexual interview is a sexual intervention. In: Innovations in oncology nursing, vol 414. Meniscus, p 2

17. Coates A, Gelski V, Bishop JF et al. (1987) Improving the quality of life during chemotherapy for advanced breast cancer N Engl J Med 317:1490–1495
18. Singer PA, Tasch ES Stockig C et al. (1991) Sex or survival: trade-offs between quality and quantity of life. J Clin Oncol 9(2):328–324
19. Schipper H (1990) Guidelines and caveats for quality of life measurement in clinical practice. Oncology 4(5):52
20. Leventhal H, Nerenz DR, Leventhal EA et al. (1991) The behavioral dynamics of clinical trials. Prev Med 20:132–146
21. Feinstein AR (1976) Compliance bias and the interpretation of therapeutic trials. In: Sackett DL, Haynes RB (eds), Compliance with therapeutic regimens. Johns Hopkins University Press, Battimore
22. Bell RL, Curb JD, Friedman LM et al. (1985) Enhancement of visit adherence in the national beta blocker heart attack trial. Controlled Clin Trials 6:89–101

Quality-of-Life Considerations in the Adjuvant Setting: Critical Review

A. Coates

ANZ Breast Cancer Trials Group, Royal Prince Alfred Hospital, Camperdown NSW, Australia

This session combined theoretical and practical considerations relevant to the measurement of quality of life (QL) in the setting of adjuvant therapy and preventive trials in breast cancer. Perhaps more importantly, by its very inclusion it underlined the importance attached to the concept of QL in clinical trials and clinical practice. In adjuvant therapy, and still more in preventive interventions, the woman who undertakes more or less toxic treatment does so in the hope of future gain. In neither case does the patient have discernible disease at the time that therapy is used; thus any morbidity incurred can be compensated only by delay of disease or death. Where alternative strategies for the pursuit of such benefits are being compared, it is important to measure the impact of each on QL.

Dr. Aaronson opened the session with a sound exposition of the classical psychometric approach to QL evaluation. He noted that, despite the obvious desirability of a standard approach and common measuring instruments, most existing data are generated with quite disparate techniques, frequently employing instruments of unknown psychometric properties. He advised that the patient should complete QL instruments, but the role of the physician in recording aspects such as performance status scales was also acknowledged. Definition of the concepts of QL remains difficult, and he stressed the necessity to restrict study to aspects relevant to the clinical situation, leading to a recommendation that the measurement of QL should be as a multidimensional construct, covering symptoms of disease, side effects of treatment, and physical, psychological, social and role functioning. For practical reasons Dr. Aaronson regarded questionnaires as preferable to interview techniques, and urged investigators wishing to measure QL in trials not to develop new measures but to choose among existing instruments with an eye to brevity and simplicity as well as established reliability and validity.

Dr. Hürny then discussed coping strategies, an important aspect of QL, and reviewed the conflicting available evidence linking coping with prog-

Recent Results in Cancer Research, Vol. 127

nosis. Methodological problems still obscure a clear answer to this question, but in studies measuring coping at more than one time point the change in coping was related to survival. The current International Breast Cancer Study Group trials that he described, in which coping is being measured prospectively, may eventually contribute important information, but preliminary analysis presented elsewhere at this conference showed little evidence of a link between coping and survival duration. Dr. Hürny also stressed the need for prospective evaluation of coping within existing clinical trials, using reliable, valid and sensitive instruments followed sequentially.

Dr. Gelber presented data on Q-TWiST, a methodology allowing comparison of QL in trials in which it was not directly measured. Essentially this approach partitions the overall survival experience of patients in a trial into discrete states and assign a relative utility to each, relative to a state without either disease symptoms or treatment morbidity. The time periods spent in each state are then corrected by the desired utility coefficient, and the results are added to obtain an overall value for average quality-adjusted survival, the Q-TWiST. One attractive feature of this approach is the potential to re-evaluate trial results using any desired utility values. Even if utilities cannot be exactly assessed, a threshold analysis may clearly show that for all plausible utility values one treatment is to be preferred and so assist in reaching a treatment decision. One can also plot the amount of quality-adjusted survival time associated with more and less intensively treated groups over time. This Q-TWiST gain function elegantly displays the future gains to be expected on average from an initial investment in toxic therapy. Dr. Gelber suggested the use of time trade-off techniques to establish appropriate utilities and thus allow a standardized comparison of treatment benefits and side effects from the patient viewpoint. In the session summary, the present author illustrated the application of the utility approach in a study of patients who had received cytotoxic adjuvant therapy [1]. These patients were willing to accept quite small increments in survival duration or probability to justify the morbidity of chemotherapy.

Dr. Schain addressed the psychological aspects of adjuvant trials but also focussed attention on the important distinctions between trials of adjuvant therapy, in which all participants have a malignant disease, and interventions designed to prevent disease, in which the large majority of treatments are given to well persons who will never contract the disease in question. She challenged the historical paternalistic approach, asserting the right of the patient to an informed input to treatment decisions. Dr. Schain advocated a modular approach to evaluation of QL, such as that of the EORTC core questionnaire and disease-specific modules. In the prevention trial setting, she noted that the patient's motivation for entering the trial, her beliefs (not necessarily true) about which arm she is on and her perception of treatment side effects together with her personal health behaviour may all influence compliance and trial endpoints. Finally, she noted that in some clinical trials such as those of hormone replacement therapy the QL endpoints are primary rather than subsidiary.

Overall, the session provided a valuable review of this vital aspect of the cost-benefit balance inherent in treating asymptomatic patients, but it also pointed to some unresolved issues. If we are to make assessment of QL routine in clinical trials, the instruments used for its measurement must be simple. This does not of course remove the requirement that they be reliable, sensitive and valid. The two approaches to this question presented at the session differ in approaches to resolving this dilemma. The psychometric school favors more complex, extensively validated instruments and seeks to convince trialists that they are really not as impractical as they seem. In contrast, a pragmatic approach pioneered by Priestman et al. [2] and followed by the International Breast Cancer Study Group [3] uses instruments selected for their practicality and seeks by the results obtained to add to the evidence for their validity. Further resolution of this question must await a future conference, but the attention paid to QL by both cannot but improve our understanding of this important dimension of clinical research and treatment.

References

1. Coates AS, Simes RJ (1992) Patient assessment of adjuvant treatment in operable breast cancer. In: Williams CJ (ed) Introducing new treatments for cancer: practical, ethical and legal problems. Wiley, London, pp 447–458
2. Priestman T, Baum M, Jones V, Forbes J (1977) Comparative trial of endocrine versus cytotoxic treatment in advanced breast cancer. Br Med J 1:1248–1250
3. Hürny C, Bernhard J, Gelber RD, Coates AS, Castiglione M, Isley M, Dreher D, Peterson H, Goldhirsch A, for the International Breast Cancer Study Group (1992) Quality of life measures for patients receiving adjuvant therapy for breast cancer: an international trial. Eur J Cancer 28:118–124

VII. Long-Term Toxicity and Economic Aspects

Long-Term Sequelae from Adjuvant Chemotherapy

P. Valagussa, A. Moliterni, M. Zambetti, and G. Bonadonna

Istituto Nazionale Tumori, Milan, Italy

Introduction

It has been estimated that 5 000 000 Americans living in 1987 have had cancer at some time during their lives, and that 3 000 000 have survived 5 years or longer, largely because of improvement in early detection techniques and the use of intensive multimodal therapies [1]. As far as operable breast cancer is concerned, the updated international overview [2] (reprinted in part in this volume) has recently confirmed that adjuvant systemic treatments can effectively reduce the 10-year risk of new disease manifestations and mortality. While worthwhile in human terms, this improvement seems moderate in size especially when findings from various chemotherapy protocols, different for drugs, doses, and intensity of treatment, are combined to produce an "average" result. It is thus important to investigate types and severity of long-term and late effects to assess the cost-benefit ratio of these treatments.

In this paper, we present the experience of the Milan Cancer Institute on late sequelae from adjuvant chemotherapy, with or without breast irradiation, following surgery for operable breast cancer.

Patients and Methods

The medical records of 1045 women admitted to three different randomized protocols initiated between December 1980 and July 1990 [3–5] were carefully reanalyzed. In the first protocol [3] a total of 90 patients with node-negative and estrogen receptor negative breast cancer were randomly allocated to either no adjuvant treatment or to the intravenous administration of cyclophosphamide (600 mg/m^2), methotrexate (40 mg/m^2), and fluorouracil (600 mg/m^2; CMF) every 3 weeks for 12 courses. The other two protocols dealt with node-positive breast cancer: 552 women with one to

Recent Results in Cancer Research, Vol. 127

three involved nodes [4] were randomized to either 12 courses of CMF (as above) or to 8 courses of CMF followed by 4 courses of doxorubicin (Adriamycin, ADM; 75 mg/m^2), while all 403 patients with more than 3 positive nodes [5] received 4 courses of ADM either before or alternated with CMF. Local-regional treatment consisted of either modified radical mastectomy or quadrantectomy plus full axillary dissection. In women subjected to conservative surgery, breast irradiation was delivered concomitantly with adjuvant chemotherapy. No other treatments were administered; in particular, none of our patients received adjuvant tamoxifen. Follow-up timing and methods were reported previously [3–5].

For the purpose of the present evaluation and in the absence of recorded sequelae, a minimum of 1 year follow-up in clinical complete remission should have elapsed from discontinuation of all treatments. A total of 798 women (76% of all patients entered in the three protocols) systematically followed in the outpatient clinic of the Division of Medical Oncology were considered suitable for this evaluation; 27 (3%) were assigned to no adjuvant treatment, 288 (36%) to CMF, and 483 (61%) to ADM plus CMF. Patients allocated to ADM but who for various reasons (refusal, 22/26; electrocardiographic abnormalities following CMF 4/26) did not receive this anthracycline were considered in the CMF group. A total of 347 women (43%) also received concomitant breast irradiation; no dose or drug adjustments were devised for these patients. The median observation time, i.e., the time elapsed from the end of all treatments to either the date of last visit or the documentation of new disease manifestations or second neoplasms, whichever occurred first, was approximately 57 months (range 6–123), and one fourth of these patients was followed for 8 years or more.

Results

Noncardiac Effects

At the time of last follow-up five women (0.6%) presented with leukocyte counts ranging between 3100 and 3400/mm^3 and 26 (3.3%) with hemoglobin levels between 9.5 and 11.8 g/dl (Table 1); thrombocytopenia, i.e., platelet fall to less than 110 000/mm^3, was not recorded. Leukopenia and hemoglobin falls were occasional episodes and were always preceded by normal values in the peripheral blood counts. Three of the 27 patients never received adjuvant chemotherapy, and 17 of 451 were not subjected to breast irradiation. Herpes zoster infection was documented in 2% of women, all of whom received adjuvant chemotherapy. Chronic or progressive liver alterations were never documented; however, eight patients (1%) showed abnormal SGPT (>2.5 normal values), which was associated with elevated SGOT values in three women.

Superficial thrombophlebitis was not considered as a complication of cancer chemotherapy. Thrombotic events were documented in two patients;

Table 1. Noncardiac effects from adjuvant chemotherapy with or without breast irradiation

	%
Leukocytes 3100–3400/mm^3	0.6
Hemoglobin 9.5–11.8 g/dl	3.3
Herpes zoster infection	2.0
Liver function tests >2.5 × normal	1.0
Thrombotic complications	0.3
Irradiation-related fibrosis	
Lung	3.2
Breast	3.7
Skin	14.1
Second neoplasms	1.4
Myelodysplastic syndrome	0.1
In situ cancers	0.4

one postmenopausal woman aged 62 years at surgery died of a cerebrovascular stroke 31 months later. In a premenopausal patient aged 43 years at the time of surgery a cerebrovascular stroke occurred 16 months later; postmortem examination detected the presence of massive pulmonary embolism. No other episodes of venous or arterial thrombosis were recorded.

Radiation-related fibrosis was not a major complication (Table 1). Eleven asymptomatic patients (3.2%) showed radiological signs of lung fibrosis which was always mild and reversible. Moderate to severe cases of breast and skin fibrosis were reported in 3.7% and 14.1%, respectively; however, ADM-related skin reactions were never documented.

Eleven of the 798 patients (1.4%) developed a second malignancy, including three in situ or basal cell carcinomas. In only one patient did we document signs of myelodysplastic syndrome, 38 months after surgery.

Amenorrhea and Increase in Body Weight

The frequency of amenorrhea was evaluated in 508 patients still menstruating at the time of local-regional treatment. As reported in Table 2, permanent cessation of menses was documented in 76.5% of women given adjuvant chemotherapy as compared to 8 of 14 (57.1%) in the control group. Amenorrhea following adjuvant chemotherapy was age related; all women aged over 45 years at surgery became amenorrheic, compared to 86% of those between 41 and 45 years and 49.5% of those between 36 and 40 years. Only 2 of 48 (4.2%) patients aged under 36 years at surgery and given adjuvant chemotherapy showed permanent cessation of menses more than 6 years after treatment discontinuation. It is worth mentioning that 11 women (2.2%) developed reversible amenorrhea (cessation of menses for 3–6 months) during or immediately after adjuvant chemotherapy; all were

Table 2. Frequency of amenorrhea in menstruating patients

	Adjuvant treatment (n = 494)	No adjuvant treatment (n = 14)
	%	%
No amenorrhea	21.3	42.9
Reversible	2.2	0
Permanent		
≤18 months after surgery	66.4	7.1
>18 months after surgery	10.1	50.0

still menstruating after a median follow-up of 44 months (range 9–79). By contrast, 50 patients (10.1%) in the adjuvant treatment group who continued to menstruate during chemotherapy developed permanent cessation of menses at a median time of 3 years from surgery (range 20–96 months); their median age at the time of amenorrhea was 44 years (range 38–51). Similarly, 7 of 14 women not treated with adjuvant chemotherapy became amenorrheic more than 3 years after surgery, at a median age of 50 years (range 42–53).

Following adjuvant chemotherapy the median increase in body weight was 3.5 kg (range −9 to +19) in premenopausal women, regardless of whether (3 kg) or not (4 kg) amenorrhea was documented. In postmenopausal patients the median increase in body weight was 2 kg (−11 to +15). Due to the paucity of information, no attempts were made to correlate these findings to either endocrinological dysfunctions, psycological effects, or dietary habits.

Cardiac Effects

In our series of patients, 483 women (61%) were given ADM to a maximum cumulative dose of 300 mg/m^2, while 347 (43%) received breast irradiation (50 Gy plus a boost of 10 Gy over 4–6 weeks) as part of breast conserving treatment. Cardiac abnormalities were documented in a total of 94 patients (11.8%) within a median of 17 months after surgery (range 6–120) and of 6 months (range 0–100) from the end of all treatments. Table 3 presents the frequency of these complications as a function of the type of adjuvant chemotherapy, breast irradiation, and age at surgery. As can be seen, regardless of the type and severity of cardiac effects, adjuvant chemotherapy per se did not appear to play an important role, whereas irradiation, particularly when delivered to the left breast (26.6%) and associated with ADM (31.2%), increased the frequency of cardiac disturbances. In addition, frequency of cardiac effects was twice as high (19.9%) in women aged over

Table 3. Cardiac effects as a function of adjuvant chemotherapy, breast irradiation, and age at surgery

	n	%
Total	94/798	11.8
No adjuvant treatment	3/27	11.1
CMF	29/288	10.0
ADM and CMF	62/483	12.8
No breast irradiation	29/451	6.4
Breast irradiation	65/347	17.7
Left breast	47/177	26.6
CMF	11/63	17.5
ADM	34/109	31.2
Age at surgery		
≤55 years	66/657	10.0
>55 years	28/141	19.9

55 years at surgery (an age group which excludes all but two premenopausal women) as in younger patients (10.0%). Among the 94 patients who presented cardiac effects, 30 (31.9%) had pre-existing risk factors at surgery (arterial hypertesion alone or associated to metabolic dysfunctions in 25, heart disease in 5), and 6 had minor aspecific electrocardiographic changes at surgery.

Table 4 summarizes the types and course of cardiac effects. Of the four women who developed ADM-related cardiotoxicity, three also received irradiation to the left breast, two had a previous history of heart disease, and one showed aspecific electrocardiographic changes at surgery. At the time of the present analysis, two patients have died 32 and 86 months later, respectively. Of the remaining two women, one remains alive and disease free at 66 months; the other is alive at 75 months with a second ovarian cancer treated with paraplatin. Only one episode of acute myocardial infarction was documented 113 months from surgery in a patient aged 48 years and who had not received adjuvant ADM or irradiation. She is presently alive, with osseous metastases documented 5 months after myocardial infarction.

A total of 35 women (4.4%) showed abnormalities of the ST-T tract in the absence of other clinical and laboratory signs. These abnormalities were documented more frequently in patients given irradiation to the left breast (11.3%); this was particularly true when ADM was part of the adjuvant program (irradiation to the left breast: ADM 15.6% versus CMF 3.2%). Twenty-five of these women were evaluated after a minimum follow-up of 18 months in clinical complete remission from their breast cancer and in 92% (23/25) ST-T abnormalities completely recovered.

Fifty-four women (6.4%) presented other cardiac abnormalities, among whom 16 (2%) developed ischemic heart disease, 16 (2%) cardiac arrythmia, and 3 (0.4%) pericarditis. Risk factors at surgery were present in 21 patients

Table 4. Type and course of cardiac effects (n = 94)

Type	n	%	Risk factors	ADM	Irradition to left breast	Comments
Cardiotoxicity	4	0.5	2	4	3	Deaths: 2 (32 and 86 months) Alive: 2 (66 and 75 months)
Acute myocardial infarction	1	0.1	–	–	–	Disease progression after 5 months
Abnormal ST-T tract[a]	35	4.4	7	23	20	RT to left breast and ADM (15.6%); RT to left breast and CMF (3.2%); transient in 92%
Others	54	6.8	21	35	24	RT to left breast (13.6%), with no difference between CMF (14.3%) and ADM (12.8%); age >55 years (16.3%); Improved in 52.5%

[a] In the absence of other clinical and laboratory signs.

(38.9%). These abnormalities were more frequent following irradiation to the left breast (13.6%) and in women aged over 55 years at surgery (16.3%). By contrast, the type of adjuvant treatment did not seem to play an important role, with two abnormalities documented in 27 (7.4%) patients not subjected to adjuvant systemic treatment, 6.2% following CMF alone, and 8.1% after the ADM-containing regimen. In women given irradiation to the left breast, the frequency of these myocardial alterations was 14.3% after CMF and 12.8% following ADM. Despite prompt institution of appropriate treatment, the increase in severity of these abnormalities was documented in 5% and no change in 42.5% of patients.

Discussion

It is well known that apart from acute toxicity potentially curative multimodal treatments may produce long-term sequelae that occur as chronic problems after cessation of therapy or as late effects surfacing months to years later. Sequelae can result from direct injury to tissues caused by irradiation and/or drug treatment, complications from surgery, or persistent immunologic deficits caused by the underlying disease or its therapy. Long-term survivorship of adult cancers is a relatively new phenomenon, and information on late treatment effects is scarse. This is especially true for patients with operable breast cancer, despite the fact that modern adjuvant systemic programs were begun almost 20 years ago. Published series are generally small in numbers or in follow-up time [6] or deal with one particular treatment effect [7, 8]. Thus, the incidence of late complications may be underestimated (or overestimated).

To assess the type and frequency of long-term complications, we analyzed a series of 798 women entered into three randomized protocols carried out at the Milan Cancer Institute [3–5] and followed for a median time of about 5 years while patients remained in continuous complete remission; one fourth of these patients were followed for 8 years or more.

Apart from cardiac effects we documented no other sequelae. In particular, despite the administration of methotrexate, we observed no chronic or progressive liver alterations. Irradiation-related fibrosis of the breast was not a major problem. In only 11 women (3.2%) did we detect mild lung fibrosis, which was asymptomatic and promply reversible in all instances. As far as second cancers were concerned, only one patient developed a myelodysplastic syndrome, while four ovarian cancers, two gastrointestinal carcinoma, and one papillary thyroid cancer were documented. Overall, these findings are consistent with our previous observation on second malignancies following adjuvant CMF [8, 9]. Thrombotic complications have been reported to occur after adjuvant chemotherapy with or without combined tamoxifen [10–12]. In our series, we documented only two episodes of cerebrovascular stroke (0.3%), one occurring in a premenopausal woman 16 months after surgery. No other episodes of venous or arterial thrombosis were detected.

Among the various growth-inhibiting compounds utilized in the treatment of malignant diseases, doxorubicin has the greatest potential for cardiotoxicity [13]. The incidence of clinically apparent chronic cardiomiopathy is clearly dose related. Potentially fatal acute effects include pericarditis-myocarditis, conduction disturbances, and arrhythmia; transient electrocardiographic abnormalities may occur, but they are usually harmless. Also, therapeutic irradiation can lead to ischemic heart disease, and data from animal models suggest two pathogenic mechanisms: microvascular and macrovascular arterial damage [14]. The frequency of cardiac complications is related to dose, dose rate, irradiated volume, and radiotherapy technique. Cardiac damage appears to progress for several years after cessation of radiotherapy.

In our series of patients, 61% of whom received an ADM-containing regimen and 43% postoperative breast irradiation, cardiac effects of different types and severity were documented in a total of 11.8% of patients. Four patients (0.8%) developed ADM-related cardiotoxicity, which was fatal in two patients, 32 and 86 months later. Three women received full-dose ADM (300 mg/m^2), while in one patient cardiotoxicity was documented after two courses. Overall, the incidence of this toxic effect was similar to that reported by investigators at M.D. Anderson Cancer Center after adjuvant chemotherapy with fluorouracil, doxorubicin, and cyclophosphamide (FAC) [15].

Of particular interest is the frequency of abnormalities in the ST-T tract in the absence of other clinical and laboratory signs. This cardiac effect was more frequently observed after the administration of concomitant irradiation to the left breast and ADM (15.6%). In our experience, these changes became reversible in almost all patients, but continuous follow-up is mandatory. Fifty-four (6.8%) additional patients developed other cardiac alterations (including ischemic heart disease in 16, cardiac arrythmia in 16, pericarditis in 3). Irradiation to the left breast (13.6%) and age over 55 years at surgery (16.3%) seemed to play a major role, while the type of adjuvant treatment per se did not seem to be an inducer of these effects (CMF 6.2%, ADM 8.1%; following radiotherapy to left breast: CMF 14.3%, ADM 12.8%). It is worth mentioning that these abnormalities were also documented in 2 of 27 women (7.4%) not subjected to adjuvant chemotherapy. Based on these findings, a detailed analysis is in progress, and additional laboratory investigations will be carried out also in patients not receiving adjuvant chemotherapy.

In conclusion, apart from cardiac effects, for which the exact contribution of other factors such as age, life-style, preexisting risk factors, irradiation doses, and techniques still remain to be fully assessed, adjuvant chemotherapy appears devoid of important long-term sequelae, at least during the first 5–10 years. However, continuous follow-up is mandatory, both to help prevent and to manage late iatrogenic complications as well as to assess their actual incidence. How should the recognition of late complications change our approach in the adjuvant treatment of breast cancer? Drug selection and appropriate radiotherapeutic techniques remain important. Nonetheless, the choice of treatment should not be based merely on the potential risk of developing late complications. Cure remains the primary aim also in high-risk operable breast cancer, although in a fraction of patients this disease can be managed for a few years once relapse has occurred. The international overview [2] has proven that both endocrine and cytotoxic adjuvant treatments significantly reduce the annual odds of disease recurrence and death. While for endocrine manipulations these reductions reflect average results which can be achieved with these modalities, to further improve treatment outcome there is still ample room for optimally designed short-term and full-dose adjuvant cytotoxic regimens.

References

1. American Cancer Society (1988) Cancer facts and figures. American Cancer Society, New York
2. Early Breast Cancer Trialists' Collaborative Group (1992) Systemic treatment of early breast cancer by hormonal, cytotoxic or immune therapy: 133 randomised

trials involving 31 000 recurrences and 24 000 deaths among 75 000 women. Lancet 339:1–15, 71–85
3. Zambetti M, Bonadonna G, Valagussa P et al. (1992) CMF for node-negative and estrogen receptor-negative breast cancer. Natl Cancer Inst Monogr 11: 79–85
4. Moliterni A, Bonadonna G, Valagussa P et al. (1991) Cyclophosphamide, methotrexate, and fluorouracil with and without doxorubicin in the adjuvant treatment of resectable breast cancer with one to three positive axillary nodes. J Clin Oncol 9:1124–1130
5. Buzzoni R, Bonadonna G, Valagussa P et al. (1991) Adjuvant chemotherapy with doxorubicin plus cyclophosphamide, methotrexate, and fluorouracil in the treatment of resectable breast cancer with more than three positive axillary nodes. J Clin Oncol 9:2134–2140
6. Love RR, Wiebe DA, Newcomb PA et al. (1991) Effects of tamoxifen on cardiovascular risk factors in postmenopausal women. Ann Intern Med 115: 860–864
7. McDonald CC, Stewart HJ, for the Scottish Breast Cancer Committee (1991) Fatal myocardial infarction in the Scottish adjuvant tamoxifen trial. Br Med J 303:435–436
8. Valagussa P, Bonadonna G (1993) Carcinogenic effects of cancer treatment. In: Peckham M, Pinedo H, Veronesi U (eds) Oxford textbook of oncology. Oxford University Press, Oxford (in press)
9. Valagussa P, Tancini G, Bonadonna G (1987) Second malignancies after CMF for resectable breast cancer. J Clin Oncol 5:1138–1142
10. Weiss RB, Tormey DC, Holland JF et al. (1981) Venous thrombosis during multimodal treatment of primary breast carcinoma. Cancer Treat Rep 65: 677–679
11. Levine MN, Gent M, Hirsh J et al. (1988) The thrombogenic effect of anticancer drug therapy in women with stage II breast cancer. N Engl J Med 318:404–407
12. Saphner T, Tormey DC, Gray R (1991) Venous and arterial thrombosis in patients who received adjuvant therapy for breast cancer. J Clin Oncol 9: 286–294
13. Tokaz LK, von Hoff DD (1984) The cardiotoxicity of anticancer agents. In: Perry MC, Yarbro JW (eds) Toxicity of chemotherapy. Grune and Stratton, Orlando, pp 199–226
14. Corn BW, Trock BJ, Goodman RL (1990) Irradiation-related ischemic heart disease. J Clin Oncol 8:741–750
15. Hortobagyi GN, Buzdar AU, Marcus CE et al. (1986) Immediate and long-term toxicity of adjuvant chemotherapy regimens containing doxorubicin in trials at M.D. Anderson Hospital and Tumor Institute. Natl Cancer Inst Monogr 1: 105–109

Long-Term Toxicity of Tamoxifen

L.E. Rutqvist

Oncologic Centre, Karolinska Hospital, 104 01 Stockholm, Sweden

Introduction

Since tamoxifen was introduced as a treatment for breast cancer in the early 1970s several tens of thousands of patients worldwide have been treated with the drug. The introduction of long-term tamoxifen as an adjunct to primary surgery, particularly in patients with low-risk tumors, means that there will be a growing number of long-term survivors who have been exposed to the drug for several years. The absolute benefit with adjuvant treatment appears to be relatively small – although potentially clinically wortwhile – in low-risk subgroups. In this setting even relatively infrequent adverse side effects could potentially offset the treatment benefit. This may also apply to chemopreventive treatment in previously healthy women aimed at decreasing their risk of developing breast cancer.

Because of the large number of treated women our knowledge about side effects of tamoxifen is much greater than for all other types of endocrine breast cancer treatment. However, most of the large adjuvant studies have not included a prospective collection of data on side effects, and information on infrequent adverse events is still limited. In general, tamoxifen has only few and relatively mild acute side effects, such as hot flushes, gastrointestinal disturbances, vaginal discharge, and menstrual irregularities in premenopausal women [1]. More serious adverse effects are rare. Most of them, such as thrombembolism and second cancer, are probably related to the agonistic estrogenic effects of tamoxifen which in recent years have been demonstrated in several human tissues including the liver and pituitary gland [2]. Estrogenic agonism may also have beneficial effects, such as decreased blood levels of cholesterol and prevention of osteporosis [3, 4]. The reported ocular toxicity of tamoxifen, on the other hand, does not have an endocrine mechanism [5]. It may be related to the structual similarity of tamoxifen to compounds such as choroquine which have well-documented ocular side effects.

Recent Results in Cancer Research, Vol. 127

Thrombembolic Events

Many reports have suggested an association between long-term tamoxifen and thrombembolic events [1, 6–8]. Some studies have suggested that the mechanism may be a decrease in antithrombin III levels [9, 10], whereas others do not demonstrate such an effect [11, 12]. Decreased antithrombin III levels have been observed in women taking oral contraceptives, and the putative thrombembolic effects of tamoxifen are therefore probably related to its agonistic estrogenic effects.

Data from controlled trials using adjuvant tamoxifen in early-stage breast cancer indicate a significant increase in thrombembolic events in the tamoxifen group, although the increase appears to be moderate [1, 13]. In a joint analysis of seven consecutive trials by the Eastern Cooperative Oncology Group the increase with tamoxifen was similar to that observed with adjuvant chemotherapy [13]. The greatest increase in thrombembolic disease was observed in patients treated with combined chemohormonal treatment.

Other Cardiovascular Effects

Epidemiological studies have indicated that in postmenopausal women the administration of estrogens results in reduced cardiovascular morbidity and mortality [14]. Estrogen replacement therapy is associated with a decrease in serum cholesterol and low-density lipoproteins and with an increase in high-density lipoproteins. Tamoxifen therapy has been shown to be associated with similar changes. In 1984 Rössner and Wallgren [3] demonstrated a 20% decrease in serum low-density lipoprotein cholesterol after 2 months of treatment. More recently these results have been confirmed and expanded by other authors [15].

In the Scottish Adjuvant Tamoxifen Trial [16] there was a significantly decreased incidence of myocardial infarctions among patients in the tamoxifen group. However, other trials of similar size have not demonstrated such a benefit [17].

In the 10-year update of the Oxford overview of all available adjuvant tamoxifen trials, information was available from about two thirds of the 40 included trials on whether the observed deaths were due to breast cancer or to other causes [18] (reprinted in part in this volume). There was a 12% reduction in non-breast cancer deaths ($p = 0.05$) associated with tamoxifen. More detailed information on cause-specific mortality was available only from four individual trials. The total number of vascular deaths in these studies was 179. The analysis suggested a 25% reduction in such deaths among the tamoxifen-treated patients ($p = 0.06$).

Table 1. The incidence of endometrial hyperplasia at hysteroscopy in postmenopausal women treated with long-term tamoxifen, according to cumulative dose of tamoxifen (from [20])

Cumulative dose	Patients (n)	Hyperplasia	
		n	%
<9 g	18	1	6
9–15 g	13	3	23
>15 g	15	6[a]	40

[a] Includes two cases with adenocarcinoma.

Second Cancers

Epidemiological studies have indicated associations between estrogens and the occurrence of several types of cancer, such as endometrial, liver, and breast cancer. In view of the complex mechanism of action of tamoxifen – with both agonistic and antagonistic estrogenic effects – tamoxifen may theoretically also be related to the occurrence of these types of cancer.

Endometrial Cancer

The estrogenic effecs of tamoxifen in the genital tract of postmenopausal women result in an increase in the karyopycnotic index (KPI) of the vaginal epithelium, vaginal discharge, endometrial hyperplasia and polyps [19, 20]. An increase in the KPI can be observed after only 4–8 weeks of treatment. The occurrence of endometrial hyperplasia, on the other hand, appears to be related to the cumulative dose of tamoxifen. In a study based on findings at hysteroscopy in postmenopausal women the incidence of endometrial hyperplasia was 40% in women treated to a cumulative dose of more than 15 g, compared to 6% in women with a cumulative dose of less than 9 g (Table 1) [20]. A cumulative dose of 15 g corresponds to a schedule of 20 mg daily for about 2 years.

It has been hypothesized that the risk of endometrial hyperplasia and endometrial cancer with tamoxifen may be related to the daily dose of tamoxifen, with little or no risk with daily doses of 20 mg as opposed to 30–40 mg. However, there are no clinical data to support that hypothesis. Estrogenic effects in the female genital tract – as evidenced by an increase in the KPI – have also been demonstrated in women treated with a daily dose of 20 mg [19].

In vitro, tamoxifen has been shown to stimulate the growth of endometrial cancer cells [21]. In the Stockholm Adjuvant Tamoxifen Trial there was a

Table 2. Summarized description of three Scandinavian randomized trials of adjuvant tamoxifen in early breast cancer on the relative risk (RR) of endometrial cancer (tamoxifen versus control group)

Study	Patients (*n*)	Tamoxifen schedule	Median follow-up	RR of endometrial cancer (95% C.I.)[a]
Stockholm Trial [22]	1846	40 mg 2–5 years	5 years	6.4 (1.4–28)
Danish Breast Cancer Group [23]	1710	30 mg 1 year	8 years	3.3 (0.6–32)
South Swedish Breast Group [24]	719	30 mg 1 year	9 years	2.2

[a] The information on endometrial cancer was in all three trials obtained from population-based cancer registers.

significant increase in endometrial cancer among the tamoxifen patients compared to the control patients corresponding to a relative risk of 6.4 [22]. In that trial the daily tamoxifen dose was 40 mg and the allocated duration 2 or 5 years. The increase in endometrial cancer was most pronounced in the 5-year group, but there was some increase also in the 2-year group.

There has been some controversy over the fact that significant increases in endometrial cancer have not been reported from any of the large adjuvant tamoxifen trials other than the Stockholm trial. However, few of these studies have included a prospective collection of data on second primaries other than contralateral breast cancers. Nor have such data been available from population-based cancer registries, except for the Stockholm trial and other studies carried out in the Scandinavian countries. Therefore, there is probably a considerable underreporting of second primaries and a corresponding lack of statistical power to detect a difference between the treated and control groups in many of the currently available trials of more long-term adjuvant tamoxifen.

Table 2 summarizes results from the three Scandinavian studies on adjuvant tamoxifen that have so far reported endometrial cancer incidence rates based on information obtained from population-based cancer registers. The treatment time (1 year) was shorter, and the daily dose of tamoxifen (30 mg) was lower in both the Danish and the South Swedish trials than in the Stockholm trial [23, 24]. Despite these differences all three trials show increased relative risks of endometrial cancer.

The association between tamoxifen and endometrial cancer can today be regarded as clearly established, but the absolute size of the relative risk with different schedules remains unclear. There is also uncertainty as to the clinical relevance of the association. Preliminary clinical data suggest that endometrial cancers induced by tamoxifen in general are highly differentiated tumors with a good prognosis (Stockholm Breast Cancer Study Group, unpublished data); thus they probably do not offset the benefit with adjuvant tamoxifen for early breast cancer even in subgroups with a low risk of disease recurrence.

Liver Cancer

Tamoxifen induces liver cancer in laboratory animals [25]. In the western world primary liver cancer is a relatively rare disease. In the Swedish female population the incidence is about 4.5/100 000 whereas the incidence of breast cancer is about 110/100 000. This implies that large populations are necessary to provide reliable estimates of incidence. Most information on cancer incidence during long-term tamoxifen comes from adjuvant studies of breast cancer patients. In such studies there is a risk of primary liver cancer being incorrectly diagnosed as breast cancer metastasis. Moreover, few such studies have included a prospective collection of data on second cancers other than contralateral breast cancers. Therefore there is probably a considerable underreporting of liver cancer in the currently available literature on long-term tamoxifen use.

With two exceptions, there are no case reports in the literature of liver cancer associated with long-term tamoxifen use. However, in the Stockholm Adjuvant Tamoxifen Trial there were two cases, both among patients in the tamoxifen group [22]. The cancers were diagnosed 20 and 46 months after initiation of treatment. The first patient was allocated to 2 years of tamoxifen and the second to 5 years. The potential association of these cancers to tamoxifen remains controversial. The expected incidence of liver cancer in the tamoxifen group, based on general population incidence rates during the period of follow-up, was 0.5, thus the estimate of the relative risk for the tamoxifen patients was about 4. However, this estimate was of course far from statistical significance due to the small number of cases.

Breast Cancer

Estrogens are considered to act as promotors of initiated breast cells in the development of breast cancer. This suggests that the risk of the disease may be reduced by the prophylactic use of tamoxifen, provided that the drug actually has a predominantly antagonistic estrogenic effect on breast epithelium.

At present there are no data on the ability of tamoxifen to decrease breast cancer incidence in previously healthy women, but several adjuvant trials in early-stage breast cancer show a decreased incidence of second, contralateral breast cancers among the tamoxifen-treated patients (Table 3). However, such data are to some extent uncertain because it can be argued that some contralateral cancers represent recurrences from the patients' first

Table 3. Second primary breast cancers in selected randomized adjuvant tamoxifen trials

Trial	n	Tamoxifen	Control	p[a]
NSABP B-14 [1]	2644	28	52	<0.01
CRC [36]	2230	22	25	NS
Premenopause		13	8	NS
Postmenopause		8	16	0.08
Scottish trial [16]	1312	13	23	<0.05
Premenopause		2	3	–
Postmenopause		7	17	–
Stockholm trial [37]	1846	33	52	<0.05

[a] Tamoxifen versus control group.

cancer rather than new, primary malignancies. Therefore, until a decreased incidence of breast cancer with tamoxifen is demonstrated in controlled trials including previously healthy women, the chemopreventive ability of the drug should only be regarded as tentative. Moreover, in the CRC trial [36] there was no decrease in second breast cancers among premenopausal patients. A differential effect could theoretically be due to the difference in serum estrogen levels between pre- and postmenopausal women.

Ovarian Cancer

No study has demonstrated a statistically significant increase in ovarian cancer among patients treated with tamoxifen. However, tamoxifen has been associated with the development of ovarian cysts [26, 27]. This could possibly be related to increased serum levels of estrogens during treatment of premenopausal women. The clinical relevance of these observations remain controversial.

Effects on Bone Mineral Density

Bone demineralization and subsequent osteporosis in postmenopausal women has been associated with the decrease in sex steroid levels that occurs after the menopause. Several studies indicate that estrogen replacement therapy in postmenopausal women preserves bone mineral density (BMD) and decrease the risk of fractures of both the vertebrae and hips [28]. Theoretically, the antiestrogenic properties of tamoxifen could accelerate the normal rate of bone loss. However, clinical studies indicate that tamoxifen in postmenopausal women has mainly estrogenic properties in bone, as indicated by a 20%–30% decrease in serum ostecalcin levels after

2–3 months of tamoxifen therapy [4]. Osteocalcin is a bone matrix protein synthesized by proliferating osteblasts. It can be used as a marker for bone mineral metabolism. Estrogen replacement therapy has been shown to reduce ostecalcin levels to about 50% of pretreatment levels.

Direct measurements of BMD using single- or dual-photon absorptiometry in patients treated with long-term tamoxifen have generally not shown differences in comparison with untreated controls [4, 29]. If anything, tamoxifen may possibly have preserved BMD.

Most of the clinical studies of long-term tamoxifen and BMD have concerned postmenopausal patients. Estrogenic agonistic effects of tamoxifen may predominate in a low-estrogen environment, as is the case in postmenopausal women, whereas antagonistic effects may be more important in the premenopausal, high-estrogen environment. Only few data are available on BMD in premenopausal patients treated with long-term tamoxifen [27].

Ocular Effects

Tamoxifen is structurally related to compounds such as chloroquine which have well-documented ocular side effects. Reported effects of tamoxifen include retinopathy with hemorrhage, keratopathy with corneal ulceration, and optic neuritis [30–33]. Some of these effects may be reversible if the drug is discontinued. Some case reports of ocular toxicity have concerned patients treated with high daily doses (>70–80 mg/m^2) or high cumulative doses of tamoxifen (>90 g). However, similar ocular effects have also been reported in patients treated with standard daily doses (20–40 mg) and at low cumulative doses (7–8 g) [33].

Ocular effects with tamoxifen are rare and therefore probably do not impair the clinical usefulness of tamoxifen in the adjuvant situation, where there is a clearly established benefit in terms of recurrence-free and overall survival. However, none of the large-scale trials of long-term tamoxifen has included a prospective evaluation of ocular toxicity, and there are therefore no reliable data on the cumulative incidence of such effects.

Tamoxifen-Stimulated Tumor Growth

Conventionally the effect of tamoxifen has been described as antiestrogenic through a competetive binding of the drug to estrogen receptors in the tumor cells. However, the tamoxifen-receptor complex binds to DNA, which may explain the partial agonistic estrogenic effects observed in many human tissues. In fact, tamoxifen has been shown to stimulate the growth of experimental MCF-7 tumor cell lines that have acquired tamoxifen resistance [34]. Osborne et al. recently showed that this phenomenon was assoicated with decreased tumor levels of tamoxifen and an increased ratio of the *trans-*

to *cis*-isomer of the tamoxifen metabolite 4-OH tamoxifen in the tumor cells [35]. The *cis*-isomer is less potent and may even have predominant estrogenic properties.

Tamoxifen-induced tumor cell growth has thus been demonstrated in experimental tumors in laboratory animals. Whether it also occurs in human breast cancer is unknown. It has been hypothesized that the withdrawal response occasionally seen after cessation of tamoxifen may be related to this phenomenon.

These observations highlight the importance of ongoing controlled trials of longer versus shorter treatment with adjuvant tamoxifen in early-stage breast cancer. At present there are no data from such trials showing a benefit with extending the treatment beyond 2 years. Such a benefit may be counterbalanced by tamoxifen-induced tumor cell growth in patients whose tumors have acquired resistance to tamoxifen during the treatment period.

Summary

Long-term tamoxifen has generally only few and usually mild adverse side effects. More serious, potentially life-threatening toxicities are rare. Aside from the ocular effects, most documented side effects appear to be related to the estrogenic properties of tamoxifen, for instance, thrombembolic disease and endometrial cancer. On the other hand, these properties may also be beneficial, for instance, they may contribute to a decreased risk of cardiac disease and osteoporosis. The potential association between tamoxifen and other possibly estrogenic side effects such as liver cancer and tamoxifen-induced tumor growth in patients with acquired tamoxifen resistance remain controversial.

References

1. Fisher B, Costantino J, Redmond C et al. (1989) A randomized clinical trial evaluating tamoxifen in the treatment of patients with node-negative breast cancer who have estrogen-receptor-positive tumors. N Engl J Med 320:479–484
2. Fornander T, Rutqvist LE, Wilking N, Carlström K, van Schoultz B (1992) Estrogenic effecs of adjuvant tamoxifen in postmenopausal breast cancer. Eur J Cancer (in press)
3. Rössner S, Wallgren A (1984) Serum lipoproteins and proteins after breast cancer surgery and effects of tamoxifen. Atherosclerosis 52:339–346
4. Fornander T, Rutqvist LE, Sjöberg HE, Blomqvist L, Mattsson A, Glas U (1990) Long-term adjuvant tamoxifen in early breast cancer: effect on bone mineral density in postmenopausal women. J Clin Oncol 8:1019–1024
5. Jackson IM, Litherland S, Wakeling AE (1991) Tamoxifen and other antiestrogens. In: Powles TJ, Smith IE (eds) Medical management of breast cancer Cambridge University Press, Cambridge, pp 51–59
6. Hendrick A, Subramanian VP (1980) Tamoxifen and thrombembolism JAMA 243:514–515

7. Lipton A, Harvey HA, Hamilton RW (1984) Venous thrombosis as a side effect of tamoxifen treatment. Cancer Treat Rep 68:887–889
8. Nevasaari K, Heikkinen M, Taskinen PJ (1978) Tamoxifen and thrombosis. Lance 2:946–947
9. Enck RE, Rios CN (1984) Tamoxifen treatment of metastatic breast cancer and antithrombin-III levels. Cancer 53:2607–2609
10. Rieche K (1986) Die Beeinflussung des funktionellen Antithrombin III im plasma durch Tamoxifen und Aminoglutethemid. Krebsmedizin 7:60–63
11. Jordan VC, Fritz NF, Tormey DC (1987) Long-term adjuvant therapy with tamoxifen: effects on sex hormone binding globulin and antithrombin III. Cancer Res 47:4517–4519
12. Auger MJ, Mackie MJ (1988) Effects of tamoxifen on blood coagulation. Cancer 61:1316–1319
13. Saphnerr T, Tormey DC, Gray R (1991) Venous and arterial thrombosis in patients who received adjuvant therapy for breast cancer. J Clin Oncol 9: 286–294
14. Barrett-Connor E, Bush TL (1989) Estrogen replacement therapy and coronary heart disease. Cardiovasc Clin 19:159–172
15. Love RR, Newcomb PA, Wiebe DA et al. (1990) Effects of tamoxifen therapy on lipid and lipoprotein levels in postmenopausal patients with node-negative breast cancer. J Natl Cancer Inst 82:1327–1332
16. Breast Cancer Trials Comittee, Scottish Cancer Trials Office (1987) Adjuvant tamoxifen in the mangement of operable breast cancer: the Scottish trial. Lancet 2:171–175
17. Rutqvist LE, Cedermark B, Glas U et al. (1992) Randomized trial of adjuvant tamoxifen in node negative postmenopausal breast cancer. Acta Oncol (in press)
18. Early Breast Cancer Trialists' Collaborative Group (1992) Systemic treatment of early breast cancer by hormonal, cytotoxic, or immune therapy, 133 randomised trials involving 31 000 recurrences and 24 000 deaths among 75 000 women. Lancet 339:1–15, 71–85
19. Boccardo F, Bruzzi P, Rubagotti A, Nicolo G, Rosso R (1981) Estrogen-like action of tamoxifen on vaginal epithelium in breast cancer patients. Oncology 38:281–285
20. De Muylder X, Neven P, de Somer M et al. (1991) Endometrial lesions in patients undergoing tamoxifen therapy. Int J Gynaecol Obstet 36:127–130
21. Satyaswaroop PG, Zaino RJ, Marbel R (1984) Estrogen-like effecs of tamoxifen on human endometrial carcinoma transplanted into nude mice. Cancer Res 44:4006–4010
22. Fornander T, Rutqvist LE, Cedermark B, Glas U, Mattsson A, Silfverswärd C, Skoog L, Somell A, Theve T, Wilking N, Askergren J, Hjalmar ML (1989) Adjuvant tamoxifen in early breast cancer: occurrence of new primary cancers. Lancet 1:117–120
23. Andersson M, Storm HH, Mouridsen HT (1991) Incidence of new primary cancers after adjuvant tamoxifen therapy and radiotherapy for early breast cancer. J Natl Cancer Inst 83:1013–1017
24. Rydén S, Fernö M, Möller T et al. (1992) Long-term effects of adjuvant tamoxifen and/or radiotherapy. The South Sweden Trial. Acta Oncol (in press)
25. Fentiman IS, Powles TJ (1987) Tamoxifen and benign breast problems. Lancet 2:1070–1072
26. Boccardo F, Rubagotti A, Bruzzi P et al. (1989) Tamoxifen vs chemotherapy vs chemotherapy plus tamoxifen in stage II ER+ breast cancer patients. Preliminary results of the GROCTA trials (Abstr). Proceedings of the 5th European Conference on Clinical Oncology (ECCO-5): Federation of European Cancer Societies, London

27. Powles TJ, Hardy JR, Ashley SE et al. (1989) A pilot trial to evaluate the acute toxicity and feasability of tamoxifen for prevention of breast cancer. Br J Cancer 60:126–131
28. Weiss NS, Ure CL, Ballard JH et al. (1980) Decreased risk of fractures of the hip and lower forearm with postmenopausal use of estrogen. N Engl J Med 303:1195–1198
29. Love RR, Mazess RB, Tormey DC et al. (1988) Bone mineral density in women with breast cancer treated with adjuvant tamoxifen for at least two years. Breast Cancer Res Treat 12:297–301
30. Ashford AR, Donev I, Tiwari RP, Garret TJ (1988) Reversible ocular toxicity related to tamoxifen therapy. Cancer 61:33–35
31. Kaiser-Kupfer MI, Kupfer C, Rodrigues MM (1981) Tamoxifen retinopathy: a clinicopathologic report. Ophtalmology 8:89–93
32. Griffiths MF (1987) Tamoxifen retinopathy at low dosage. Am J Ophtalmol 104:185–186
33. Vinding T, Nielsen NV (1983) Retinopathy caused by treatment with tamoxifen in low dosage. Acta Ophtalmol (Lopenh) 61:45–50
34. Gottardis MM, Robinson SP, Jordan VC (1988) Estradiol-stimulated growth of MCF-7 tumors implanted in athymic mice: a model to study the tumoristatic action of tamoxifen. J Steroid Biochem 30:311–314
35. Osborne CK, Coronado E, Allred DC et al. (1991) Acquired tamoxifen resistance: correlation with reduced breast tumor levels of tamoxifen and isomerization of *trans*-4-hydroxytamoxifen. J Natl Cancer Inst 83:1477–1482
36. Abram WP, Baum M, Berstock DA et al. (1988) Cyclophosphamide and tamoxifen as adjuvant therapies in the management of breast cancer. Preliminary analysis by the CRC Adjuvant Breast Trial Working Party. Br J Cancer 57:604–607
37. Rutqvist LE, Cedermark B, Glas U et al. (1991) Contralateral primary tumors in breast cancer patients in a randomized trial of adjuvant tamoxifen therapy. J Natl Cancer Inst 83:1299–1306

New Endocrine Agents for the Treatment of Breast Cancer

R.C. Coombes[1], M. Jarman[2], M. Dowsett[3], S.K. Chander[1], M.G. Rowlands[2], E.Di Salle[4], and T.J. Evans[1]

[1] Department of Medical Oncology, Charing Cross Hospital, Fulham Palace Road, London W6 8RF, UK
[2] Drug Development Section, Institute of Cancer Research, Cotswold Road, Belmont, Sutton, Surrey SM2 5NG, UK
[3] Department of Molecular Endocrinology, Royal Marsden Hospital, Fulham, London, SW3 6JJ, UK
[4] Department of Endocrinology, Farmitalia Carlo Erbo, Milan, Italy

Introduction

Over the past 6 years we have focused on developing improved drugs for the treatment of human breast cancer. The use of tamoxifen is well established in both advanced disease and in the adjuvant setting, but patients still suffer from side effects such as the tumour flare phenomenon, and remissions obtained are of relatively short duration. For this reason we have developed a new antioestrogen, pyrrolidino-4-iodotamoxifen (PIT), details of which have recently been published [1]. Other endocrine agents act by inhibiting oestrogen synthesis, and these include aminoglutethamide. However, inhibition of oestrogen synthesis is often incomplete, and side effects are severe. Our efforts have therefore also centred on the development of new, more potent and less toxic aromatase inhibitors. Examples include 4-hydroxy androstenedione [2], pyridoglutethimide [3] and exemestane [4].

Finally, another source of oestradiol (E_2) is via oestrone sulphatase, which converts oestrone sulphate (E_1S) to oestrone (E_1), which can then be metabolized to E_2. We have carried out studies to characterise this enzyme, and we have examined ways of inhibiting its activity with the hope of developing inhibitors that could be used either alone or in conjunction with aromatase inhibitors.

Pyrrolidino-4-iodotamoxifen (Idoxifene)

PIT was synthesised by R. McCague in the laboratory of M. Jarman. We have evaluated it in the oestrogen receptor (ER) binding assay, on the growth of cancer cells in vitro and on the growth of nitrosomethylurea (NMU)-induced rat mammary tumours in vitro as well as its intestinal effects and effects on vaginal cornification [1].

Recent Results in Cancer Research, Vol. 127

Oestrogen Receptor Binding Assays

ER binding affinities of the new antioestrogen were compared to those of tamoxifen. Receptor binding curves were used to calculate the relative binding affinities. Tamoxifen, 4-iodotamoxifen (4-IT) and PIT had ER binding affinities of 5, 12.5, and 12.5-fold increase with respect to that of E_2. The analogues 4-IT and PIT both showed 2.5-fold greater affinity for ER than did tamoxifen.

Effect of Analogues on the Growth of Breast Cancer Cells In Vitro

The effect of varying concentrations of the analogues alone on the growth of MCF-7 cells was compared after 3 and 7 days. At $10^{-5} M$ all analogues were completely cytotoxic after 3 days of treatment. The highest level of inhibition, compared with that of the control, for all the analogues was observed at $10^{-5} M$ after 3 days of treatment (tamoxifen, 38.7%; 4-IT, 35.2%; PIT, 58.7%). After 7 days of treatment at $10^{-6} M$ there was a reduced but significant inhibition produced by all the analogues, compared with the control ($p = >0.001$). At doses of 10^{-8} and $10^{-7} M$ after both 3 and 7 days of treatment there was also a significant inhibition of growth. Although PIT showed a reduction in the level of inhibition at 10^{-7} and $10^{-8} M$ after 3 and 7 days, the effect was to superior to both tamoxifen and 4-IT ($p = >0.001$). With E_2 alone a 22.4-fold increase in cell number was observed compared with the control.

The effect of the analogues on the inhibition of E_2-stimulated growth of MCF-7 cells was also studied. Again, a dose of $10^{-5} M$ was cytotoxic after 3 days of treatment. Maximal growth inhibition was seen at $10^{-6} M$ after 7 days of treatment. At this dose tamoxifen and 4-IT produced 44% and 48% inhibition, respectively, of the E_2-induced proliferation; PIT produced 65% inhibition. There was no significant difference between tamoxifen and 4-IT in their levels of inhibition at a dose of $10^{-6} M$ ($p = 0.15$). However, a comparison between tamoxifen and PIT showed that the latter was a significantly more effect inhibitor (by 1.5-fold) than tamoxifen ($p = 0.006$). At doses of 10^{-7} and $10^{-8} M$ tamoxifen and 4-IT had little effect on the E_2-stimulated growth of MCF-7 cells. However, PIT was still effective and produced 51% inhibition at 10^{-7} but was without effect at $10^{-8} M$.

Reversal of Antioestrogen Inhibition by Oestradiol

The inhibitory effects of the antioestrogens on the oestrogen-stimulated growth could be reversed by removing the drug after 3 days and treating with $10^{-8} M$ E_2 alone for 4 days. This indicated that the inhibitory effect of the antioestrogens was reversible.

Effect of Antioestrogens on MDA-MB-231 Cells

The effect of the various drugs on the growth of the ER-negative cell line MDA-MB-231 was investigated (Table 1). None of the compounds had any effect on cell numbers after 7 days compared with untreated controls. No growth stimulation of MDA-MB-231 was observed with E_2.

In Vivo Studies of Tamoxifen Analogues

The NMU-induced rat mammary tumour model was used to investigate the antiproliferative activities of the various antioestrogens. In a preliminary single-dose study, PIT produced tumour regression in 83% of rats. In a subsequent dose-response experiment PIT caused regression in 91.7% of rats at doses of both 1 and 2 mg/kg; this was significantly different from the control (1 mg, $p = 0.006$; 2 mg, $p = 0.0007$). In a third comparative study among tamoxifen, 4-IT and PIT at doses of 1 mg/kg all three drugs inhibited tumour progression compared with the control at 28 days (Kruskal-Wallis = >H = 8.61; $p = <0.02$). The greatest percentage of reduction in tumour volume was achieved in the order: PIT > tamoxifen > 4-IT. Although there was no significant difference between tamoxifen and PIT in decreasing total tumour volume, in this particular study PIT was effective in causing some degree of tumour regression in all rats, whereas tamoxifen caused tumour regression in only 75% of animals; the remaining 25% of rats showed tumour progression. Overall in the three studies, PIT caused regression in 92% of rats, which was significantly greater than that caused by tamoxifen.

The effect of the various agents, either alone or together with oestradiol benzoate (E_2B) on uterine weight in immature rats was also examined. E_2B alone produced a 3.7-fold increase in uterine weight. Tamoxifen given alone subcutaneously at doses up to 10 mg/kg stimulated an average uterine growth of 123 mg/100 g body weight, compared with the control of 65.2 mg/100 g body weight (1.9-fold increase). When administered together with E_2B, it failed to inhibit completely the uterotrophic action of E_2B. The 4-IT analogue also resulted in partial agonist effects, as an increase in uterine weight of 108 mg/100 g body weight was recorded at the highest dose compared with the control 1.7-fold increase. However, the increase in weight with 4-IT was less than that observed with tamoxifen. Doses of 1 and 10 mg/kg PIT alone both resulted in a 1.3-fold increase in uterine weight compared with the control (1 mg/kg, $p = 0.018$; 10 mg/kg, $p = 0.006$). When given with E_2B, it produced a dose-dependent inhibition of the uterotrophic action of E_2B. At 10 mg/kg PIT completely blocked the effect of E_2B. This study showed that PIT had the lowest uterotrophic activity, which was significantly lower by 1.4- and 1.27-fold compared with tamoxifen and 4-IT, respectively ($p = 0.030$).

The ability of 4-IT and PIT to inhibit tamoxifen uterotrophic activity was investigated. Although both PIT and 4-IT showed some effect on inhibiting tamoxifen-stimulated uterine weight, this was not significant ($p = 0.3$) between 1 and 10 mg/kg. The uterotrophic activities of the various antioestrogens were also examined. Tamoxifen alone was highly uterotrophic at 0.1 mg/kg whereas PIT and 4-IT showed minimal uterotrophic activity at this dose but were highly uterotrophic at 10 mg/kg. Neither tamoxifen and 4-IT were able to block the E_2 effect. PIT, however, showed a dose-dependent inhibition of the E_2 stimulation but was unable to block the effect completely at the highest dose.

Tamoxifen also displayed oestrogenic activity, as indicated by vaginal cornification at 0.5 mg/kg and was completely cornifying at 20 mg/kg in adult ovariectomised rats. However, in contrast, 4-IT and PIT did not show any oestrogenic activity at 0.5 mg/kg but did so at 5 mg/kg. Full cornification was observed at 50 mg/kg with 4-IT and PIT Control animals, given E_2 only, showed cornified smears from the fourth to the eighth day inclusive. At doses much below those required to induce vaginal cornification, tamoxifen and 4-IT both displayed antioestrogenic activity. They produced a dose-dependent inhibition of E_2 stimulation but were unable to completely block the effect at 10 mg/kg. However, PIT was able to completely block the E_2-induced cornification in a dose-dependent manner. Inhibition caused by PIT at 10 mg/kg was significantly different from tamoxifen and 4-IT ($p = 0.0009$).

These data indicate that PIT has a higher affinity for the ER than tamoxifen, as well as a more potent effect in vitro. It still has partial agonist activity, but less than tamoxifen. Clinical trials with PIT are currently in progress.

Aromatase Inhibitors

4-Hydroxyandrostenedione has been the subject of several recent reviews [5] and is not described further in this review. More recently, we have examined exemestane (FCE 24304) in a phase 1 study [6]. Exemestane has been shown by the work of Di Salle to be a potent aromatase inhibitor [4].

Experimental Studies

In in vitro studies with human placental aromatase, exemestane was found to inhibit aromatase with an IC_{50} of 42.5 nM, which is similar to that of 4-hydroxy androstenedione. The potency of exemestane is about 40 times higher than for aminoglutethamide (IC_{50} of 1754 nM).

In vivo exemstane has been compared to 4-hydroxyandrostenedione in its activity on ovarian aromatase activity. Exemestane reduced ovarian aromatase after both subcutaneous and oral treatment, showing ED_{50} values of 1.8 and 3.7 mg/kg respectively. 4-Hydroxyandrostenedione was effective when given parenterally (ED_{50} of 3.1 mg/kg) whereas by the oral route it caused marginal enzyme inactivation. Exemestane has no binding affinity for the ER and only very low affinity for the progestin glucocorticoid and mineralocorticoid receptors (RBA × 0.1%). It also shows very low binding affinity to androgen (0.25%) and progestin receptors (0.25%).

Clinical Studies

A phase I trial in healthy postmenopausal volunteers has been conducted to assess the tolerability and aromatase inhibitory effect of exemestane after a single oral dose [6]. Reduction in plasma E_1, E_2 and E_2S and in urinary total E_1 and E_2 was taken as evidence of aromatase inhibition. In the first part of the study, exemestane was administered at the dose of 25, 50, 200, 400 and 800 mg, respectively, in five successive cohorts of three subjects each. Plasma and urinary oestrogens were assayed at baseline and for 48 h after drug administration; in the 800-mg cohort the sampling period was extended to day 7. In the 25–400 mg dose range, for which endocrine measurements were performed for only 48 h, a clear, non-dose-related, suppression of oestrogens was initially observed at 8–24 h in plasma and at 24–28 h in urine; at 48 h the effect on plasma levels was still increasing, oestrogen suppression being 60%–23% of basal values for E_2, 52%–38% for E_1, and 38%–22% for E_1S. In general, the endocrine effects seen at 400 mg were not more evident than those at 25 mg. At the highest tested dose of 800 mg, at which endocrine measurements were extended up to 7 days, the maximal reduction in oestrogen levels was observed at day 4, reaching 10% of basal values for E_1S and undetectable levels for E_1 and E_2; a similar degree of suppression was still present on day 7.

To determine the threshold dose for endocrine efficacy, the study was subsequently enlarged to doses of 0.5, 5, 12.5 and 25 mg in 14 additional volunteers (three or four subjects per dose), with an extended sampling period, up to 5–8 days. The dose of 0.5 mg was ineffective. Suppression of all plasma estrogens (to 60%–47% of basal values on day 3) was observed starting from 5 mg and was more pronounced and longer lasting with increasing doses. At 25 mg the maximal suppression was observed at day 3: plasma oestrogen fell to 35% (E_1) and 39% (E_2) and 28% (E_1S) of basal values, these suppressions still persisting at day 5 post-treatment.

No changes were observed in other hormonal parameters (cortisol, aldosterone, dehydroepiandrosterone sulphate, 17-hydroxyprogesterone, follicle-stimulating hormone and luteinising hormone), which were determined in the highest dose group of each part of the study (800 and 25 mg). No clinically relevant side effects or alterations in laboratory parameters were observed up to the maximum exemestane dose of 800 mg.

These data suggest that exemestane is a very potent, selective and orally active aromatase inhibitor in post-menopausal women.

Inhibition of Oestrone Sulphatase

Plasma levels of E_1 and E_2 in postmenopausal women are very low; however, and oestrogen concentration in breast tumour tissues is of an order of magnitude higher than in the plasma [8], suggesting local intratumoural production of oestrogens in breast tumour cells from precursor substrates. Although the predominant source of oestrogen production in postmenopausal women is considered to be the extraglandular conversion of androstenedione to E_1 by peripheral tissues catalysed by the aromatase enzyme [9], E_1S is the most abundant oestrogen in peripheral blood [10]. The plasma E_1S level is higher in postmenopausal women with breast cancer than in normal postmenopausal women [11]. Although the E_1S itself is unable to bind to the ER and stimulate a biological response, studies involving MCF-7 cell lines have shown that the E_1S can be taken up by these cells and hydrolysed to the unconjugated E_1 in sufficient amounts to stimulate a biological response [12].

In addition, a comparative study of intratumoural aromatase and sulphatase activities in breast cancer cells showed that under enzyme-saturating conditions, the capacity of the sulphatase pathway in forming E_1 is one million-fold greater than the aromatase pathway, and even at the physiological concentration of substrate the sulphatase enzyme appears to be at least ten times more important than the aromatase enzyme. Therefore the sulphatase pathway is likely to be an important means of local production of biologically active oestrogens in breast carcinoma tissue [13].

We therefore considered it pertinent to further characterise the E_1 sulphatase enzyme in human placenta and human breast carcinoma and investigate its inhibition by both naturally occurring and synthetic steroids and by antiendocrine agents currently in use for the management of human breast carcinoma.

The inhibition of placental E_1 sulphatase by antiendocrine drugs and their major metabolites was investigated. Danazol was the most potent inhibitor in this group, although only 20% inhibition was seen at the maximum concentration used ($50\,\mu M$). None of its major metabolites had any significant effect, and none of the other compounds in this group had any significant (>10%) inhibition at $50\,\mu M$ (Table 1). Twenty-four naturally occurring and synthetic steroids were similarly investigated for potential inhibition (Table 2). Of the oestrogens, significant inhibition was seen in the presence of $50\,\mu M$ E_1 (41%) and $50\,\mu M$ E_2 (42%), but – 2-hydroxyoestradiol and 2-methoxyestrone were inactive. Of the unconjugated androgens only 5α-androstane-3α,17β-diol had any significant activity (37% inhibition with $50\,\mu M$ inhibitor).

The most potent inhibitors of E_1 sulphatase examined all had a sulphate group in the 3 position of the steroid ring. The compound with the greatest activity (87% inhibition at $50\,\mu M$) was 5α-androstene-3β,17β-diol-3-sulphate. In each case where both a 3-sulphated steroid and its unconjugated parent

Table 1. Inhibition of placental estrone sulfatase by antiendocrine drugs

Compound	% Inhibition	
	10 μ*M* inhibitor	50 μ*M* inhibitor
Aminoglutethimide	8	0
Pyridoglutethimide	3	0
Danazol	14	20
Ethisterone	7	0
17-Hydroxy-2-(hydroxyl)17α-pregna-1,4-dien-20-yn-3-one	0	0
17-Hydroxy-2α-(hydroxymethyl)-17α-pregna-4-en-20-yn-3-one	7	0
Tamoxifen	8	10
4-Hydroxytamoxifen	0	0
N-Desmethyltamoxifen	0	0
Cis-Tamoxifen	0	6
4-Hydroxyandrostenedione	7	5
Diethylstilboestrol	8	4
FCE 24304	6	0

Each value is the mean of duplicate determinations at each of two time points, and all values are within 10% of the mean value shown. Any result >10% is regarded as significant.

steroid were investigated, the sulphated compound was more potent. In contrast, considerably less inhibition was seen with the 17-sulphated steroids and with the disulphated steroids. It is likely that the 3-sulphated steroid compounds act as alternative substrates as they demonstrate competitive inhibition on Lineweaver-Burk plots which would support this hypothesis.

Bulky chemical groups in the 3 position, such as an acetate group, result in greater inhibition than seen in the presence of the corresponding unconjugated parent steroid. However, even in the presence of a sulphate group in the 3 position, modifications elsewhere in the steroid molecule lead to modification of inhibitory activity. The presence of a sulphate group at the 17 position, an aldehyde group at the 19 position, a keto group at the 11 position, and a methoxy or hydroxy group at the 2 position all considerably reduce sulphatase inhibition.

A sample of the compounds which had been screened on the placental enzyme were investigated on the human breast carcinoma enzyme. Again the most potent inhibitor (75% at 50 μ*M*) was 5-androstene-3β-17β-diol-3-sulphate. Significant inhibition was also seen with the other compounds screened.

It is anticipated that these screening inhibition studies of human placental tissue, with selection of the most potent inhibitors for evaluation on human

Table 2. Inhibition of placental estrone sulfatase by steroid compounds

Compound	% Inhibition	
	10 μ*M* inhibitor	50 μ*M* inhibitor
Estrogens		
17β-Oestradiol	13	42
Oestrone	20	41
2-Hydroxyoestradiol	0	0
2-Methoxyestrone	0	1
Androgens		
5-Androsten-3β-17β-diol-3-acetate	31	38
5α-Androstane-3α,17β-diol	20	37
Testosterone	6	5
Dehydroepiandrosterone	0	14
5α-Androstene-3β,17β-diol	13	6
Dihydrotestosterone	0	0
Sulphated steroids		
5-Androsten-3β,17β-diol-3-sulphate	58	87
Pregnenolone-3-sulphate	33	77
17β-Oestradiol-3-sulphate	26	52
Dehydroepiandrosterone sulphate	23	50
Androsterone-3-sulphate	11	47
Cholesterol-3-sulphate	15	43
5β-Pregnene-3α,20α,diol-3-sulphate	0	43
Oestriol-3-sulphate	13	12
5β-Androstan-3α-ol-17one-3-sulphate	8	18
5β-Androstan-3α-ol-11,17dione-3-sulphate	0	5
Androst-5-en-3β-17one-19al-3-sulphate	13	0
5-Androstene-3β,17β-diol-17-sulphate	8	24
17β-Oestradiol disulphate	0	0
Androst-5-ene-3β,17β-diol-disulphate	13	16

Each value is the mean of duplicate determinations at each of two time points, and each value is within 10% of the mean. Any result >10% is regarded as significant.

breast carcinoma tissue enzyme will lead to the rational design of a potent E_1 sulphatase inhibitor, which may be a useful novel endocrine agent in the management of human breast cancer.

References

1. Chander SK, McCague R, Luqmani Y, Newton C, Dowsett M, Jarman M, Coombes RC (1991) Pyrrolidino-4-iodotamoxifen and 4-iodotamoxifen, new analogues of the antiestrogen tamoxifen for the treatment of breast cancer. Cancer Res 51:5851–5858
2. Coombes RC, Goss P, Dowsett M, Gazet J-C, Brodie A (1984) 4-Hydroxyandrostenedione in treatment of postmenopausal patients with advanced breast cancer. Lancet 2:1237–1239
3. Dowsett M, MacNeill F, Mehta A, Newton C, Haynes B, Jones A, Jarman M, Lonning P, Powles TJ, Coombes RC (1991) Endocrine, pharmacokinetics and clinical studies of aromatase inhibitor 3-ethyl-3-(4-pyridyl) piperidine-2, 6-dione ("pyridoglutethimide") in postmenopausal breast cancer patients. Br J Cancer 64:887–894
4. Di Salle E, Giudici D, Ornati G, Briatico G, d'Alession R, Villa V, Lombardi P (1990) 4-Aminoandrostenedione derivatives; a novel class of irreversible aromatase inhibitors. Comparison with FCE 24304 and 4-hydroxyandrostenedione. J Steroid Biochem Mol Biol 37:369–374
5. Coombes RC, Wilkinson JR, Bliss JM, Shah P, Easton DF, Dowsett M (1991) 4-Hydroxyandrostenedione in the prophylaxis of *N*-methyl-*N*-nitrosourea induced mammary tumourigenesis. Br J Cancer 64:247–250
6. Coombes RC (1991) Clinical studies with 4-hydroxyandrostenedione in advanced breast cancer. In: Coombes R., Dowsett M (eds) 4-Hydroxyandrostenedione—a new approach to hormone-dependent cancer. Royal Society of Medicine Services, London.
7. Di Salle E, Ornati G, Giudici D, Lassus M, Evans TRJ, Coombes RC (1992) Exemestane (FCE 24304), a new steroidal aromatase inhibitor. Proc eedings of the 4th International Congress on Steroid Hormones and Cancer J Steroid Biochem Mol Biol 43:137–143
8. Millington DS (1975) Determination of hormonal steroid concentrations in biological extracts by high resolution mass fragmentography. J Steroid Biochem 6:239–245
9. Grodin JM, Siiteri PK, McDonald PC (1973) Source of estrogen production in postmenopausal women. J Clin Endocrinol Metab 36:207–214
10. Loriaux D, Ruder H, Lipsett M (1971) The measurement of estrone sulfate in plasma. Steroids 18:463–472
11. Prost O, Turrel MO, Dahan N, Craveur C, Adessi GL (1984) Estrone and dehydroepiandrosterone sulfatase activities and plasma estrone sulfate levels in human breast carcinoma. Cancer Res 44:661–664
12. Pasqualini JR, Gelly C, Nguyen BL, Vella C (1989) Importance of estrogen sulfates in breast cancer. J Steroid Biochem 34:155–163
13. Santner SJ, Feil PD, Santen RJ (1984) In situ estrogen production via the estrone sulfatase pathway in breast tumours: relative important versus the aromatase pathway. J Clin Endocrinol Metab 59:29–33
14. Carlstrom K, Doberl A, Pousette A, Rannevik G, Wilking N (1984) Inhibition of steroid sulfate activity by danazol. Acta Obstet Gynaecol Scand Suppl 123: 107–111

Financial Costs, Benefits, and Patient Risk Preferences in Node-Negative Breast Cancer: Insights from a Decision Analysis Model

B.E. Hillner

Division of General Medicine, Department of Internal Medicine, Medical College of Virginia, Virginia Commonwealth University, Richmond, VA 23298-0170, USA

Introduction

Since the 1988 National Cancer Institute Clinical Alert [1], treating node-negative breast cancer patients outside the context of a clinical trial has been actively debated. To address this controversial question, we developed a decision analysis model to explore the effectiveness of adjuvant therapy in node-negative women at different levels of recurrence risk [2]. Decision analysis is one of a variety of techniques used to gather, analyze, and synthesize information. Other tools include randomized clinical trials, meta-analysis, database analysis, expert reviews of the literature, and consensus panels. Using these methods, a physician or policy maker ideally reaches a conclusion that will be translated into a clinical care or health care policy recommendation. Where does decision analysis fit into this hierarchy? It is an analytic tool that uses a decision tree which incorporates data from each of these sources to concurrently consider "apples and oranges," for example, the trade-offs that must be made in the risks and benefits of any health care intervention [3]. Ideally, decision analysis "quantifies the qualifiers" and provides an integrated view of a specific question. Breast cancer is a fertile area for decision analysis since the key ingredients are identifiable and quantifiable: clear definitions of the disease and its natural history, definable benefits and risks with different modes of therapy, competing alternative approaches, and controversy.

Materials and Methods

The Model. We used a Markov process to calculate the cumulative outcomes for two groups of women with stage I node-negative, estrogen receptor negative breast cancer: one receiving chemotherapy and one being untreated. We addressed two questions: (a) For an individual woman, what

Recent Results in Cancer Research, Vol. 127

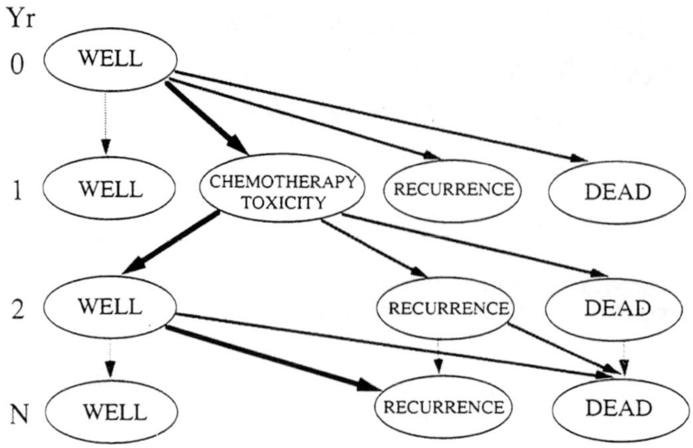

Fig. 1. Markov simulation. *Black arrows*, the movements of a single woman receiving chemotherapy (through an abridged version of the Markov model); *gray arrows*, potential movements; *ovals*, states of health at the beginning of each year. At year 0, everyone is in the well oval. From the well oval, movement into any of the other ovals in possible. Chemotherapy toxicity can be entered only during year 1. After entering the cancer recurrence oval, no one can return to the well oval. Cancer recurrence can occur during any year. The probability of cancer recurrence is reduced with chemotherapy (from [2])

is the size of the benefit from chemotherapy? (b) From a societal perspective, what is the cost for each year of life gained by chemotherapy? The model simulates a clinical trial of a large number of patients over several decades. The reasons for using a Markov (or state transition) model were the relatively long time frame and the time-dependent nature of the events considered. Our model followed women until the age of 90 or death. Since the chance or probability to disease recurrence, death, and chemotherapy toxicity are time dependent, the relative value of these events depends on both *whether* and *when* they occur. For example, even if cancer does return, it is desirable to delay its recurrence for as long as possible. Figure 1 shows an abbreviated version of the Markov model of prognosis used. Each year we counted by taking a computer snapshot of the position of each women and assigning credits to the women in each state. These snapshots were similar to interim points during a clinical trial. We adjusted the credit to reflect the quality of life for having spent the year in a specific health state. We then totaled the credits for each of the years to calculate the average quality-adjusted life expectancy.

Assumptions. One of the benefits and curses of decision analysis is that one must be explicit about the assumptions used to construct a model. Three assumptions should be emphasized. First, the annual probability of the first recurrence of breast cancer is constant. Second, chemotherapy alters only the probability of first recurrence of breast cancer. This appears to be true unless recurrences occurs soon after chemotherapy. Third, chemotherapy is equally effective (or ineffective) for high-risk and low-risk cancers. Although uncertain at the time of our original analysis, the 1992 meta-analysis confirmed this assumption [4].

Natural History. The initial estimated risk of breast cancer recurrence of 4% per year for the untreated women corresponds to an 80.4% disease-free survival at 5 years [5, 6]. This assumes that a definitive risk stratification cannot be carried out.

Benefits and Risks of Chemotherapy. The baseline relative risk reduction or benefit from multidrug chemotherapy in node-negative patients was 30% in disease-free survival [7]. Hence, the recurrence rate would be 4% per year in untreated women and 2.8% per year in treated women. The absolute risk reduction would be 1.2% per year. Prior to the publication of Early Breast Cancer Trialist' Collaborative Group updated meta-analysis (reprinted in part in this volume) there was uncertainty if the preliminary results of a significant reduction in relapse-free survival would subsequently lead to a later gain in overall survival. The recent meta-analysis of almost all randomized clinical trials shows that chemotherapy alters the risk of recurrence for at least the first 5 years after therapy [4]. Thereafter, no additional benefit accrues. Our original report used a similar 5-year limitation in the effect of chemotherapy. The toxicities of therapy would occur only during the year in which it was given. Minor and major toxicities were considered that would reduce a patient's quality of life and required unscheduled physician visits. Only major toxicity required hospitalization.

Endpoints. The endpoints of the analysis were of three types: a "hard" endpoint (survival), a "soft" endpoint (quality of life), and a societal economic endpoint (costs). A change in overall survival is self-explanatory. Quality of life or health status is a major concern of women both during treatment and is associated with the different stages of the natural history of breast cancer. Levine et al. [8] and Gelber et al. [9] have carried out pioneering work in determining the quality of life of women with stage I or node-positive cancer. Unfortunately, directly translating their work into values usable in the model was not feasible due to the 1-year cycle period and the multiple recurrence states modeled. Therefore, using a linear analog scale and clinical vignettes, we assigned a relative quality-of-life value to each of the health states using a survey of our oncology staff. For example, a woman who develops her first recurrence of breast cancer during the year contributes only 70% of a year to the cohort's net credits. We admit that this approach is suboptimal, arbitrary, and provider-centric, but the assigned values were internally consistent.

Table 1. Baseline results: chemotherapy group results or benefit (5 years) compared with no therapy (relative efficacy of chemotherapy of 30%)

	45-year-olds	60-year-olds
QALY	11.03	9.49
Benefit in QALY	0.43	0.34
Overall survival (years)[a]	19.5	14.7
Benefit in overall survival (years)	0.92	0.64
Expected life expectancy without breast cancer (years)	35.8	22.5
Benefit in median survival (years)	1.0	0.8
Cost per QALY saved	$15 400	$18 800

QALY, Quality-adjusted life years.
[a] Overall survival is not quality adjusted and not discounted.

Time Perspective. One strength of our model, unlike others such as the Q-TWiST [9], is that the time value of the health states is considered. Our model address this issue by discounting the benefits and costs of therapy at a rate of 5% per year. Discounting refers to the additional current value in either health status or money present today compared to benefits or dollars in the future [10].

Cost Analysis. An economic assessment was made in which the direct health care costs were estimated for each group. We were initially quite frustrated since no reports of the costs of chemotherapy used in various clinical trials could be found. Similarly, our medical center could not provide a unified statement of charges for a typical 6-month course of adjuvant chemotherapy. Therefore, based on individual patients, we worked with our billing office to estimate a typical nonprotocol patient charges (as a surrogate for costs) for physician, laboratory, office, and hospital services. The costs of care for disease recurrence and terminal care were estimated from Medicare data that were inflation adjusted and our own "best guess' estimates [11]. Whether Medicare data from 1974–1981 are reflective of current trends in the types and location of care cannot be assessed.

Results and Discussion

Table 1 shows the results for groups of 45- and 60-year-old women. Readers can choose their own preferred endpoint: quality-adjusted life expectancy, survival, or change in median survival. The benefits to the 60-year-old women are all lower due to shorter average life expectancy and greater chance of death from noncancer causes.

What if one disagrees with the baseline assumptions? To answer such questions, a sensitivity analysis or "what if" analysis was performed. A wide variety were carried out to assess different chemotherapy efficacies, toxicities, and costs; tumor biology; and patient risk preferences. These sensitivity analyses are discussed elsewhere [2].

Is chemotherapy worthwhile? The answer may depend on whose perspective is being considered: that of the patient or that of society. The minimal benefit sufficient to undergo therapy appears to depend on when patients are asked. In an important but preliminary study, Simes et al. [12] found that 90% of Australian women *after receiving* adjuvant chemotherapy for breast cancer would do so again if therapy would provide an additional 2 years of survival or a 10% increase in the chance of being alive after 5 years. A subsequent report by Slevin et al. [13] of 100 English men and women with newly diagnosed solid tumors (primarily lung cancer) were studied *before receiving* chemotherapy. The median benefit for these patients was an additional 3 months of survival for a mild treatment and 12 months for an intensive treatment. These benefit thresholds were assessed by sensitivity analyses in the form of patient questions. We found that the level of benefit from chemotherapy of about 1 year is very close or exceeds the typical woman's threshold for choosing chemotherapy.

A patient's attitude toward risk is usually expressed in a more declarative form. Two prototypic examples are: "Chemotherapy scares me as much as cancer" and "I will do anything to prolong my life and avoid the return of cancer." For the former woman, her quality of life during chemotherapy would be very low. Her discount rate would be high, indicating that present health has much greater value than future years. For the latter woman, her quality of life during chemotherapy would be minimally reduced since her aim is to maximize the chance of preventing a recurrence. Her discount rate would be low to zero, suggesting that future years of good health are of equal value to current health. By adapting the quality-of-life adjustment and the discount rate, the model can adjust its assumptions for each of these women.

Cost-effectiveness analysis is based on the economic principle that choices must be made between alternative ways of using limited resources. From a societal perspective, what does chemotherapy cost compared to other medical activities? The cost per quality-adjusted life year is the health economist's tool for making comparisons between disease types [14, 15]. In general, interventions which have a cost-effectiveness comparable to or less than hemodialysis or hypertension are broadly accepted in the United States. Table 2 shows the costs associated with other accepted interventions or procedures.

A variety of improvements can be made in the model. In the future, combinations of prognostic factors will be used to better define recurrence

Table 2. Cost-effectiveness comparisons of common medical interventions

Strategy	Cost per year of life saved ($)
Transplantation for acute nonlymphocytic leukemia [20]	10 000
Coronary artery bypass grafting for three-vessel coronary disease [21]	13 000
Continuous zidovudine for early HIV + [22]	7 000–70 000
Medical therapy for moderate hypertension [23]	25 000–35 000
Maintenance renal dialysis [23, 24]	35 000–45 000
Chemotherapy for node-negative breast cancer	5 100–57 000
Mammography for women aged under 50 [25]	160 000
Intravenous immune globulin in chronic lymphocytic leukemia [26]	6 000 000

risk. Such a multifactorial risk analysis should be linked to a prediction algorithm to estimate the recurrence probability at a variety of relevant time horizons. This assumes that the relative efficacy of therapy is constant and independent of the prognostic factors. Although the natural history of metastatic cancer is fairly well defined, further improvements are needed. For example, studies stratifying patients by their extent of disease and response to therapy could be assessed using meta-analysis [16]. This was a major recommendation of the Institute of Medicine's effectiveness initiative [17]. Such work will improve this model and a separate model that we have developed simulating the use high-dose chemotherapy with autologous bone marrow transplantation support compared with standard chemotherapy in early metastatic breast cancer [18].

The cost data used were the best available but were relatively crude. Although most individuals are aware of the difference between cost and charges for services, we would be happy to obtain accurate, real-time charges! The cost accounting in the United States for a specific disease and treatment varies widely in quality and accessibility. In general, one can obtain high-quality data from a single medical center for inpatient care and pharmaceutical expenses. The quality of data are inconsistent if care is given primarily in the outpatient setting or is given by multiple providers or at multiple sites. Relatively poor-quality data can be obtained for non-hospital-based hospice care. Similarly, if care is staggered over several years, changes in health insurance providers due to relocating, switching companies, or type of insurance may lead to incomplete estimates. Limited access due to the commercial nature of insurers in the United States limits the strength of any estimate, particularly for non-Medicare women. In general, a new attitude of cooperation – not confrontation – is needed with the third-party payers in order to monitor the costs accrued. Such cooperation is absolutely necessary since the majority of adjuvant therapy and preterminal care is provided in the outpatient area. Large prepaid health plans in the United States may be able to lead the way in this area. In addition, the national cooperative oncology groups should include accounting and reporting of costs associated with their clinical trials.

If the model is an accurate representation of the natural history of breast cancer, it can be modified to other subgroups of women with breast cancer and other types of treatment. We have modified the model in a preliminary report to estimate the cost-effectiveness of adjuvant chemotherapy and tamoxifen versus tamoxifen alone in postmenopausal women who have one to three positive axillary nodes and estrogen receptor positive breast cancer [19].

The acid test of any model is whether it changes information exchange, provider actions, or patient outcomes. It is too early to determine whether our model will do any of these. We anticipate that the influence of decision analysis will grow in parallel with the desire for greater scrutiny of outcomes as part of the clinical effectiveness movement. By providing explicit structure and quantification, decision analysis will help guide future research in all areas of medicine. We hope clinicians will understand the basic principles of decision analysis and use these reports as another key data source to guide their provision of clinical care.

References

1. National Cancer Institute (1988) Clinical alert May 16–18. National Cancer Institute, Bethesda
2. Hillner BE, Smith TJ (1991) Efficacy and cost effectiveness of adjuvant chemotherapy in women with node-negative breast cancer. A decision-analysis model. N Engl J Med 324:160–168
3. Pauker SG, Kassirer JP (1987) Decision analysis. N Engl J Med 316:250–258
4. Early Breast Cancer Trialists' Collaborative Group (1992) Systemic treatment of early breast cancer by hormonal, cytotoxic or immune therapy. Lancet 339: 1–15, 71–85
5. Rosen PP, Groshen S, Saigo PE, Kinne DW, Hellman S (1989) A long-term follow-up study of survival in stage I (T1N0M0) and stage II (T1N1M0) breast carcinoma. J Clin Oncol 7:355–366
6. Carter CL, Allen C, Henson DE (1989) Relation of tumor size, lymph note status, and survival in 24,740 breast cancer cases. Cancer 63:181–187
7. NIH Consensus Conference (1991) Treatment of early-stage breast cancer. JAMA 265:391–395
8. Levine MN, Guyatt GH, Gent M et al. (1988) Quality of life in stage II breast cancer: an instrument for clinical trials. J Clin Oncol 6:1798–1810

9. Gelber RD, Goldhirsch A, Cavalli F (1991) Quality-of-life-adjusted evaluation of adjuvant therapies for operable breast cancer. The International Breast Cancer Study Group. Ann Intern Med 114:621–628
10. Eisenberg JM (1989) Clinical economics: a guide to the economic analysis of clinical practices. JAMA 262:2879–2886
11. Baker MS, Kessler LG, Urban N, Smucker RC (1991) Estimating the treatment costs of breast and lung cancer. Med Care 29:40–49
12. Simes RJ, Cocker K, Glasziou P, Coates AS, Tattersall MH (1989) Costs and benefits of adjuvant chemotherapy for breast cancer: an assessment of patient preferences (Abstr). Proc Am Soc Clin Oncol 8:52A
13. Slevin ML, Stubbs L, Plant HJ et al. (1990) Attitudes to chemotherapy: comparing views of patients with cancer with those of doctors, nurses, and the general public. Br Med J 300:1458–1460
14. Detsky AS, Naglie T (1990) A clinician's guide to cost-effectiveness analysis. Ann Intern Med 113:147–154
15. Drummond MF, Stoddart GL, Torrance GW (1987) Menthods for the evaluation of health care programmes. Oxford University Press, Oxford, pp 39–72
16. Gelber RD, Goldhirsch A (1986) The concept of an overview of cancer clinical trials with special emphasis on early breast cancer. J Clin Oncol 4:1696–1703
17. Institute of Medicine (1990) Breast cancer: setting priorities for effectiveness research. Institute of Medicine, Washington
18. Hillner BE, Smith TJ, Desch CE (1992) Efficacy and cost-effectiveness of autologous bone marrow transplantation in metastatic breast cancer – estimates using decision analysis while awaiting clinical trial results. JAMA 267:2055–2061
19. Hillner BE, Smith TJ (1992) Estimating the efficacy and cost-effectiveness of tamoxifen compared to tamoxifen plus chemotherapy in node-positive, estrogen receptor positive postmenopausal women (abstract). Proc Am Soc Clin Oncol 10:60
20. Welch HG, Larson EB (1989) Cost effectiveness of bone marrow transplantation in acute nonlymphocytic leukemia. N Engl J Med 321:807–812
21. Weinstein MC, Stason WB (1982) Cost-effectiveness of coronary artery bypass surgery. Circulation 66 Suppl 3:III56–III66
22. Schulman KA, Lynn LA, Glick HA, Eisenberg JM (1991) Cost effectiveness of low-dose zidovudine therapy for asymptomatic patients with human immunodeficiency virus (HIV) infection. Ann Intern Med 114:798–802
23. Edelson JT, Weinstein MC, Tosteson ANA, Williams L, Lee TH, Goldman L (1990) Long-term cost-effectiveness of various initial monotherapies for mild to moderate hypertension. JAMA 263:407–413
24. Garner TI, Dardis TI (1987) Cost-effectiveness analysis of end-stage renal disease treatments. Med Care 25:25–34
25. Eddy DM (1989) Screening for breast cancer. Ann Intern Med 111:389–399
26. Weeks JC, Tierney MR, Weinstein MC (1991) Cost effectiveness of prophylactic intravenous immune globulin in chronic lymphocytic leukemia. N Engl J Med 325:81–86

Long-Term Toxicity and Economic Aspects: Critical Review

K.W. Brunner

In adjuvant therapy cost-benefit considerations must weigh not only short term toxicities and psychological distress against gain in survival time, but also subacute and late toxicities. In addition, the financial cost per years of life gained by various medical interventions must also be considered to an increasing degree.

Dr. Velagussa presented data on subacute and late toxicity from 728 breast cancer patients treated with adjuvant chemotherapy in Milan observed over a median period of 57 months. Second neoplasms are the main concerns of present adjuvant chemotherapy (rare in the Milan series). Other late effects include: amenorrhea with unknown late consequences, reversible radiotherapy-related lung fibrosis, and cardiac toxicities, especially after treatment with anthracyclines and irradiation of the left breast. In the future we must look very carefully for a possible increase in late sequelae, especially late second neoplasms, with the combined use of radio- and chemotherapy in the conservative, breast conserving therapy of node-positive breast cancer.

Dr. Rutqvist presented an overview of available data on possible unfavorable as well as favorable late effects of long-term treatment with tamoxifen. Most documented undesired and some possibly beneficial effects of tamoxifen appear related to the agonistic estrogenic properties of tamoxifen. Undesired side effects include an increased incidence of thromboembolic disease, especially in combination with chemotherapy, and of endometrial cancer, reported mainly in studies using more than 20 mg tamoxifen daily. An increase in the incidence of liver cancer and tamoxifen-induced tumor growth stimulation in patients with acquired tamoxifen resistence remain controversial. The presumed tumor-stimulating effects of tamoxifen are possibly more than compensated by a decrease in the incidence of contralateral breast cancer. On the other hand, the agonistic estrogenic effects of tamoxifen may have beneficial effects, contributing to a decreased risk of cardiac disease, especially myocardial infarction, and of osteoporosis. The

Recent Results in Cancer Research, Vol. 127

reported ocular effects (retinopathy with hemorrhage, keratopathy and optic neuritis) are probably rare and may be related to a structural relationship to compounds such as chloroquine. Documented and suspected unfavorable as well as favorable effects of long-term adjuvant therapy with tamoxifen highlight the importance of carefully controlled clinical trials of longer versus shorter application of tamoxifen.

Dr. Hillner presented a model of decision analysis to assess the potential trade-offs between financial costs, benefits, risks, and patient preferences.

Table 1. Summarizes different factors contributing to medical and economic costs and benefits from which a balance must be drawn.

I. *Costs*
  A. Medical
    Acute toxicity (1% deaths?)
    – Psychosocial stress, anxiety (drugs)
    Subacute toxicity
    – Thromboembolism (chemotherapy)
    – Hair loss
    Late toxicity from chemotherapy
    – Amenorrhoe: osteoporosis(?) heart disease(?)
    – Organ toxicity (drugs or radiotherapy): heart, lung
    – Second cancers(?) (Melphalan)
    Late toxicity from endocrine therapy
    – endometrial cancer(?) (tamoxifen)
  B. Economic
    Cost of adjuvant chemotherapy
    Cost of early and late complications

II. *Benefits*
  A. Medical
    1. Increased survival time without toxicity or symptoms from recurrent disease – depends on:
      – Gain in disease-free survival
      – Nodal status
      – Pre- or postmenopausal
      – Estrogen and progesterone receptors, other risk factors
      – Toxicity of the treatment
      – Subjective judgment about possible gains: 6 months–several years
    2. Possible gains from tamoxifen
      – Myocardial infarction ↓
      – Osteoporosis ↓
      – Contralateral breast cancer ↓
  B. Economic
    Prevented cost for medical care for time of delayed relapse or cure

III. *Balance*
  Cannot be calculated in a purely objective way
  Depends upon subjective judgments about possible gains by individual patients and physicians
  Attempts to calculate sociomedical and socioeconomic benefits are useful but cannot be a guideline for decisions in individual patients

Using baseline assumptions in this model, the authors found that adjuvant chemotherapy increases quality-adjusted life expectancy and survival by a substantial amount and at a cost comparable to or lower than most other therapeutic interventions in medicine. The use of such models may become increasingly important in the future for decision making and for the distribution of resources by public health authorities. It remains controversial, however, whether such considerations could or should be used as a main guideline for physicians' decisions in caring for individual patients.

VIII. Conclusion

Adjuvant Therapy of Primary Breast Cancer: Closing Summary

J.H. Glick[1], R.D. Gelber[2], A. Goldhirsch[3], and H.-J. Senn[4]

[1] University of Pennsylvania Cancer Center, Philadelphia, PA, USA
[2] Dana Farber Cancer Institute, Boston, MA, USA
[3] Ospedale Civico, Lugano, Switzerland
[4] Kantonsspital Oncology Center, St. Gallen, Switzerland

Introduction

Adjuvant therapy for stage I and II breast cancer remains in evolution as new data emerge from controlled randomized trials and from the overview analysis by the Early Breast Cancer Trialists' Collaborative Group [4] (reprinted in part in this volume; referred to below as the Overview). The Fourth International Conference on Adjuvant Therapy of Primary Breast Cancer, held in St. Gallen, Switzerland, in February, 1992, brought together breast cancer experts from all over the world to present their most recent data and to discuss the remaining challenges that confront both clinicians and basic scientists.

The data presented at the 1992 St. Gallen Conference allow us to revisit the treatment recommendations made at the 1985 and 1990 NIH Consensus Development Conferences, as well as those made at the 1988 St. Gallen meeting [1–3]. The timing of the 1992 St. Gallen Conference was fortunate in that the 10-year data from the Overview had recently been published. Four distinct overviews were conducted to evaluate whether adjuvant therapy with tamoxifen, chemotherapy, ovarian ablation, or immunotherapy, either alone or as part of combined modality treatment, reduced the risk of recurrence and death. Eligible randomized trials included those started before January 1985 in which the modality under study was the only difference between treatments received by two randomized groups of patients. Data were available for 75 000 women randomized in 133 clinical trials. The specific positive findings that attracted attention were based on 30 000 women in tamoxifen trials, 1800 women below the age of 50 years in ovarian ablation trials and 11 000 women in combination chemotherapy trials.

It was clear that the 10-year Overview data presented by Peto and colleagues greatly influenced the participants at the 1992 St. Gallen Conference. The Overview conclusions included demonstration of statistically highly

Recent Results in Cancer Research, Vol. 127

significant reductions in the annual rates of both recurrence and of death produced by tamoxifen in both node-negative and node-positive patients by ovarian oblation for patients aged under 50 years and by combination chemotherapy for those under age 50 and those 50–65 years of age [4]. With tamoxifen and combination chemotherapy, the avoidance of recurrence is chiefly during the first 5 years, but the avoidance of mortality is highly significant during both the first and second 5 years; therefore the cumulative differences in survival are large both at 5 and then at 10 years. Indirect comparisons show that long-term tamoxifen (e.g., 2 years or even 5 years) is significantly more effective than tamoxifen treatment programs of shorter duration. Between ages 50 and 69, direct comparisons show that chemotherapy plus tamoxifen is superior to chemotherapy alone for both recurrence and mortality, and better than tamoxifen alone for recurrence. In women aged under 50, chemotherapy and ovarian oblation appear, by indirect comparison across two separate overviews, to be of comparable efficacy. The 30%–40% proportional risk reductions that can be produced by combined chemoendocrine therapy in middle age are similar for node-positive and for node-negative patients, while the absolute improvement in 10-year survival is about twice as great for the node-positive patients [4]. Thus, the conclusions from the 10-year Overview analysis clearly influenced the treatment recommendations made at the 1992 St. Gallen Conference, which are discussed in a later section. The timeliness of this Conference is illustrated by the remarkable lack of conflict from different investigators, who, using their own data and those from the 10-year Overview, came to similar conclusions regarding the 1992 St. Gallen treatment recommendations.

Conference Highlights

The role of currently accepted and new prognostic factors was a subject of active debate. There was broad acceptance that tumor size, axillary lymph node status, hormone receptors, and histopathology are important prognostic factors. Both Clark and McGuire, and Dressler stressed the importance of determining S phase by flow cytometry as an important prognostic factor for node-negative patients. While S phase determination by flow cytometry is broadly accepted in the United States as a routinely used prognostic variable for node-negative patients, Silvestrini from the NCl in Milan did not confirm the value of S phase as determined by flow cytometry for these patients. Instead, Silvestrini argued that the [^{3}H]thymidine labeling index is the most important indicator of relapse. Clark and McGuire discussed the prognostic significance of overexpression of the tumor suppressor gene p53 in node-negative patients. The incidence of p53 mutations, as determined by immunohistochemistry, was observed in 50% of patients and independently predicted early recurrence in node-negative patients. Klijn et al. discussed the prognostic value of the epidermal growth factor receptor (EGF-R) and concluded that EGR-R negative patients have improved disease-free and overall survival. However, they observed that the prognostic value and best cutoff level of EGF-R remain open to question. Baum observed that prognostic factors help in the selection of patients most likely to benefit from adjuvant therapy, and that they are also of value for biological subdivisions of disease to determine qualitative interactions with specific therapies. Despite the proliferation of new prognostic factors each year, the St. Gallen Conference participants concluded that only the number of axillary lymph nodes involved, tumor size, age or menopausal status, histopathology, and hormone receptor status should be routinely used at this time.

Data presented at the Conference continue to demonstrate that breast conservation therapy (lumpectomy and radiation therapy) achieves equal 10-year overall survival as compared with modified radical mastectomy. Thus, lumpectomy and radiotherapy offer equal efficacy with less morbidity and are the preferred local treatment for most patients with early stage breast cancer. Margolese (this volume), reporting data from the NSABP, noted a 40% rate of local breast recurrence at 9 years in patients who were treated with lumpectomy alone. However, there was no difference in overall survival between the lumpectomy alone as compared to lumpectomy and radiotherapy patients. A very low incidence of breast recurrence has been observed in recent NSABP trials in which chemotherapy was used in addition to radiotherapy to the conserved breast. For patients with a tumor no greater than 1.0 cm in size, the NSABP trial demonstrated no significant difference in local breast recurrence rate between lumpectomy alone as compared to lumpectomy plus radiotherapy. Thus, controversy remains as to whether there is a subgroup of patients with smaller tumors (i.e. $\leq$1 cm), who can be treated with lumpectomy alone and spared the cost and possible morbidity of radiation therapy.

Bonadonna et al. discussed the Milan trial using primary systemic (neoadjuvant) chemotherapy for operable breast cancer. The primary aim of this trial was to increase the frequency of breast conservation treatment in patients with an initial tumor of at least $\geq$3 cm. In this series of 227 patients, 82% had tumors initially measuring between 3.0–5.0 cm at the time of entry to study, while only 18% of patients had tumors larger than 5.0 cm. Bonadonna and colleagues administered three or four cycles of chemotherapy prior to surgery. The surgical technique included either lumpectomy or quadrantectomy for tumor sizes measuring less than 3 cm and mastectomy for tumors greater than 3 cm. Definitive radiotherapy was then administered. Although 91% of patients in this trial subsequently underwent breast conservation surgery, and only 9% required mastectomy, Fisher observed that 75%–80% of this series of patients would have been eligible for initial lumpectomy in the NSABP trials.

Harris and Recht discussed the integration of primary radiotherapy and adjuvant chemotherapy. In a small retrospective series, they observed that significant delays in the initiation of radiotherapy, in order to allow the delivery of chemotherapy before radiation, may increase the rate of local recurrence in the treated breast. However, the small number of patients in this retrospective analysis makes this conclusion tenuous at this time. Thus, the optimal sequencing of definitive radiation and chemotherapy remains an open question.

Kurtz also reviewed factors influencing the risk of breast recurrence following lumpectomy and radiation. He noted that patients aged under 35 incur a significant increased risk of local recurrence as compared to older patients. There was no influence of menopausal status, location of the primary in the breast, tumor size, axillary node status, or hormone receptors in predicting an increased local breast recurrence. Patients with an extensive intraductal component did have a significantly increased rate of local failure.

Peto reviewed the data from the Overview and commented on the importance of these data as follows. The definitive effect of adjuvant therapy on 10-year survival is clearly demonstrated. The additional mortality benefit was seen between years 5 and 9 with the addition of tamoxifen. Ovarian oblation in patients aged under 50 produced similar effects in the reduction of recurrence and mortality to those seen with combination chemotherapy. Tamoxifen was effective in women aged over 50 in significantly improving both relapse-free survival and overall survival for all women, even those who are estrogen receptor poor. There was a definite reduction in mortality from hormonal treatment in node-negative patients. The administration of tamoxifen significantly reduced the incidence of contralateral breast cancers.

Bonadonna, in a separate contribution, then critically reviewed the endocrine data from the 10-year Overview. He recommended tamoxifen alone only for estrogen receptor positive, node-negative patients and was not impressed by the tamoxifen data for estrogen receptor poor patients. Bonadonna commented that, to improve treatment outcome, he recommended the use of both tamoxifen and chemotherapy as partners due to the known tumor heterogeneity of breast cancer. For the majority of patients requiring adjuvant therapy, either node-negative or node-positive, Bonadonna recommended sequential treatment with chemotherapy for 6 months followed by tamoxifen for at least 3 years. Baum remarked that the 10-year Overview data provide clear evidence that chemotherapy is standard treatment for premenopausal patients with positive axillary lymph nodes, while tamoxifen remains the standard therapy for postmenopausal patients with positive lymph nodes. However, Baum admitted that the Overview data now raised uncertainties in his mind about the role of adjuvant chemotherapy in node-positive postmenopausal patients. Gelber and Goldhirsch recommended that the arithmetic construct of the Overview be broken up to distinguish single-modality from combined-modality treatment effects. By using trials which evaluated treatments actually given (for example, chemoendocrine therapy versus chemotherapy or endocrine therapy alone), they concluded that chemoendocrine therapy appears to provide the best chance of success although, even with all of the Overview results, additional trials are needed to define the patients who benefit and the best way to combine modalities. They stressed the importance of the Overview for stimulating international collaboration and identifying questions for future clinical trials which will improve patient care.

The role of high-dose chemotherapy in high-risk node-positive patients with at least ten positive axillary nodes was discussed by Abeloff. Using a dose-intensive 16-week regimen developed at Johns Hopkins University, Abeloff reported a 53% disease-free survival with a median follow-up of 40 months in this subgroup of patients. The data from Peters at Duke University were also reviewed by Abeloff. With a median follow-up of 2 years in 85 eligible patients treated with standard adjuvant chemotherapy, followed by high-dose chemotherapy and bone marrow transplantation, the Duke group observed 72% 5-year event-free survival. Although these data are provocative, there was general agreement at the St. Gallen meeting that the role of adjuvant high-dose chemotherapy and bone marrow transplantation remain investigational and should not be used outside the context of the randomized controlled clinical trial.

Tormey et al. reviewed the data from several randomized trials conducted by the Eastern Cooperative Oncology Group. These trials addressed particularly the role of long-term tamoxifen for at least 5 years versus shorter courses of tamoxifen (i.e., 1 year). The studies demonstrated that long-term tamoxifen is associated with a significantly longer time to recurrence than the shorter term tamoxifen regimens. However, there are no survival differences noted as yet in these trials.

Fisher [5] reviewed the NSABP data on node-positive patient who were defined as nonresponsive to tamoxifen, based on definitions in older NSABP studies which included selection criteria using age and progesterone receptor status. Doxorubicin and cyclophosphamide administered every 21 days for four cycles achieved equivalent disease-free and overall survival to conventional adjuvant chemotherapy of cyclophosphamide, methotrexate, and 5-fluorouracil (CMF). In tamoxifen-responsive, estrogen receptor positive patients doxorubicin and cyclophosphamide were administered concurrently with tamoxifen (ACT) and were compared to tamoxifen alone. The ACT regimen achieved significantly improved 5-year disease-free survival (70%) compared to tamoxifen alone (60%; $p = 0.002$) as well as significantly improved 5-year overall survival (ACT 87% versus 76% with tamoxifen alone; $p = 0.002$). The data from this NSABP trial, when viewed in the context of the 10-year Overview analysis, was influential in the proactive treatment recommendations for chemotherapy in postmenopausal patients made at the St. Gallen Conference.

The NSABP trials in node-negative patients were also reviewed by Fisher, who presented the 7-year data from the B-13 trial, which randomized patients with estrogen receptor negative tumors to methotrexate and 5-fluorouracil versus a no-treatment control arm. At 7 years there remains a highly significantly improved disease-free survival on the chemotherapy arm for both pre- and postmenopausal patients. Although no difference in overall survival for all patients entered on this trial was observed, in the subgroup of patients aged 50 years or older there was a significant improvement in overall survival. An additional important observation was made by Fisher concerning tumors measuring 1 cm in size or smaller. With methotrexate and 5-fluorouracil, 90% of these patients were disease-free at 7 years compared to only 75% in the control arm. The relatively poor prognosis for patients with smaller tumors was at variance with the data presented at 1990 NIH Consensus Conference [2]. Patient selection factors for those entering this NSABP trial may explain this apparent discrepancy.

Fisher [5] also presented updated data on the tamoxifen versus placebo trial in node-negative, estrogen receptor positive patients. Significant improvement in both disease-free and overall survival at 7 years was noted for patients in the tamoxifen arm. The benefit with tamoxifen was also seen for patients with smaller tumors ($\leq$1.0 cm). In the latter subgroup of patients only 78% of the placebo-treated patients were disease-free at 7 years. Thus, Fisher was unable to confirm the data of Rosen et al. [6] on patients with tumors measuring 1.0 cm or smaller, who were reported to have a 86% 20-year disease-free survival.

Jordan and Wolf used a laboratory model to describe the survival advantage observed in patients taking adjuvant tamoxifen. In their model, tamoxifen initially inhibits estrogen-stimulated growth of MCF-7 breast cancer cells transplanted into athymic mice. However, in animals transplanted with MCF-7 tumors and treated with tamoxifen for up to 1 year they observed tamoxifen-stimulated tumor growth. At 4 years, these tamoxifen-stimulated tumors still maintained estrogen receptors, but the replacement of tamoxifen with physiological circulating levels of estradiol caused the immediate and total regression of established tumors. Jordan and Wolf suggested that during adjuvant treatment with tamoxifen tumor cells are initially prevented from growing during the 1st year, but that clones of tamoxifen-stimulated tumor cells eventually emerge. The benefit from tamoxifen comes when treatment is stopped, and the circulating estradiol kills tamoxifen-dependent disease. This provocative laboratory observation has not yet been tested in clinical trials but remains a new avenue of investigation.

The long-term toxicities of adjuvant chemotherapy (CMF with or without doxorubicin) were reviewed by Valagussa et al. With a median follow-up of 52 months, virtually no long-term leukopenia was noted, while 2% of patients had a hemoglobin level of less than 12 g. Venous thrombosis was observed in only 0.6% of patients undergoing chemotherapy. However, drug-related amenorrhea was a common finding and was observed in 69% of patients. There was no significant increase in the incidence of second neoplasms, which were observed in 0.9% of chemotherapy-treated patients. In addition, the incidence of doxorubicin-related cardiotoxicity was only 0.8%, while radiotherapy-related lung fibrosis was noted in 3.4% of patients.

Gelber et al. discussed how to compare the quality of life of breast cancer patients in clinical trials. They argued that this is best done within randomized trials using the Q-TWiST technique based on time with and without specific types of toxic effects of therapy or with and without symptoms of recurrent disease as endpoints. They discussed methods to define the emotional adjustment which concerns almost every patient faced with the diagnosis of breast cancer. This type of adjustment represents the main reason for discrepancies between the way in which patients in various clinical situations cope with disease and treatment. Their methodology facilitates the comparison of treatment benefits and subjective side effects from the patient's point of view. This methodology could be adopted in current and future trials of adjuvant therapy, particularly where the differences in treatment outcome are expected to be of small biological value.

Hillner discussed the financial costs, benefits, and the role of patient risk preferences. He described a model that uses the results of available randomized controlled trials in node-negative patients to assess the potential clinical and financial effects of the universal use of adjuvant chemotherapy. Using baseline assumptions, Hillner found that chemotherapy increases quality-adjusted life expectancy and survival at a cost comparable to most medical interventions. The model highlights the need for greater study of patient preferences and the need for accurate cost accounting for oncologic therapies and the role of patient preferences.

Conclusions: The 1992 St. Gallen Treatment Recommendations

The 1985 and 1990 NIH Consensus Conferences as well as the recent 10-year Overview from the Early Breast Cancer Trialists' Collaborative Group present a wealth of data indicating that adjuvant chemotherapy and hormonal therapy are effective treatments for breast cancer patients with both positive and negative axillary lymph nodes [1, 2, 4]. However, there remains considerable debate regarding the use of adjuvant therapy in many common situations in clinical practice. Although optimal therapy has not been defined for any subset of patients, it is unfortunate that fewer than 5% of all such patients in the United States are actually entered into a clinical trial of adjuvant therapy. This is also true for most of Europe. Thus, practicing oncologists and their patients are continually faced with a therapeutic dilemma as to which node-negative patients should be observed, and which should be treated with adjuvant therapy outside the setting of a clinical trial. In addition, much controversy remains regarding which subsets of node-positive patients should receive chemotherapy, hormonal manipulation, or both modalities. Outside the context of a clinical trial, and based on the research data presented at the 1992 St. Gallen Conference, which included the recently available data from the 10-year Overview, we can summarize the treatment recommendations made at the 1992 St. Gallen meeting (Table 1).

Table 1. 1992 St. Gallen recommendations for the adjuvant treatment of breast cancer

	Premenopausal	Postmenopausal	Elderly
Node-negative			
Minimal/low risk	Nil or Tam	Nil or Tam	Nil (?)
Good risk	Tam	Tam	Tam
High risk			
HR-negative	CTX	CTX ± Tam	Tam (CTX if tolerated)
HR-positive	CTX ± Tam	Tam ± CTX	
Node-positive			
HR-negative	CTX	CTX ± Tam	CTX (?) or Tam
HR-positive	CTX ± Tam	Tam ± CTX	Tam

HR, Hormone receptor; Tam, tamoxifen; CTX, chemotherapy.

Node-Negative

Minimal/Low Risk

Within the node-negative group of patients, a minimal/low-risk category can be defined which includes patients with noninvasive tumors (ductal carcinoma in situ), incidentally discovered small invasive tumors detected by mammography or by microscopic examination of tissue removed because of benign breast disease or because of in situ breast carcinoma. In addition, patients with tubular, colloid (mucinous), and papillary tumor types are included in this subgroup because of their low risk of recurrence. For patients described in this minimal/low risk category, observation without adjuvant therapy remains the current treatment recommendation. However, the benefits of tamoxifen for this subgroup of patients remain to be determined by ongoing clinical trials. If, after explaining the potential risks and benefits from the administration of tamoxifen to a given patient in this subgroup, the individual patient decides that tamoxifen provides an expected benefit, the administration of tamoxifen in this setting is not unreasonable and remains a viable option.

The 1990 NIH Consensus Panel concluded that, in general, patients with tumors no greater than 1 cm in diameter have an excellent prognosis, with less than a 10% recurrence rate at 10 years; adjuvant therapy was therefore not indicated for this subgroup of patients [2]. The data presented at the 1992 St. Gallen Conference were less definitive and more controversial regarding the benefits of adjuvant therapy for patients with tumors measuring 1 cm in size or smaller. Consequently, the 1992 St. Gallen treatment recommendations leave open the options of observation versus 5 years of tamoxifen as potential treatments for patients with tumors of this size. The decision to use adjuvant therapy in a patient with small tumors should follow a thorough discussion with the patient regarding the likely risk of recurrence without adjuvant therapy, the expected reduction in risk with adjuvant therapy, toxicities of therapy, and the impact on quality of life. Even small absolute benefits in terms of reduction in disease recurrence and mortality may be viewed by patients as an important benefit. In this case, adjuvant therapy, particularly with tamoxifen, for patients with these small tumors is indicated.

Good Risk

A good-risk subgroup is defined as those patients with an approximately 85%–90% chance of remaining disease-free at 5 years. This category includes patients whose tumor is larger than 1 cm but no greater than 2 cm and is estrogen receptor positive. Patients in this category would also have good nuclear grade tumors. Based on the Overview data there was remarkable consensus that this group of good-risk patients should be treated with tamoxifen. This proactive treatment recommendation applies to premenopausal, postmenopausal, and elderly patients. Tamoxifen should serve as the control arm for future clinician trials in the good-risk subgroup. Thus, for the first time, a general recommendation to use adjuvant tamoxifen is made for the good-risk subgroup of node-negative patients.

High Risk

A high-risk subgroup of node-negative patients is also defined on the basis of well-known and accepted prognostic factors. This group includes patients with unequivocally estrogen receptor negative tumors which are at least 1 cm in size, estrogen receptor positive tumors larger than 2 cm in diameter, and nuclear grade III (poor) tumors. The presence of any one of these unfavorable prognostic parameters justifies the use of adjuvant therapy outside the setting of a clinical trial. Additional prognostic factors such as high S phase as determined by flow cytometry can be added to the prognostic profile to guide the clinician and the individual patient. In addition to the consideration of these well-known prognostic factors, the physician must evaluate the patient's general medical condition and psychosocial status before deciding on a therapeutic recommendation.

Therefore, virtually all patients in the high-risk group should receive some form of adjuvant systemic therapy. All of the recent major clinical trials demonstrate significant prolongation of disease-free survival with either tamoxifen or chemotherapy for this subgroup of patients. Evidence of significant prolongation of overall survival is beginning to emerge from these individual trials as well. Moreover, the 10-year Overview data, while not subdivided on the basis of risk factors, provides strong evidence that node-negative patients should receive some form of adjuvant therapy.

The 1992 St. Gallen treatment recommendations for node-negative high-risk breast cancer patients are as follows.

1. All premenopausal, node-negative, high-risk patients should receive adjuvant chemotherapy irrespective of their estrogen receptor status. For receptor positive patients in this subgroup, the combination of chemotherapy and tamoxifen also must be considered but needs to be compared prospectively to chemotherapy alone for this subset of patients. Outside the context of a clinical trial, for the premenopausal receptor-positive, node-negative patient, either chemotherapy alone, chemotherapy plus concurrent tamoxifen, or chemotherapy followed sequentially by tamoxifen are appropriate treatment options. For the premenopausal receptor-negative patient, adjuvant chemotherapy remains the treatment of choice at this time.

2. For postmenopausal, node-negative, high-risk patients the primary therapeutic modality depends on estrogen receptor status. For patients in this category who are estrogen receptor positive, tamoxifen remains the mainstay of treatment. There is increasing evidence both from individual trials and from the Overview data that tamoxifen combined with chemotherapy for this subgroup of patients may have additional benefit. Thus, the combination of tamoxifen plus chemotherapy is a reasonable alternative to tamoxifen alone for this subgroup. For postmenopausal patients in the high-risk node-negative category who are estrogen receptor negative, adjuvant chemotherapy is indicated as standard treatment. The role of tamoxifen when added to chemotherapy in these receptor-negative patients remains controversial and is under current investigation.

3. For the elderly patient in the node-negative high-risk group, tamoxifen appears to be of benefit irrespective of estrogen receptor status. However, it can be envisioned that chemotherapy could be administered to selected older receptor-negative patients with excellent performance status and in good general medical condition who are at high risk for recurrence despite their node-negative disease. In this subset of patients, full-dose chemotherapy might well be indicated.

It is now apparent that all patients with node-negative breast cancer should have an oncological consultation at the time of diagnosis so that the patient and her physician can discuss the patient's prognostic profile and the available therapeutic options as well as the risk versus benefit ratio. Although the patient should be urged to participate in one of the many available clinical trials, it must be recognized that the vast majority of patients are treated outside the context of a clinical trial. In this situation, a physician should recommend adjuvant chemotherapy with or without tamoxifen for all node-negative high-risk patients, tamoxifen for the overwhelming majority of patients in the good risk category, and observation versus tamoxifen for patients in the minimal/low-risk subgroup. Thus, the treatment recommendations made at St. Gallen in 1992 support the general recommendations made in the controversial 1988 NCI Clinical Alert [7].

Node-Positive

All patients with node-positive breast cancer should receive some form of adjuvant therapy, according to the treatment recommendations made at the 1992 St. Gallen Conference.

1. For premenopausal, node-positive patients who are either hormone receptor positive or negative, adjuvant chemotherapy remains the standard of care and should be administered to all patients. In the receptor-negative patient in this category, chemotherapy alone is the treatment of choice. For premenopausal receptor-positive patients, the addition of tamoxifen to chemotherapy remains a viable treatment option. In these patients, it is not known whether tamoxifen should be administered concurrently with chemotherapy or sequentially after the chemotherapy is completed. Although ovarian ablation achieves a relative reduction in the annual odds of recurrence and mortality of approximately 25%, the 1992 St. Gallen Conference does not recommend the routine use of ovarian ablation outside the context of a clinical trial. The role of ovarian oblation, particularly achieved using luteinizing hormone releasing hormone agonists such as Zoladex, either by itself or compared to chemotherapy alone, or in addition to chemotherapy for premenopausal, receptor-positive, node-positive patients is under active investigation.

2. For postmenopausal, node-positive, hormone receptor positive patients, tamoxifen remains the accepted treatment. However, data from both the NSABP and the 10-year Overview provide increasing evidence of the added benefit of chemotherapy when given in addition to tamoxifen for this subgroup of patients. Again, the proper sequencing of chemotherapy and tamoxifen remains to be defined.

3. For postmenopausal, node-positive, hormone receptor negative patients, there is a clear consensus favoring adjuvant chemotherapy. The strong recommendation for adjuvant chemotherapy made at the 1992 St. Gallen Conference represents for the first time a broad international consensus on the use of chemotherapy as standard treatment for this group of patients. In this subset of receptor-negative patients, there is increasing evidence that tamoxifen may be added to chemotherapy to improve disease-free and overall survival. Therefore, the addition of tamoxifen to chemotherapy for this subgroup of patients remains an increasingly viable treatment option to be studied in clinical trials.

4. For the elderly, node-positive, hormone receptor positive patient, tamoxifen remains clearly the standard of care. For the elderly patient with node-positive, receptor-negative breast cancer, the option of adjuvant chemotherapy must be considered if the patient's general medical condition warrants the administration of full-dose chemotherapy. Alternatively, tamoxifen could be administered to this subset of receptor-negative elderly patients.

It now appears in 1992 that almost all patients with clinical and pathological stage I or II breast cancer, regardless of age, menopausal, nodal, or receptor status, will benefit from some form of adjuvant chemotherapy and/or hormonal therapy in terms of both improved disease-free survival and overall survival. Thus, the 1992 St. Gallen treatment recommendations confirm and expand on the guidelines suggested at the time of the last St. Gallen Conference in 1988 [3]. Although further clinical investigation is imperative, it is now incumbent upon each physician to apply the known adjuvant therapeutic regimens broadly, so as not to deny any patient the specific benefits of adjuvant therapy that have already been demonstrated.

References

1. NIH Consensus Conference (1985) Adjuvant chemotherapy for breast cancer. JAMA 254:3461–3463
2. NIH Consensus Conference (1991) Treatment of early-stage breast cancer. JAMA 265:391–395
3. Glick JH (1988) Adjuvant therapy for breast cancer. J Nat Cancer Inst 80: 471–475
4. Early Breast Cancer Trialists' Collaborative Group (1992) Systemic treatment of early breast cancer by hormonal, cytoxic, or immune therapy: 133 randomized trials involving 31 000 recurrences and 24 000 deaths among 75 000 women. Lancet 339:1–5, 71–85
5. Fisher B (1992) The recent NSABP experience and strategies. Proceedings of the 4th International Conference on Adjuvant Therapy of Primary Breast Cancer, St. Gallen
6. Rosen PP, Groshen S, Saigo PE et al. (1989) Pathological prognostic factors in stage I (T_1 N_0 M_0) and stage II (T_1 N_1 M_0) breast carcinoma. J Clin Oncol 7: 1239–1251
7. National Cancer Institute (1988) Clinical alert. National Cancer Institute, Bethesda